Praise for
REGENERATE

"Sayer Ji holds the reader's hand like a great guide to explore the exciting twists and turns of the new biology of the human body. Beyond highlighting the body's tremendous power of healing and regeneration, Sayer provides easy-to-understand steps to make this happen for everyone who follows his guidelines. A great guide to a new regenerated you!"

— STEVEN R. GUNDRY, M.D.
New York Times bestselling author of *The Longevity Paradox* and *The Plant Paradox*, and medical director of The Centers for Restorative Medicine, Palm Springs and Santa Barbara, California

"Sayer Ji's *Regenerate* is a must-read for anyone who wishes to understand the exciting implications of the New Biology, the awe-inspiring power of the human body to heal itself in face of adversity, and how to practically apply the cutting-edge science to one's life."

— DR. MARK HYMAN
founder of The UltraWellness Center and
New York Times bestselling author of *Food*

"*Regenerate* leverages leading-edge science to show how we can actually change the expression of our DNA to build resilience and reverse the biological clock of degeneration that we've all come to expect. This is powerful, deeply validated, but nonetheless user-friendly information that will clearly pave the way for health."

— DAVID PERLMUTTER, M.D.
#1 *New York Times* bestselling author of *Grain Brain* and *Brain Wash*

REGENERATE

REGENERATE

UNLOCKING YOUR BODY'S
RADICAL RESILIENCE THROUGH
THE NEW BIOLOGY

Sayer Ji

HAY HOUSE, INC.

Carlsbad, California • New York City
London • Sydney • New Delhi

Published in the United States by: Hay House, Inc.: www.hayhouse.com®
Published in Australia by: Hay House Australia Pty. Ltd.: www.hayhouse.com.au
Published in the United Kingdom by: Hay House UK, Ltd.: www.hayhouse.co.uk
Published in India by: Hay House Publishers India: www.hayhouse.co.in

Indexer: Joan Shapiro
Cover design: Jason Gabbert
Interior design: Charles McStravick

Library of Congress has cataloged the earlier edition as follows:

Names: Ji, Sayer, author.
Title: Regenerate : unlocking your body's radical resilience through the new biology / Sayer Ji.
Description: 1st edition. | Carlsbad, California : Hay House, Inc., 2020. |
Identifiers: LCCN 2019058756 (print) | LCCN 2019058757 (ebook) | ISBN 9781401956387 (hardback) | ISBN 9781401956400 (ebook)
Subjects: LCSH: Self-care, Health. | Alternative medicine. | Rejuvenation.
Classification: LCC RA776.95 .J52 2020 (print) | LCC RA776.95 (ebook) | DDC 613--dc23
LC record available at https://lccn.loc.gov/2019058756
LC ebook record available at https://lccn.loc.gov/2019058757

Tradepaper ISBN: 978-1-4019-6526-6
E-book ISBN: 978-1-4019-5640-0
Audiobook ISBN: 978-1-4019-5639-4

11 10 9 8 7 6 5 4 3 2
1st edition, March 2020
2nd edition, August 2021

Printed in the United States of America

This product uses papers sourced from responsibly managed forests. For more information, see www.hayhouse.com

This book is dedicated to Kelly Brogan,
my beloved wife and partner, who, like
a Force of Nature, turned my life upside down
and inside out the moment I knew she existed.
The alchemical crucible of our immense love
inspired in me the courage to face and move
beyond my deeply held fears, perceived
limitations, and stories, and tap into the
unlimited potential for physical and spiritual
regeneration which I now know is buried
deep within us all as a birthright.

CONTENTS

INTRODUCTION

*R*egenerate means to rejuvenate, revitalize, and renew. These words hold great promise, especially for so many of us who feel something is wrong, most often in our bodies but increasingly in our souls. We yearn for a feeling of peace, wholeness, and vitality, but experience our bodies as the fallible and vulnerable structures we have been made to believe them to be. In fact, we have been designed to naturally draw strength, energy, and healing from deep within rather than to succumb like clockwork to the "inevitable" downward spiral of biological time. On the cellular level, our bodies have the innate power and ability to reverse damage, regenerate, and restore a directly felt experience of well being we have lost.

This isn't just wishful thinking. A significant number of new studies in biomedical science confirms that our bodies are radically resilient and that all we need to do to reclaim our health and vitality is to eliminate sources of interference with our bodies' innate, robust self-regenerating capacity. Our physical form represents eons of adaptation to and mastery over constantly changing conditions, including powerful forces of environmental and biological adversity. Our bodies have emerged from this crucible with veritable superpowers, not the least of which is our seemingly magical and irrepressible capacity for radical resilience.

The New Biology offers a revolutionary and breathtaking vision of the body as resilient, intelligent, and seamlessly interwoven with the larger universal patchwork. As you read this book, you will learn how to engage your body's self-healing mechanisms and unleash your cells' regenerative powers.

On a molecular level, every cell in your body is undergoing a constant process of coming into and out of being, much like the flicker of a flame, and doing it so perfectly that we only experience ourselves on a macroscopic level as immutable, relatively unchanging organisms. Yet there are trillions of changes and microadjustments occurring every moment in each cell, completely regenerating damaged and diseased tissue.

On the most basic level, regeneration follows from removing what the body does not need and adding back what it does.

In **Part I: Your Body and the Miracle of Regeneration**, you will learn about the secret relationship between human and plant evolution, your genes, and the most common health regenerators and disruptors. Contrary to popular dogma, your DNA is not your destiny. You are in the driver's seat and your choices—from the food you eat to your interactions with nature—powerfully impact your health. You will learn about the regenerative powers of your cells and how to optimize them for healing and longevity. You will pick up some fundamental scientific knowledge, like how microRNAs, the potent messengers in food that communicate directly with your cells, can orchestrate your gene expression, and how telomeres, the noncoding pieces of DNA at the end of your chromosomes, directly influence your experience of aging.

Part II: Rethinking Chronic Disease, Prevention, and Healing offers startling new information about the Western Pattern Diet—the archetypal grain-centric, chemically processed, industrialized food staples and preferences that emerged in the post–World War II era that has since been exported from the United States to almost every nation in the world—and its connection to the emergence of chronic conditions that accelerate aging and adversely impact both the length and quality of life, including cancer, Alzheimer's, cardiovascular disease, and metabolic syndrome, clusters of health conditions referred to as "diseases of affluence" and all representing a short-circuiting of the regenerative processes within your body. Because fear is a major impediment to successful healing, Part II addresses the psycho-emotional dimension of cellular degeneration and the role the medical establishment plays in perpetuating these trends.

Part III: Regenerate Rx provides you with a road map to better health. You will learn how to detox from the Western Pattern Diet and heal with the foods of the ancestral diet. You will learn how to optimize the effects of the ancestral diet with natural supplements for long-term results and use nature's abundant energy sources to encourage the regenerative process, strengthening your body from the inside out. You will plunge into the joy of intentional movement and learn time-tested techniques for improving your sleep and diffusing stress to decelerate the aging process and help neutralize the underlying conditions that foster chronic disease.

Whether you are seeking to improve your quality of life, reverse a chronic condition, or harmonize your body with your ancestral and evolutionary healing mechanisms, using the principles of the New Biology will transform your body, mind, and soul, and enhance your ability to truly feel deeply alive and well again—experiences that I believe are your natural birthright.

MY OWN JOURNEY OF HEALING

While today I find myself easily amazed at the extreme intelligence and resilience of the the human body, it took many years for me to experience its vitality firsthand. I came into this world as a sickly infant, and during my journey to recovery, I felt so saddled with hopelessness and dependency on medications that I often doubted that I would make it to adulthood. Yet, in so many ways, I am stronger now than I have ever been. I've gone from being an over-weight inactive asthmatic with a bum hip to a marathon-running natural health advocate who hasn't used a medication of any kind for decades.

My struggle to overcome disease started when I was six months old, at our doctor's office, where my big sister was getting a checkup while my mother held me in her arms. The nurse observed my pale skin and heard my shallow, wheezy breathing, and, instead of fetching my sister, she whisked me from my mother's arms for clinical evaluations and tests. That day, I was diagnosed with severe bronchial asthma and thereafter spent most of my childhood on a never-ending merry-go-round of doctor's appointments and hospital stays, struggling with a multitude of overlapping health issues, from recurrent colds to chronic allergies to severe "asthma attacks" requiring emergency trips to the hospital, at times as often as twice a week.

I received all the vaccines customary at the time—the first battery of which coincided exactly with the onset of my asthma—and was given powerful medications like antibiotics and steroid inhalers, which I continued to take throughout my childhood. When things got really bad, my parents would rush me to the nearest emergency room for an injection of epinephrine, an anxiety-provoking rush of adrenaline intended to dilate the bronchial passageways during an acute asthma attack. Between these shots, my vaccinations, and immunotherapy injections for allergies, I sometimes felt like a human pincushion. But even though my bathroom medical cabinet was overflowing, no remedy lasted, because the root causes of these episodes—which no one seemed to be searching for at the time—remained unaddressed.

When I was six, I had my adenoids removed, an immune organ, whose removal has now been linked to a range of diseases of the upper respiratory tract and increased risk of infectious/parasitic diseases later in life.[1] When I was 12 and 13, I underwent two major surgeries for a relatively rare bone and hip joint condition called slipped capital femoral epiphysis, a condition that we now know occurs more frequently in asthmatics whose exposure to inhaled corticosteroids has had the unintended effect of disrupting normal bone and cartilage development. Given my physical limitations (to this day, my right femur bone is half an inch shorter than my left) and general lack of vitality, it was often difficult for me to play with the other kids or participate in school gym classes. I was overweight, unfit, and desolate. I felt like an outcast imprisoned within the dilapidated confines of my body. Sometimes my respiratory challenges were so bad that I had difficulty walking up the stairs.

When I was 17, my doctor assured me and my parents that if I had surgery on my sinuses, my breathing would improve. But the surgery left me with worsening nasal obstructions and chronic sinus infections that made it even more difficult to breathe.

These early life experiences of riding the medical merry-go-round left me deeply traumatized, prompting me to disassociate from my body, where so much physical and emotional pain was stored. Not only did modern medicine fail to significantly help me; it seemed to be, at times, actively torturing me. In retrospect, I see how my growing sense of powerlessness was reinforced by a medical system that believed chronic health conditions like asthma were outside one's sphere of control. Asthma was said to simply "run in the family," as if it were a settled matter of shoddy genetics.

At least a dozen doctors examined and treated me as a child and young adult, and not one investigated the environmental conditions, diet, toxicant burden, or mind-body-emotion connection as upstream triggers of my symptoms. It wasn't until my first year in college, when I was exposed to an entirely new realm of alternative health ideas and practices, that I considered the possibility that my asthma had been caused by dietary, behavioral, and emotional factors.

When I learned that cow's milk, far from being the calcium-rich elixir of health that millions have been encouraged to believe, has "mucus-forming properties," I decided to test the idea on myself by removing milk and cheese from my diet. The result was, and has continued to be, nothing less than miraculous. Within days, my lifelong asthma went into complete remission. After 17 years of nonstop asthma medication usage, I put it away—for good. The symptoms of asthma never came back unless I inadvertently consumed even the smallest amount of dairy products. (The one exception is clarified butter, or ghee, dairy products that are made safe by the removal of the antigenic casein protein.)

After a life defined and circumscribed by medical complaints, I felt simultaneously wronged and liberated. Even more exciting than being able to breathe again was realizing that I am not biologically destined to be weak and flawed. Thereafter, I began to deconstruct and question the medical institutions that everyone, myself included, held as the ultimate authorities on health.

I would eventually learn that cow's milk contains white, sticky proteins, such as A1 β-casein, and powerful, gene-impacting microRNA molecules, packaged in little particles called exosomes, that are intended for bovine calves. The biological pathways[2] that cow's milk activated in my body presented the symptoms of asthma. Asthma, on some level, was my body trying to communicate a profound mismatch between my body's needs and the inadequacies of the conventional Western diet that I was consuming. The symptoms were not the enemy but were instead harbingers of the solution.

Later, I learned that other gastrointestinal symptoms (such as constipation and acid reflux) that had plagued me were caused not by bad genes or bad luck but by our biological incompatibility with gluten-containing grains like wheat. From that point onward, I became so absorbed by connections between adverse medical conditions, food, and the body's untapped potential for healing that it eventually became my life's work. So far, I have amassed a database of over 10,000 researched health topics that I share with the world via my brainchild, GreenMedInfo.com. I created GreenMedInfo.com with the intention to provide both cynics and believers with the published, empirically validated proof of what countless individuals have experienced firsthand: the transformative power of self-healing through nutrition, nature, and holistic medicine. To help expand public access to an entire arsenal of untapped modalities long revered by ancient medical systems.

To promote informed consent and medical freedom around every allopathic treatment. And most pivotally, to enable you to recapture autonomy in your life and to become the master of your own health destiny.

The New Biology revolution is happening quickly but so quietly that it flies under the radar of most conventional medical and pharmaceutical professionals. In fact, it's been happening in the annals of the most respected medical journals for more than two decades. However, you don't need a science degree to understand or apply the findings. This book distills my gleaned knowledge about how to ignite your body's natural healing powers—the very same ones that Hippocrates described when he said, "Natural forces within us are the true healers of disease."

I'm writing this book in the hopes that I can help others who are experiencing persistent symptoms or sickness to pause and consider that their bodies, far from being flawed, are sending a message that something they are consuming, breathing, or thinking is toxic or biologically incompatible with wellness. Symptoms are the body's way of signaling distress, lack of equilibrium, and its desperate need for support. To truly heal, it's time to feed, nurture, and tend to your symptoms as you would a crying baby rather than silencing and suppressing them.

As you modify the lens through which you explore your symptoms, two truths will percolate to the surface. First, your birthright is health rather than disease and debility. And second, your illness is an opportunity for consciousness-awakening insights and radical transformation. Wherever you may be on your life's journey, every day you can make choices and decisions that will help make your body more capable of regeneration and radical resilience. Let me show you how.

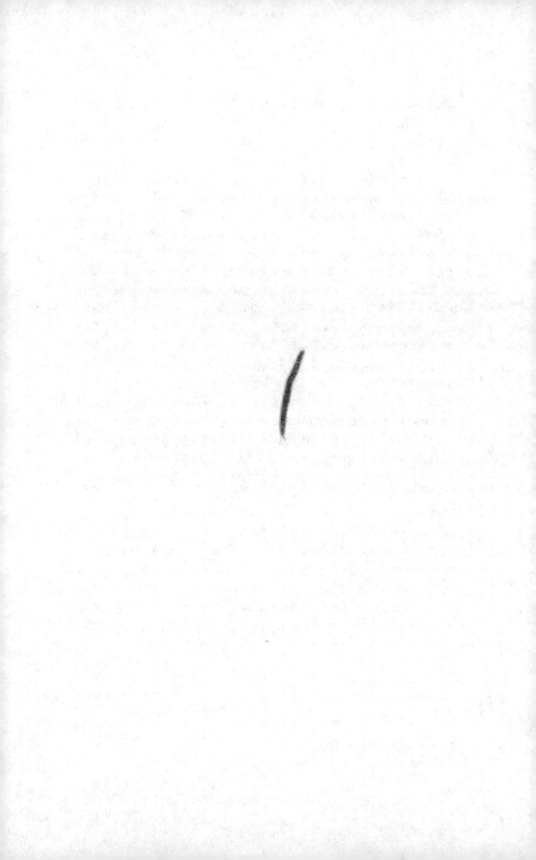

PART ONE

YOUR BODY
AND THE
MIRACLE OF
REGENERATION

THE TRUTH ABOUT
YOUR GENES,
FOOD AS INFORMATION,
AND YOUR BODY'S
ALCHEMICAL PHYSIOLOGY

CHAPTER ONE

THE NEW BIOLOGY REVOLUTION

DNA, MicroRNA, and the Gene Expression Connection

I f you are like most dis-eased Americans, you aren't feeling so well. You may have been diagnosed with at least one chronic disease—diabetes, hypertension, arthritis, or acid reflux being the most common—or suffering in silence from numerous other common afflictions like depression and anxiety.

Statistics issued by the Centers for Disease Control (CDC) rank chronic disease as the leading cause of death and disability in the United States today. According to the CDC, 7 out of every 10 deaths are caused by chronic diseases, and an astounding 75 percent of our annual health care expenditure is directed at managing this ever-expanding epidemic.[1] I am betting that you're not interested in a lifelong commitment to popping prescription pills as a method of palliative management. And I hope you don't think that your body is inherently defective and destined to be broken beyond repair. Instead, I'm here to tell you that there is another way, and new science substantiates that promise with intelligent, elegant, and sophisticated research.

To understand the source of my optimism about your body's potential, consider how far your body has come. The cells of your body exist because of an incredibly resilient germline lineage that has been replicating in all living things since the beginning of biological time on this Earth, and possibly much further back. These germline cells—sperm in men and ova in women—represent a quasi-immortal and unbroken biological thread of a near-infinite number of cell divisions connecting us to the last universal common ancestor (LUCA), which is estimated to have emerged some 3.5 to 3.8 billion years ago in the vicinity of the hydrothermal vents on the primordial ocean floor.

Relative to the somatic, or body, cells to which they give rise, these germline cells are "deathless" in the sense that their biological information has been transmitted from generation to generation for billions of years without interruption and will continue to be passed down through our offspring and descendants to come. The stem cells produced from their union are instrumental in renewal and regeneration of damaged cells in your body right here, in this instant. No pharmaceutical intervention will ever come close to the self-healing abilities of the stem cells contained within every tissue of your body.

The fundamental takeaway, as we will explore, is that your body contains a seed of immortality—and this is not a metaphor but literal. It is manifested in the tireless regenerative capacities of your many stem cells and has access to a near-limitless amount of energy that comes from a source beyond the caloric content of your food. This is the core of the New Biology, a scientific revolution that is radically changing our understanding of the human body. With the New Biology, a diagnosis doesn't have to be a lifelong sentence. Drugs are not your only viable option. The exquisitely intelligent healing properties of the right kinds of food and your body's ability to harvest its own inner reservoir of regenerative energy are far more powerful than any medical prescription that you've been issued. This is not what the multi-billion-dollar, fee-for-service, profit-driven medical-pharmaceutical-industrial complex wants you to know. With the primary objective of generating a perpetual cycle of revenue by selling drugs, they are driven to create lifetime users rather than promote wellness.

The good news is that our drug-based disease management system is largely replaceable by open-source, biocompatible (made of the same natural compounds as your body), freely extracted botanical medicine as well as dietary and lifestyle intervention. The highly empowering message—that your body can regenerate and heal itself of the most feared diseases of our time—is no longer being trumpeted only by herbalists and energy medicine practitioners; it has now also been accredited by medical professionals.

The Birth of the New Biology

When I was in college, inhaler-free for the first time after having removed cow's milk products and wheat from my diet, I was excited to learn more about the reasons why such a minor dietary change could result in what amounted to a full remission of a lifelong and, at times, life-threatening condition. I chose to dive deep into science and medicine but found that superficial exploration of the diet-health relationship alone could not explain my experience. Food, after all, was never designated a significant role beyond its calories and nutrient count. It is the constant questioning of such deep-seated assumptions that led me down the rabbit hole into the study of philosophy, a discipline that entails systematically deconstructing and deprogramming all areas of human knowledge and experience. Through the help of incredible professors, especially my mentor, the great American philosopher Dr. Bruce Wilshire, and our shared interest in a special branch of empirically grounded philosophy known as phenomenology, I turned my attention to scientific and medical literature and started to notice a new way of thinking on the subject of the body and healing. It may not have been validated fully through the old scientific methods, but it was compelling enough to demand further inquiry. This is what led me down the path to the material and concepts that inspired the creation of this book.

In the decades since then, I have been especially wary of the rise and increasing ideological dominance of "scientism," the belief that all forms of knowledge should be judged by the long-held assumptions and methods of the physical and biological sciences and that what cannot be proven on these terms is not relevant or does not exist.

To truly grasp the specter of scientism, which materialized during the 17th-century Scientific Revolution, we must understand how that movement elevated rationale, logic, and reasoning at the expense of other human faculties such as creativity, imagination, intuition, and direct experience. The accompanying idea that science alone has access to the ultimate, objective truth ignores the implicit biases, conflicts of interest, competing agendas, and cultural ideologies that have influenced the outcomes of medical research and even the development of scientific language itself.

Scientism leads to what I call "medical monotheism," or the belief that there is only one true and right way to interpret and practice medicine, whereas alternative or competing methods are deemed heretical and steeped in quackery, despite the evidence of their being safer, more effective, and more readily available. This groupthink approach has entrenched itself within the biomedical establishment, making it career suicide for any professional to cite research or findings that defy or disprove popular medical opinion, much less apply alternative modalities like homeopathy or nutritional interventions instead of the establishment's prescribed standard of care. The medical establishment will go to enormous lengths to prove that natural medicine is ineffective at best and dangerous at worst. In our time, physicians have been indoctrinated and trained to match conditions with drugs and play symptom whack-a-mole, often making it impossible to discern patterns that have not already been stamped for approval by their peers. This is what is often called "consensus medicine" or "eminence-based medicine," which is based upon the often arbitrary and agenda-driven agreements of a group of highly influential individuals who have "always done it this way" instead of using the evidence at hand.

The maligning of anything but pill-for-an-ill medicine dates back to the 19th century, when natural medicine fell from grace. Back then, chiropractors and doctors who practiced natural healing methods, including hydropaths, naturopaths, and homeopaths, were preeminent over other medical professions. They became a relic in the aftermath of the Flexner Report, published in 1910. This survey to assess the American medical educational system, commissioned by the council of the American Medical Association (AMA), demonized these healers as quacks and charlatans. In order to gain a monopoly over the medical landscape, the AMA spearheaded a systematic smear campaign to delegitimize schools of medical practice that did not advocate drug-based treatments in their curricula, giving legal credence and institutional sanction only to medical schools that did.

This homogenization in licensure and medical education coincided with the funding of the earliest medical schools by oil magnate John D. Rockefeller and the rise of petroleum-based pharmaceutical drugs, in which Rockefeller had a vested financial interest and which became the bedrock of allopathic medicine (a form of medicine that focuses on suppressing symptoms of disease with drugs and surgery, in neglect of addressing their root causes). With these developments, medical doctors, formerly relegated to lower rungs on the social ladder, ascended the hierarchy to the position they now occupy—idolized as the guardians of privileged knowledge.

In theory, the cornerstone of the medical establishment's approach is "evidence-based medicine," or conclusions that were reached and treatment algorithms that were enacted based on well-designed, well-conducted research. The reality is that the scientific literature itself is fraught with controversy, as articulated by Richard Horton, editor-in-chief of *The Lancet*, who stated, "The case against science is straightforward: much of the scientific literature, perhaps half, may simply be untrue."[2] Likewise, the former editor-in-chief of the high-impact journal the *New England Journal of Medicine* arrived at similar conclusions: "It is simply no longer possible to believe much of the clinical research that is published, or to rely on the judgment of trusted physicians or authoritative medical guidelines. I take no pleasure in this conclusion, which I reached slowly and reluctantly over my two decades as an editor."[3]

Industry funding is a major impediment to unbiased results, as analyses have shown that industry-sponsored trials report positive outcomes significantly more often than trials financially backed by the government, nonprofits, or nonfederal organizations.[4] In a publication, bias known as the "file drawer" phenomenon, negative and null trials, or results that are unfavorable to drugs are more likely to be suppressed.[5] There is also widespread rigging of data—deliberate manipulation of outcomes and use of statistical sleight-of-hand—wherein the outcomes of trials are being corrupted by commercial interests.[6] And then there is the issue of industry bribery of journal editors. One retrospective observational study revealed that 50.6 percent of journal editors accept payments from industry sources, with an average payment of $28,136 and some payments approaching half a million dollars, meaning that the editors of the most influential journals in the world, who steer the scientific dialogue, are effectively on the take.[7] In addition, a 2007 national survey published in the *New England Journal of Medicine* found that 94 percent of physicians had ties to the pharmaceutical industry, with physicians receiving free meals, reimbursement for medical education or professional meetings, consulting, lecturing, and enrolling patients in clinical trials.[8]

The influence of pharmaceutical reps, who have been shown to maneuver the direction of physician prescribing practices, cannot be underestimated either. If many medical doctors and researchers are bought, if tampering with and distorting research findings is ubiquitous, and if publication of studies favors promising candidate drugs,[9] the edifice of evidence-based medicine begins to crumble. When the judge and jury are bought off, it is no longer possible to trust the recommendations that are established as standard of care.

Given these tactics, it takes a discerning eye to wade through the catacombs of scientific databases, analyze study methodology, ascertain study quality, assess conflicts of interest, and separate the proverbial wheat from the chaff. Thanks to my librarian mother and biology professor father, I was, early on, made familiar with resources like MEDLINE, the government database of over 30 million citations for biomedical literature, which offered me my first glimpse into high-quality peer-reviewed research around my own health issues. And perhaps thanks to this background, I had an uncanny knack for finding non-industry-funded clinical pearls within the immense ocean of published literature containing promising information that conventional medicine was unenlightened about, or even actively suppressing.

Ultimately, I made this deep digging into and re-examination of medical literature my life's work, spending thousands of hours as an informed health advocate and activist, sifting through hundreds of thousands of studies to find, index, and share information that would arm me and others. My goal was always to explore, find, and share the science of natural healing. This involves shining a spotlight on the unintended, adverse effects of conventional medical drugs and practices, known as iatrogenesis, while also uncovering natural, evidence-based alternatives that work in harmony with human physiology.

My ultimate purpose is to help people regain confidence in their bodies' self-healing abilities and to underscore that when it comes to the majority of complaints, all the medicine you need has resided within you all along. Most people that I interact with are at least curious about alternatives to pharmaceutically driven allopathic medicine—but they do not want to, nor should they, take my or anyone else's information on faith alone. Just as they are growing increasingly skeptical of the advice and treatment algorithms of conventional, drug-based medical doctors, they are also leery of falling prey to the latest fad supplement or tabloid diet. Beyond anecdotal evidence, people want robust scientific evidence and strategies that can help them.

So much of the medical literature today is obscured by the highly technical and esoteric "medicalese." My mission is to help readers overcome this barrier. On GreenMedInfo.com, you will find a database of biomedical literature covering over 10,000 different health topics, with over 50,000 citations from high-quality scientific literature. These articles are authored by respected, established experts and are indexed for easy access and searchability, including by medical condition and therapeutic substances and actions. Also included in the database is a compendium of my own writing that translates innovative new research into common language.

It still amazes me how many people around the world have come to use our website—over 150 million visits in total—since its humble beginnings as a passion project from my home garage back in 2007. In order to maintain a zone free of conflict of interest as best as I can, I have chosen to run the site without ads. Still, despite the growing popularity of independent sites like my own, people find themselves overwhelmed by the immense volume of often conflicting health information on the Internet. Now more than ever, we need trusted sources of information who can reduce the noise-to-signal ratio and who can deliver simplicity out of the teeming mass of complexity and contradiction.

You now have in your hands my life's work and vision, a product of two decades of perpetual research, relentless inquiry, and rigorous self-exploration. Here you will find pivotal concepts that I find truly exhilarating and revolutionary, including key findings of the New Biology and New Biophysics.

Put simply, the New Biology unveils three foundational facts about human health that have highly empowering implications:

1. **DNA does not control your destiny.** Epigenetic factors, or factors beyond the control of your genes (such as diet, lifestyle, environmental exposures, and mindset), almost exclusively determine your life-span and quality of life.

2. **Food is not just fuel and building blocks for the body; it's also a messaging system that delivers**

critical information to the body. In fact, certain foods and lifestyle practices can unlock immense self-regenerative energetic resources within your cells, optimizing DNA expression and making them more important in affecting your health than any other single factor.

3. **The cells of your body are capable of seemingly miraculous feats.** Your cells access "free energy" from the environment, facilitating low-energy nuclear transformation of elements and radical self-regeneration through recruitment of stem cells derived from an ancient, nearly immortal cell line. When properly directed through diet and lifestyle, they can reverse both chronic disease and biological age.

Let's begin by rethinking the idea that has been drilled into all of us since grade school: that DNA is your personal blueprint for your health and disease destiny.

DNA Is Not a Blueprint

Since you first gazed upon textbook images of the DNA double helix, comprising two strands winding around one another in a twisted ladder, you have probably believed what you were taught: that DNA is a blueprint, as if your body were a car and enfolded in the DNA were instructions for how to build the chassis, engine, and windshield wipers. In Western medicine, the locus of causality and the sphere of blame are turned inward: the body is viewed as a passive recipient of genetic instructions and disease as primarily a matter of hereditary misfortune.

A person with breast cancer might resign herself to the explanation that her diagnosis was the result of "bad genes." However, in Eastern cultures and ancient medical systems, such as Indian Ayurvedic medicine and traditional Chinese medicine, there is an intuitive appreciation for the way environmental variables inter-sect with individual constitution and decisions to produce disease. They attribute disease origin to a combination of factors, such as temperament, diet, and lifestyle habits, and envision disease as the by-product of imbalances operating at a larger scale, including fluctuations in climate, the seasons, and the cosmos. Psychosocial factors, such as discord in families and community, also play a role. In contrast, the determinism of modern science undermines efforts at self-healing and regeneration through its fatalistic view of human biology as being at the mercy of our genetic code.

When I first met my friend Jennifer, she was in her late 20s, and her health was on a steep decline from cystic fibrosis. She is considered to have one of those rare and damning genetic con-ditions, having been born with a mutation of the cystic fibrosis transmembrane conductance regulator (CFTR) gene. She was on antibiotics and steroids, saddled with skin, respiratory, and diges-tive problems, and chronically underweight. She also suffered from Type 1 diabetes subsequent to pancreatic damage, a major complication of cystic fibrosis.

Jennifer decided to radically shift her diet away from pro-inflammatory foods, such as wheat, dairy, and sugar. Instead, she consumed an abundance of green, leafy vegetables, good fats, and targeted supplements, including broad-spectrum enzymes and probiotics, which gave her body relief from the increased mucus production that is symptomatic of cystic fibrosis. She incorporated blood sugar–stabilizing foods, exercise, and mind-body techniques into her regimen and ate functional foods like turmeric, soy, and cayenne. Rodent studies had shown "miraculous" partial or full correction of the CFTR gene product misfolding when subjects were exposed to the phytochemicals found in these plants.

Changing these lifestyle factors has been exactly how Jennifer continues to defy the odds. The average life-span of someone with this kind of genetic variation is only 37 years. Today, at 49, Jennifer is alive, highly functional, and healthier. And she is just one example.

THE PROBLEM WITH THE
GENES—CAUSE—DISEASE MODEL

Tens of thousands of people worldwide who have been diagnosed as having chronic, progressive, or incurable ailments defy the odds, demonstrating the regenerative potential of the human body. And we shouldn't be surprised. The New Biology reveals that it is no longer accurate to assert that our genes cause disease any more than it is correct to claim that DNA is sufficient to account for all the proteins in the human body. The DNA-as-blueprint assumption originally postulated that there should be one gene per protein, but in recent decades, through the Human Genome Project, scientists have discovered only 20,000 to 25,000 protein-encoding genes, a number that pales in comparison to the 100,000-plus proteins found in the human body. The latest estimates, in fact, have pared this number down to about 18,000. In the face of these findings, it has become impossible to maintain the simplistic concept that there is a linear, one-way path from genes to disease.[10]

Instead, the old gene-disease narrative is being supplanted by epigenetics, a school of thought that focuses on the factors "above" the genes as the primary determinant of the way in which our genetic material is interpreted, translated, and expressed. Epigenetics accounts for how a liver cell is different than a brain cell or a muscle cell. All three share the same 3 billion base pairs that make up our genetic code, but epigenetic mechanisms, such as regulatory proteins and post-translational modifications, have a great say in which genes are expressed and which are silenced, resulting in the unique phenotype, or outward appearance, of each cell.

Environmental variables can either activate or inhibit genes by influencing complex biochemical processes, and these changes can be transmitted to daughter cells upon cell division.[11] Something as simple as getting adequate B vitamins from your food will directly affect whether you can silence certain key genes necessary for health (a process known as methylation, or the attachment of one-carbon tags to DNA molecules that effectively "turns off" the expression of that gene). Moreover, a huge number of factors that are often totally within your control will influence epigenetic expression. Whether you are sedentary, pray, smoke, meditate, do yoga, eat plants, have an extensive network of social support, or are alienated from your community, all your lifestyle choices play into your risk for disease through epigenetic mechanisms. In fact, the conclusions of the Human Genome Project ushered in "nutrigenomics," a novel field of research that studies the reciprocal interaction between genes and nutrients at a molecular level. Bioactive compounds in food, for example, can modulate cellular signaling pathways, regulating key molecules like nuclear factor kappa beta (NFκB), a transcription factor that is the gateway to production of inflammatory messengers.[12]

On a smaller scale, biochemical processes encompassing the release of hormones and other cellular messengers, oxidative stress (excess free radicals), inflammation, lipid peroxidation (the "rusting" of fats), body morphology (deposition of belly fat, for example), and the proliferation of our gut microbiota exert effects on our patterns of genetic expression. Other macro-level epigenetic influences include psychological stress, socioeconomic status, geopolitical variables, educational attainment, occupational elements, urban or rural residence, and climate. These factors issue directives to our DNA and contribute to our genetic expression in either favorable or unfavorable directions. In practical terms, this means that controllable variables such as diet and lifestyle practices; exposure to pathogens, radiation, chemical contaminants, and pollutants; medical interventions; and even mind-set and emotions coalesce to determine how epigenetic factors are articulated.[13]

Rather than succumb to analysis paralysis, let this research rescue you from the clutches of a genetically divined fate. According to a recent review paper published in *PLOS ONE*, genetic factors aren't to blame in many chronic diseases.[14] Studies connect cancers of nearly all types, neurobehavioral and cognitive dysfunction, respiratory illnesses, autoimmune disorders, reproductive anomalies, and cardiovascular disease to epigenetic mechanisms.[15] The burgeoning field of epigenetics offers us a new paradigm in which nurture, not nature, can be envisioned as the predominant influence when it comes to genetic expression.

YOUR HABITS NOW AFFECT YOUR PROGENY LATER: MICRORNA AND GENE EXPRESSION

The arrival of epigenetics has overturned one of the most sacred tenets of modern genetics, the Weismann barrier, which proposes that movement of hereditary information from genes to body cells is unidirectional, and the information transferred by egg and sperm to future generations remains independent of body cells and parental experience.

Animal research has shown that parental experience is epigenetically imprinted not only onto first-generation offspring but also potentially onto a countless number of future generations. Take, for instance, one study that traced the transient exposure of pregnant rats to the insecticide methoxychlor, an estrogenic compound, and the fungicide vinclozolin, an antiandrogenic compound. Exposure to these two chemicals resulted in male infertility and decreased sperm production and viability in 90 percent of the males of all four subsequent generations that were tracked.[16] Scientists speculate that these adverse reproductive effects were mediated by changes in DNA methylation patterns in the germline cells, suggesting the transmission of epigenetic change to future generations. The authors of this research conclude, in the journal *Science*:

> The ability of an environmental factor (for example, endocrine disruptor) to reprogram the germ line and to promote a transgenerational disease state has significant implications for evolutionary biology and disease etiology.[17]

The immediate implication is that endocrine-disrupting, fragrance-laden personal care products and commercial cleaning supplies may trigger fertility problems in multiple future generations. The broader and more hopeful implications of this research, however, are that germ cells (egg and sperm) exhibit a dynamic plasticity and adaptability in response to environmental signals that can be communicated to future generations. In other words, your actions now may affect your descendants and the future of humanity for better or for worse.

Other studies indicate that characteristics of the parental sensory environment experienced before conception, such as trauma or famine, can remodel the sensory nervous system and neuroanatomy in subsequently conceived generations through epigenetics. This is best illustrated by a study in which researchers wafted the cherry-like scent imparted by the chemical acetophenone into the chambers of mice while administering electric shocks, conditioning the mice to fear the scent. Despite having never encountered the chemical before, mice in the two successive generations shuddered significantly more in its presence when compared with the control group.[18]

It has been well established that maternal famine or undernourishment in the time around conception is associated with a host of health risks in the offspring, including major affective disorders such as schizophrenia, congenital anomalies in the central nervous system, decreased intracranial volume, and higher risk for obesity, hypertension, and heart disease later in life.[19] In a similar vein, children of Holocaust survivors have shown the intergenerational effects of stress and tragedy by exhibiting altered profiles of stress hormones, which has predisposed them to anxiety, depression, and post-traumatic stress disorder (PTSD). [20]

How long epigenetic changes persist remains to be determined, but animal models provide us with clues that they endure longer than ever predicted—epigenetic memories of environmental change lasted at least 14 generations in one study of nematode worms.[21]

This body of research is game changing in that it shows that the flow of genetic information, once thought to be strictly vertical and insulated from the world, also flows horizontally and bidirectionally. New studies are overturning the conventional logic that genetic change only occurs over an elongated time range of hundreds of thousands and even millions of years. Research continues to illuminate that genetic information can be transferred through the germline cells of a species instantaneously in *real time* through the medium of exosomes.

MicroRNAs, Exosomes, and the Gene Expression Connection

Unlike messenger RNAs, whose job is to carry instructions from DNA into ribosomes where they are transcribed into proteins, microRNAs turn on and off the expression of a wide range of our genes through silencing messenger RNA.[22] MicroRNAs are transported in virus-sized exosomes, or specialized, membrane-enclosed, nano-sized vesicles secreted by all plant, animal, bacterial, and fungal cells. MicroRNAs survive the digestive process intact and function like software, altering the expression of the hardware that is our protein-coding genes. Not only are microRNAs instrumental in regulation of gene expression, but the difference in sophistication between higher life-forms such as humans relative to, say, earthworms (with whom we share about the same number of protein-coding genes: approximately 20,000) has been attributed to the higher level of RNA complexity within the so-called dark matter of the genome—which constitutes the approximately 98.5 percent of the human genome that does not code for proteins. The most important takeaway with respect to these biomolecules, however, is that our genetic and epigenetic integrity may be wholly contingent upon the gene-regulatory microRNAs imbedded in our diet.

In one groundbreaking experiment, human melanoma tumor cells genetically engineered to express genes for a fluorescent tracer enzyme were transplanted into mice.[23] Experimenters discovered that information-storing molecules containing the tracer, including exosomes, were released into the animals' blood. The exosomes were also shown to deliver RNAs to spermatozoa (mature sperm cells) and remain stored there. The implication is that the RNA carried to sperm cells by exosomes can preside over gene expression in a way that changes the observable traits and disease risk, as well as the morphology, development, and physiology of the offspring. This miRNA harbored in exosomes may be the means by which both environmental assaults and health-promoting influences are epigenetically relayed to future generations.

RADICAL RESPONSIBILITY AS THE KEY TO HEALTH

Research into microRNAs and exosomes challenges the traditional Mendelian laws of genetics and its chromosomally based theory of inheritance, which maintains that genetic inheritance occurs exclusively through sexual reproduction and that traits are passed to offspring through the chromosomes contained in germline cells and never through somatic (body) cells. This research confirms that traits that are the by-product of our lifestyle, experiences, and exposures can separate from chromosomal genes and be transmitted to progeny, resulting in persistent phenotypes (observable characteristics, traits, or diseases) that endure across generations.[24]

According to scientific literature, hazards of modern agriculture, the industrial revolution, and contemporary living— including radioactivity, heavy metals, pesticides, tobacco smoke, polycyclic aromatic hydrocarbons from vehicular exhaust, hormones, infections, and deficiencies in essential nutrients— are known or suspected drivers behind epigenetic processes.[25]

Serendipitously, however, the remedy is in nature's pharmacopeia. Exercise, mindfulness, and bioactive components in fruits and vegetables (such as sulforaphane in cruciferous vegetables, resveratrol from red grapes, genistein from soy, diallyl sulphide from garlic, curcumin from turmeric, betaine from beets, and catechins in green tea) can optimize your body's innate resilience.

The air we breathe, the food we eat, the thoughts we allow, the toxic compounds to which we are exposed, and the experiences we undergo may continue to reverberate through our progeny long after we are gone. This breathes new life into the principle of seven generation stewardship taught by Native Americans, which mandates that we consider the welfare of seven generations to come in each of our decisions. Not only should we embody this approach in practices of environmental sustainability, but we would be wise to consider how all the conditions to which we subject our bodies may translate into ill health effects and diminished quality of life for a number of subsequent generations.

Our genes have a memory, and, as Deepak Chopra says, our cells are constantly eavesdropping on our thoughts. We must reframe our relationships, our mental monologues, our narratives, and our habits in the face of this radical insight. As articulated by British geneticist Marcus Pembrey, "we are all guardians of our genome."[26]

THE PROBLEM WITH EVOLUTIONARY MISMATCH

Epigenetics account for the multiple ways in which we reside in the realm of evolutionary mismatch and the myriad means by which we have deviated from the environment in which our physiology has adapted over the course of evolutionary history. Also known as paleo-deficit disorder,[27] *evolutionary mismatch* refers to the collective deficiency of ancestral influences in the modern, industrialized landscape. Paleo-deficit disorder runs the gamut from reduced opportunities for privacy and solitude to decreased tactile contact with a variety of natural vegetation to reduced exposure to birdsong, daylight, and phytoncides, the allelochemical, volatile organic compounds emitted by plants that give the forest its characteristic aroma.[28] It is no coincidence that our career stress, our sedentary desk jobs, our sleep deficits, our processed and adulterated food, our exposure to industrial chemicals and pharmaceutical drugs, our lack of social support, and our minimal contact with nature all constitute the primary risk factors for disease.[29] These lifestyle factors, which are largely under our control, determine whether our genetic blueprints express health or disease.

Overturning the One Gene, One Disease Hypothesis

It is imperative that we reframe the way in which we perceive genetic variants, which are generically referred to as mutations. Gene mutations, also known as single nucleotide polymorphisms (SNPs), are not catastrophic curses but code adjustments that occur in at least one percent of the population and that often evolved in the interest of self-preservation. Their higher incidence implies a neutral or beneficial effect that maintains their presence in the gene pool.[30] For instance, it is widely accepted that the gene anomalies that lead to some red blood cell disorders (hemoglobinopathies) such as thalassemia and sickle cell disease may provide resistance against malarial infections.[31] Carriers of these mutations have a survival advantage in regions where malaria is endemic, which has led to persistence of this genetic signature in the human genome.

From an evolutionary medicine perspective, the CFTR gene in cystic fibrosis may similarly protect against cholera by blocking the same molecular pathway exploited by the cholera toxin that can cause severe diarrhea.[32] This would explain why an apparently highly lethal gene could survive and is still present in 5 percent of Caucasians; namely, it helps CFTR carriers survive through the reproductive window required for them to pass on their genes.

But these gene variations do not occur in a vacuum. The environment has a lot to do with how our genetic inheritance manifests. For instance, the pathological expression of the CFTR may be triggered by nutritional deficiencies (like a lack of selenium) in the womb or early in life.

In addition, approximately 20 to 30 percent of the world's population has been found to carry the HLA-DQ locus of genetic susceptibility to celiac disease on chromosome 6, yet only a small percentage—approximately 1.4 percent of people worldwide[33]—exhibit the classical symptoms of celiac disease. Research suggests that enteroviral infections, such as rotavirus, and the composition of gut bacteria may act as triggers for the expression of the celiac genes.[34] A constellation of modifiable lifestyle factors, including dietary patterns, stress levels, urban versus rural residence, having pets in the home, antibiotic treatments, use of a dishwasher compared to hand-washing dishes, and early life exposures (e.g., being born in a hospital or at home and breastfeeding duration) converge to impact our microbiota, our immune systems, and therefore the ability of "pathogenic forces" to activate these latent celiac genes.

Yet the biggest misconception revolves around the role that the breast cancer susceptibility genes, *BRCA1* and *BRCA2*, play in breast cancer risk and prognosis. Popular culture and the mainstream medical establishment target *BRCA1* and *BRCA2*, genes that interfere with the repair of radiation-induced DNA damage, as harbingers of inevitable breast cancer. This assertion has led some, including celebrity Angelina Jolie, to have their breast tissue and ovaries excised prophylactically in the hopes of avoiding an early gene-determined death. The primary justification for preemptive mastectomy and ovary and fallopian tube removal—salpingo-oophorectomy—is the belief that heredity determines risk, reflecting an ironclad faith in the inevitability of gene-driven cancer vis-à-vis a fundamentally powerless subject. Medical literature, however, is highly equivocal on the meaning of *BRCA* status.

According to the prestigious British medical journal *The Lancet Oncology*, women with either gene are not more likely to die from treatment-resistant breast cancers, such as triple-negative cancer, than other women who are diagnosed with the disease. In fact, the opposite holds true: they have higher survival rates than women without the *BRCA* mutations who were treated for breast cancer.[35] In addition, thousands of polymorphisms in the *BRCA1* and *BRCA2* genes have already been identified and characterized on a molecular level, some of which are inversely related to breast cancer risk, adding much more complexity to the picture of statistical risk and actionable treatments than is currently present in the traditional medical establishment. The "*BRCA* causes breast cancer" narrative is brought further into question by the identification of polymorphisms such as the *BRCA1* subtype *K1183R*, which paradoxically increases breast cancer survival.[36] It is therefore possible that some of these *BRCA* polymorphisms might even predispose you toward greater resilience and health and reduced breast cancer mortality despite the conventional view that *BRCA* is a monolithic, inexorably lethal "mutation" that you either have or don't.

Adding fuel to the fire, the rhetoric around *BRCA* in a cancer-phobic patient with a family history of cancer fans the flames of fear, resulting in aberrant secretion of stress hormones, which further magnifies risk in a vicious cycle.

Symptoms Aren't Life Sentences

The silver lining of this research is that you are the principle director of your body's fate, no matter your genetic endowment. Indeed, the New Biology unfolds the reality that DNA is not the locus for disease risk but a personalized resiliency warehouse. By reframing sickness through this lens, we can derive solace from the fact that every symptom manifestation, every genetic variant, and even the materialization of disease processes serves a sacred and inherent purpose. The coughing, sneezing, and runny nose that accompany a respiratory virus, for instance, are your body's attempt to expel and cleanse itself of toxicity. The fever your body produces in response to what we conceptualize as a pathogenic infection renders the body temperature inhospitable to the overgrowth of potentially virulent microorganisms; that is, the fever, in most cases, is a sign of a healthy immune system and *is* the medicine.

Genetic variants stick around the human genome because they enhance evolutionary fitness. For example, some of the genes implicated in autoimmune diseases such as celiac disease originated in Neanderthal lineages that interbred with *Homo sapiens* when primitive hominids immigrated from sub-Saharan Africa to northern Europe through western Asia.[37] The result of this interbreeding is that humans picked up many of the Neanderthal genes in a process called haplotype introgression. These same Neanderthal genetic proclivities that augment risk of autoimmune conditions also likely promote fat deposition and other metabolic and immune adaptations that optimize survival in cold climates. Thus, even detrimental genetic profiles can serve a protective purpose when viewed within the larger context.

UNLOCKING YOUR INNATE REGENERATIVE CAPACITY

Most people consider the body to be little more than a vehicle, materially distinct from the mind that resides within, passively carrying them through life and only eventually requiring the intervention of a doctor-mechanic to fix, or at least manage, the symptoms of suffering with a battery of diagnoses and medications. This reductionism is a fatalistic relic of René Descartes, the 17th-century French philosopher and mathematician who split body and soul asunder, reducing the soul to the "ghost in the machine." With this dualistic and mechanistic model, our feelings, our perceptions, our desire for meaning are relegated to an afterthought. By the same token, in the Newtonian model of physical objects, our body-machines are deemed inevitably destined for decline, frailty, and debility due to their tendency toward increasing disorder rather than order.

But we are not inanimate objects. We are living organisms, and the New Biology shows that our bodies are a veritable repository of self-healing mechanisms, always regenerating, tending to states of order against the downward spiral of entropy.

Take, for example, your small intestine. Every four to five days, your small intestine gets a new epithelial cell lining orchestrated by stem cells that have the ability to repopulate the entire intestinal tract.[38] Around every two months or so, the stratified epithelium layer of your skin, or epidermis, completely turns over as a result of the stem cells residing in the deepest, basal layer.[39] Even the prospect of cardiac cell regeneration is now a confirmed reality with the discovery of endogenous cardiac progenitor cells in the heart, blood, and bone marrow that are capable of replenishing the cells of the heart, including cardiac endothelial cells, myocytes, and smooth muscle cells.[40] Furthermore, the brain has been shown to regenerate neurons post-injury.[41]

FOOD IS INFORMATION: THE MAGIC OF HUMAN/PLANT CO-EVOLUTION

Virtually everything we are comes from the things we eat, breathe, apply to our skin, or drink. But food provides more than building blocks for the body-machine and fuel for its engines. The materialistic view that food is merely caloric content interspersed with macronutrients and micronutrients is another biological atomism relic of the Newtonian-Cartesian model. Within this view, food and life are understood from the epistemological, decompositional (bottom-up) approach, where the focus is on the indivisible and elementary vital units instead of the relationship between the units. Unfortunately, this approach obliterates the study of systems and dynamics and decimates any focus on synergy and the interactions between elements.

The New Biology has shown that food's value extends far beyond physical sustenance. Its model embraces the connectivity and proportionality embedded within our bodies and within the biosphere as a whole. Food is not just a caloric measure but an essential courier of biologically indispensable information—by way of microRNAs—on which the health and vitality of your cells depend. After eons of co-evolution with plants that provided food for our species, our biological systems are intimately intertwined. This discovery has profound implications, reinforcing the importance of eating an evolutionarily appropriate, whole foods–based diet reminiscent of what our hunter-gatherer ancestors would have eaten. The smooth operation of our physiology is literally predicated upon interfacing with microRNAs found in fruits and vegetables, as well as other ancestral foods, including grass-fed meats. (While I do not believe it is absolutely necessary to eat meat, both for ethical and physiological reasons, the therapeutic properties of high-quality, ethically raised and slaughtered meat, are undeniable, and when consumed with gratitude and moderation may be literally life-saving in certain individuals.) Today, our industrialized food culture divests us of the deeply rooted evolutionary symbiosis between the animal and plant kingdoms, as well as the biological information plants provide, putting us at greater risk for a wide range of diseases.

The Tree of Life Is Really a Web

The discoveries about microRNAs should shake up the way we think about food. One human study found that exosomal microRNAs from rice impact cholesterol receptors,[42] suggesting a new way that food can profoundly impact blood lipid profiles and cardiovascular health, as well as demonstrating that microRNA has the potential for cross-kingdom regulation of gene expression. That is, plants and animals can "talk" to one another's genes with profound impacts on their expression. This finding essentially undermines the notion that the human species is hermetically sealed off from other taxonomic kingdoms. The microRNA-mediated interkingdom communication, which involves cross talk and information sharing between bacteria and archaea (both prokaryotes) and plants and animals (both eukaryotes) confirms what Eastern cultures have known since time immemorial: we are *one* with all living things. When we deviate from our nature, we are destructive to ourselves.

In the New Biology, the distinct taxonomic categories merge into an open-ended spiral of mutualistic and reciprocal interactions. The traditional view of the tree of life as having separate and distinct branches of species falls short of the interconnected reality of life on earth. If plants communicate with animals, fungi with bacteria, and so on and so forth via microRNAs, these disparate compartments dissolve, suggesting a radical holism with all lifeforms that exist.

This new view of food as a unifying string that nourishes us *informationally* in the interdependent web of life has electrifying implications, namely that our deepest biological needs and health depend on the types and qualities of food information we are consuming. The difference between a GMO, sewage- or petrochemical-fertilizer-grown, agrochemical-sprayed, and irradiated tomato versus one grown biodynamically in natural soil, without pesticides and synthetic fertilizers, is not immediately discernible when examined through the rubric of protein, carbohydrate, mineral, or vitamin content. But when assessed from the perspective of their informational, qualitative differences, the two tomatoes are on opposite sides of the spectrum. And we can rewrite the functionality of our genomic hardware to be health-promoting or health-degrading depending on the software-like changes in our RNA profiles resulting from the food we choose to consume.

In the New Biology, food is essentially an epigenetic modifier of gene expression, contributing significantly to orchestrating which genes are turned on and which are turned off. This also means significant changes to staples within our food chain have a powerful impact on our physiological fate.

The Dangers
of Transgenic RNAi

In 2017, Dow Chemical Company, in partnership with Monsanto, America's most powerful agricultural biotechnology corporation at the time, received EPA approval to produce corn genetically modified to make an RNA-based pesticidal agent that lethally targets a metabolic pathway within the corn rootworm, known within the industry as the "billion-dollar bug." Branded as SmartStax PRO, the newly minted proprietary GMO plant produces a small, double-stranded RNA that disrupts a critical gene within the rootworm, causing its demise. Although this technology promises specificity—one RNAi molecule change equals one gene suppressed—it ignores the infinite possibilities of unintended, off-target adverse effects of transgenic RNAi that could affect human health and vitality. Even industry-sponsored research shows that hundreds of plant RNAs have a perfect complementary match to human genes as well as those of other mammals. The dire implication is that the consumption of RNAi corn could shut down dozens of essential genes required to maintain human and animal health.[43]

How the Plants You Eat
Have Your Back

The microRNA and phytochemical profiles of whole foods can differ greatly from the industrially produced foods that dominate the Western Pattern Diet. In an organically grown plant exposed to natural stressors, the levels of respective polyphenols such as resveratrol and quercetin can be magnitudes higher than in its industrially produced counterpart.

We can observe this directly in drought-stressed wild strawberries, which have a higher antioxidant capacity and phenol content[44] and taste better in contrast to the industrially produced variety. Droughts require plants to develop their inner defenses against animal herbivores, pathogenic microorganisms, and other prevailing environmental threats, which activate a repertoire of antioxidants that are highly beneficial to our bodies once we ingest them.[45] For example, one study in the *Journal of Agricultural and Food Chemistry* found organic tomatoes to contain statistically significantly higher levels of health-promoting phenolic compounds compared to conventional varieties. According to study author Rosa Maria Lamuela-Raventós, "The more stress plants suffer, the more polyphenols they produce."[46] Because nitrogenous fertilizers are not used in organic farming, the plants tend to generate higher levels of their own antioxidants.[47]

One framework for understanding this informational dimension is known as the xenohormesis hypothesis, which proposes that animals and fungi have evolved to sense signaling and stress-induced molecules in the plants they consume in order to mount a preemptive defense to environmental adversity and increase the probability of their survival.[48] Plants that produce compounds in response to impending scarcity of resources or dangerous environmental conditions, such as drought or other weather extremes, provide the animals that consume them with chemical cues, which activate resilience factors and pathways in their bodies. Nonnutritive polyphenols produced by stressed plants activate fungal and animal sirtuin enzymes, which extend the life-span of the organism that consumes the plant, suggesting that human sirtuin enzymes could also have evolved to respond similarly to plant stress molecules.[49] In this way, an interspecies system of signaling and reciprocity is established, creating an elegant evolutionary, supportive symbiosis between the seemingly divergent plant and animal kingdoms.

Taken cumulatively, this innovative body of research rolls out the red carpet for the emergence of a New Biology with trajectory-altering implications. The discovery that our bodies obtain information from food, including the very real gene-regulatory microRNAs that are embedded in all the foods we consume, has revolutionary implications for the way we understand food quality and the human body's requirements of it beyond the age-old fixation on caloric content and the measurable presence of certain minerals, nutrients, and vitamins. This also means that, with the presence of certain foundational, information-laden foods in your diet, your health will be positioned to thrive.

This notion thrusts traditional culinary practices and family recipes into a newfound light. Although often dismissed as superstition or folk medicine, food preparation techniques and ancient culinary formulas represent advanced means of self-care that have been historically refined, carefully cultivated, and passed on as ancestral wisdom. Recipes passed down through the generations are epigenetic inheritance systems, culturally encoded, time-tested instructions for what we should or should not eat, perhaps providing as much biologically critical information as the sequence of base pairs in your genome.

When we consider traditional plant-based culinary and indigenous medical practices through the lens of their informational contributions to our health, it's no wonder that food and botanical medicine provides the foundation for medical systems worldwide. A 2017 report by Kew Gardens in the United Kingdom found that 28,187 plant species are known to be used as medicines throughout the world,[50] and for good reason. Not only do they work, but, if used properly, they're safer and more accessible and are intrinsically biocompatible, working in harmony with your own biomolecules, as opposed to synthetic pharmaceuticals, the majority of which are petrochemical derivatives and recognized as foreign to your body.

Of course, plants have long been the raw material for drug development. Since 1981, in fact, of all drugs introduced since 1981, 63 percent (537 of 847 small molecule-based pharmaceuticals) were derived from natural products or had a natural product-inspired design.[51] In one sense, pharmaceutical medicine could be considered "plant-based," though the pharmaceutical industry's patent-based model almost invariably generates toxicity through the unnatural alteration of compounds. And arguably, biomedical science has played a role in validating time-honored natural remedies that have been passed down generation to generation, so much so that the vast body of folkloric medical knowledge still forms the basis for the majority of the world's primary health care system. Furthermore, "alternative medicine" modalities, which encompass the original medicine practices to which our species owes its present-day survivorship, are gaining traction, even within the walls of the patented, synthetic, and chemically based Western medical establishment.

THE EVOLUTIONARY MISMATCH OF THE WESTERN DIET

We all know the human body requires certain foods to function properly and that nutritional deficiencies can lead to serious health problems. Without the information-rich berries, vegetables, roots, tubers, and naturally raised animal products that have been part of the ancestral human diet for countless millennia, the biological rug will be pulled out from under us and lead to rapid health deterioration. Scientists call this "evolutionary mismatch." In the same way that you wouldn't expect a fish to be able to live out of water, you wouldn't expect humans to survive if they were to be suddenly extricated from their evolutionarily compatible nutritional environment.

WHEAT AS AN EXAMPLE
OF EVOLUTIONARY MISMATCH

Wheat is one of the worst offenders in the Western Pattern Diet. Not only is modern wheat hybridized to contain higher levels of gluten and the endocrine-disrupting starch known as amylopectin, contaminated with agrochemicals including pesticides and glyphosate, but from an evolutionary perspective, the seeds of cereal grasses that yielded wheat only entered the human diet 500 generations, or 20,000 years, ago. This is a mere blip on the evolutionary scale, and not nearly enough time for our physiology to adapt to their consumption in a manner that would promote health.

We are only now learning about the fragile biological system of the microbiome, the gut bacteria that regulate our metabolism and maintains our health. The introduction of grains from the grass family of plants would have been foreign to the anatomically modern humans who, according to "out of Africa" hypothesis, originated from the tropical rainforests of the African subcontinent and subsisted on insects, tubers, fruit-bearing plants, and the flesh of hunted animals. Approximately 60,000 years ago they migrated from Africa into the Northern latitudes, where vegetation would have been sparse or nonexistent during winter months. It took another 40,000 years to develop the adequate cooking and processing technology required for the consumption of grass seeds.

To a casual observer, this dietary shift might seem inconsequential. One might surmise that grains simply represented a more accessible, mass-cultivated alternative caloric fuel source of carbohydrates, protein, lipids, minerals, and vitamins. Yet replacing the roots, tubers, and forageable vegetation of the Paleolithic period with the cereal grains of the Neolithic required a dramatic shift in physiological adaptation.

In an effort to deter animals and ensure the continuance of the plant species, grass seeds were cultivated with a vast armory of antinutrients, including toxic lectins, phytates, alpha-amylase and trypsin inhibitors, and phytochemicals, which then, in turn, disrupted mammalian physiology. Although heralded since time immemorial as the "staff of life," grains could perhaps be more aptly described as a cane, precariously propping up the human body that is starved of the nutrient-dense, low-starch vegetables, fruits, edible nuts, seeds, seafood, and meats these crops have so thoroughly displaced. As a result of this shift from the ancestral Paleolithic diet to what has evolved into the contemporary Western diet, we are now running on the wrong nutritional operating system for our natural, time-tested biological hardware.

THE WESTERN DIET AS A VECTOR OF DEATH

Culturally, we are still under wheat's spell. In more ways than one, wheat resembles a drug, creating cycles of cravings and withdrawal that are often conflated with hunger. It can be argued that given the presence of pharmacologically active narcotic peptides, wheat is addictive, generating a ceaseless cycle of cravings and dependence. Twentieth-century German raw food advocate and philosopher Arnold Ehret may have been correct when he said, "We dig our graves with our teeth."[52]

For evidence of how disastrous this evolutionary mismatch has been to the health of our species, one only has to look at our present-day rates of chronic disease. Consider the statistics about disease at the turn of the 20th and 21st centuries. According to an article in the *New England Journal of Medicine*, the most common causes of death in 1900 were infections, such as pneumonia, flu, and tuberculosis. In 2010, the leading killers were heart disease and cancer. With the improvement in hygienic practices, nutrition, living conditions, and sanitation infrastructure, mortality from infectious disease declined, whereas mortality rates from chronic diseases have skyrocketed. Concurrent with the escalating rates of these chronic inflammatory conditions, our diet has become dominated by processed, manipulated, additive-laden, and laboratory-generated synthetic substances. These hyperpalatable foods, with their lab-tested combinations of salty, savory, and sweet, override normal homeostatic pathways and kick the hedonic or reward-based regulation systems into action,[53] increasing the motivational incentive to overeat and ultimately become addicted to these foods.

The Western Pattern Diet Features and Diseases

Our current harmful dietary pattern, which researchers call the Western Pattern Diet, is characterized by the following toxic foods:

- Processed, factory-farmed, GMO-fed animal products

- Conventional dairy products from grain-fed, antibiotic- and hormone-raised cows

- Highly refined grain products, including gluten-containing grains, contaminated with agrochemicals

- Industrialized vegetable oils from genetically modified corn, cottonseed, canola, and soybeans

- Trans fat–containing desserts containing refined sugars and flours

- Prepackaged foods with chemical additives, preservatives, and colorants

- Refined sugars and high-fructose corn syrup

The Western Pattern Diet contributes to many chronic diseases but has been specifically studied to determine its contribution to more than 20 distinct conditions, including various deadly cancers. In fact, it's so effective at proliferating disease and degeneration that lab researchers use it to induce disease in experimental animals. These are just some of the disease labels linked to the Western Pattern Diet:

- Acne

- Attention Deficit Disorder

- Bone fractures

- Breast cancer

- Cardiac hypertrophy (enlargement of the heart)

- Colon cancer

- *E. coli* infections

- Insulin resistance

- Lipid peroxidation (which makes the fats in your body rancid)

- Liver disease

- Low sperm count and quality

- Neurodegenerative disease

- Osteoporosis

- Oxidative stress

- Pancreatic cancer

- Prostate cancer

- Sepsis

- Types 1 and 2 diabetes

WHAT NOT TO EAT: THE WORST OFFENDERS

At a rudimentary level, food is digested, assimilated, and repackaged into the very foundations of our physiology, the biochemical machinery of our cells. What we eat, drink, and inhale, then, are critical determinants of the structural and functional integrity in our bodies. Seeds planted in fertile soil will metamorphosize into beautiful flowers, while those potted in eroded, nutrientless topsoil will be vulnerable to sickness in the form of infection and pests; our bodies are no different in the way we react to the substrate in which we grow.

But how do we mute all the contradictory recommendations in the diet-sphere to glean what may be the perfect diet? This question is the platform for a multi-billion-dollar industry of competing egos, interests, and ideals, with a never-ending procession of new fad diets and lose-weight-quick schemes bandied about year after year as the next best thing. Most adopt a strategy irrespective of ancestral heritage, biochemical individuality, or physiological landscape. Whether keto or low-carb, vegan or macrobiotic, the problem is the same: proponents are extrapolating what worked for them or what was effective for a select cohort of subjects. The nuances, complexities, exceptions, and contingencies of different human populations fall by the wayside.

Your best bet, then, is the time-tested, tried-and-true process of self-experimentation, oftentimes in the form of an "elimination diet," where you whittle your food consumption down to a blueprint of ancestrally appropriate, minimal-allergenicity, and minimal-antigenicity foods (foods least likely to provoke an immune response) for approximately a month. Then you sequentially reintroduce noncompliant foods one at a time to gauge your individual tolerance. By removing offending agents such as gluten, dairy, soy, corn, alcohol, and refined sugar from your diet, you effectively clear the static noise, enabling the messages your body dispatches in the form of food reactions to be heard loud and clear.

That being said, there is a generic template that, if followed, can deliver positive outcomes for the majority of people. The first step includes permanently removing foods that were not part of any traditional dietary culture, including genetically modified foods and foods that were produced with the use of agrochemical synthetic inputs such as petrochemically derived fertilizers and pesticides.

The second step is eliminating or reducing the consumption of cow's milk. While there is a history of animal husbandry that stretches back at least a millennium among certain populations, including Northern Europeans, the consumption of cow's milk products is a novel trend for most other ethnicities. This explains why so many adult humans of African or Native American descent do not produce the enzyme lactase for breaking down milk sugar (lactose) as adults. A more insidious culprit behind countless other adverse metabolic symptoms is a sticky protein known as A2 β-casein and the more toxic A1 form, both of which are found in the world's bovine dairy products. Even in the rare case that you find raw, organic, A2 milk from a cow, it will still contain exosomes that were intended for a calf and which may therefore disrupt normal cell-to-cell communication and epigenetic regulation in humans.[54] Through the vehicle of bovine microRNA-containing exosomes, cow's milk dairy is a Trojan horse carrying immunoregulatory cargo that tips the balance in favor of inflammation.

The final step of the template is eliminating or reducing grain-derived products. Gluten-bearing wheat, rye, and barley are particularly pernicious gateways to the "leaky gut syndrome," a condition resulting from the erosion of the intestinal barrier. These biologically incompatible foods should be removed from the diet to cultivate the conditions ideal for healing and regeneration.

Fortunately, traditional foods that were of the variety that could be foraged or hunted long before the advent of modern cultural inventions like farming and animal husbandry provide the architectural blueprint our bodies need to construct our intricate body-ecosystems from the bottom up. In ethnographic studies of remaining hunter-gatherer tribes, untouched by the influence of globalization and virtually free from the afflictions of modernity, we can witness the preservation of these health-imbuing foods and practices through the lineages, underscoring their consistently health-promoting legacy.

What to Eat: Start with Chicken Soup

One example of our evolutionarily inscribed wisdom that makes us gravitate to certain foods is our natural yearning for a steaming hot bowl of chicken soup when we have the flu. The prized peasant food of traditionally prepared chicken soup, made with bone-in animal carcass, vegetables, and herbs, is the impetus behind the newfound popularity of those bone broth bars that are cropping up across the country. Although it is oftentimes written off as a mere comfort food, chicken soup is the archetypal traditional home recipe that is an ideal and easy starting point for improving your diet.

The word *recipe* has ancient roots in Latin and originally meant "take," an exhortation by the medical doctor to the pharmacist that patients take the medicine as ordered. *Recipe* was used in the Middle Ages to mean a medical instruction or prescription, inspiring the pharmaceutical abbreviation Rx.

Chicken soup is an example of a time-tested, medicinal home recipe in all senses of the word. It helps support, optimize, and elevate our genetic expression. A paper in the journal *CHEST* found that chicken soup may elicit therapeutic effects in patients with pneumococcal pneumonia,[55] and chicken soup has also been shown to thin mucus secretions and relieve the inflammation in the upper respiratory tract that can precipitate fever, chills, muscle aches, and fatigue.[56] Its Japanese counterpart is a jellied soup known as chicken nikogori, a potent antioxidant with the ability to scavenge free radicals, which have been implicated in the unpleasant symptoms of both acute and chronic illness. Add wheat-free soy sauce to nikogori, and it's even more effective.[57] Or add ginger, one of the reigning champions in the arsenal of anti-inflammatory home remedies, which inhibits production of prostaglandins, leukotrienes, and tumor necrosis factor-α (TNF-α), biomolecules behind the cardinal signs of inflammation such as pain, redness, heat, and swelling.[58] Ginger also contains microRNAs that stimulate the growth of beneficial Lactobacillus bacteria in the gut and metabolism and reduces inflammation.[59]

Chicken soup, like virtually all food-based medicine, doesn't generally have side effects—only side benefits. It engenders a regenerative effect that stands in stark juxtaposition to the degeneration induced by synthetic chemicals produced by drug companies. Chicken soup contains easily assimilated protein found in the tendons, ligaments, and other flexible tissues that are often degraded during the cooking process, and it is a good source of easily absorbed minerals, including magnesium, calcium, potassium, silicon, sulfur, and phosphorous. In addition, it is rich in collagen and glycosaminoglycans like hyaluronic acid, glucosamine, and chondroitin sulfate, all of which elicit regenerative effects in joints, tendons, ligaments, and other connective tissues.

Chock-full of glutamine, the preferential fuel source of the cells lining the gastrointestinal tract, chicken soup helps to heal leaky gut syndrome. Bone broth generated from simmering the bone-in carcass for several hours contains glycine, an amino acid that is the prerequisite for the synthesis of our nucleotides, neurotransmitters, and the master antioxidant of our bodies, glutathione, as well as an important component of the bile and gastric acid required to emulsify dietary fats and break down proteins, respectively. Another amino acid liberated from the gelatin in bone broth, proline, is a prerequisite for wound healing and the fine-tuned construction of your connective tissue, as well as your skin, cartilage, bone, and vascular system.[60]

In the case of acute disease, functional foods like chicken soup can support our bodies in their endeavor to heal—promoting resolution of acute illness and setting the stage for reversal of the pathogenesis of chronic illness. Other foods can send your genes the equivalent of healing "text messages," providing a schematic and guide map for what your body has always known how to do—*heal*.

You'll learn all about these regenerative foods in this book. You'll also learn about targeted foods tailored for regeneration of specific organs, including the heart, brain, gut, pancreas, and liver. You will become familiar with the degenerative habits, activities, and environmental factors that you should avoid, and you will be directed to participate in the ones that stabilize your genome as well as your epigenome. Armed with this information, taking charge of your body—and navigating back home to yourself—will become second nature.

CHAPTER TWO

FOOD AS INFORMATION

Living Water, Epigenetic Pathways, and the Wisdom of the Ancestral Diet

Food delivers powerful healing properties that scientists have spent decades analyzing in detail. Take an apple, for example. This amazing fruit is brimming with pharmacologically (or better yet, nutrigenomically) active compounds, most notably ascorbic acid, also known as vitamin C. Another compound it contains is phlorizin, over a dozen polyphenols, potent antioxidants concentrated in the skin of the apple and known to elicit multitargeted effects that reduce the impact of high blood sugar in animal models.[1] But this strictly material layer of nutritional analysis barely touches the surface when it comes to appreciating the informational complexity of food.

Apples contain structured water molecules with a hexagonal crystalline configuration (H302) that's halfway between liquid and crystal. Named "the fourth phase of water" by Washington University professor Dr. Gerald Pollack, the micro-clustering pattern of structured water is capable of holding and transmitting both energy and information.[2] In fact, all raw plant, animal, fungal, and bacterial cells contain this structured water, each with a configuration as unique as a snowflake, assuming it has not been desiccated and denatured through cooking, processing, or the gamma irradiation-based food preservation process known as "cold pasteurization." "Raw" is a key word here. Raw fruit juice has a high concentration of naturally structured water, which accounts for a good portion of the anecdotal and scientific evidence regarding its healing benefits. Processed juice, on the other hand, is said to contain dys-information (dys- is a word-forming element meaning "bad, ill; hard, difficult; abnormal, imperfect,") that may misdirect the expression of our genes and harm our physiology.[3]

Virtually all water in uncooked and unprocessed plant food possesses beneficial genetic-expression-modifying information. This is a profound departure from looking at water as a fundamentally material, inert bystander in biological systems, as has been the case for centuries. Additionally, within the biological tissue of which they are composed, all foods contain the noncoding RNA molecules known as microRNAs, which affect the expression of the majority of genes in our bodies and stimulate biological pathways conducive to our species's health and wellness. Packaged in exosomes, which are roughly the size of a virus (~65 nanometers), microRNAs survive digestion, whereupon they penetrate systemic circulation in the body and affect the structure and function of all our tissues.

One example of the healing potential of microRNAs comes from a study of Chinese honeysuckle (*Lonicera japonica*), a traditional remedy for colds and flus. An animal study demonstrated that a microRNA isolated from this honeysuckle is delivered straight to the lungs, the area of active influenza infection, via the bloodstream. Once there, it targets and inhibits the replication of influenza A virus.[4] The authors of the study additionally proposed that ingestion of the Chinese honeysuckle decoction confers medicinal benefits by enhancing the dietary uptake of other microRNAs.

With every bite of food you take, you are deliberately choosing which messages you want to send to your genome. By simply being thoughtful and intentional with the foods you eat, you can remove interference in the moment-to-moment cellular regeneration that should *and will* naturally occur.

In this chapter you'll learn how regenerative foods communicate on the smallest levels, through micromolecules and via your microbiome. To understand the major role of these tiny players, let's go back to DNA and reexamine its role as the code at the center of life.

RETHINKING THE ROLE DNA PLAYS IN OUR HEALTH

Since the 19th century, when Charles Darwin revolutionized humanity's perception of its evolutionary past, present, and future, we've been taught that all organisms are separate from one another and locked into a ruthless system of survival of the fittest. This competitive arms race for resources, territory, and self-preservation yields two distinct groups: winners and losers. In this model, our genes are independent players, hermetically sealed within the chromosomes and concerned only with the solitary task of propagating themselves to the next generation. DNA (deoxyribonucleic acid) is the conductor of this abstract symphony of life, in which our place—and our fate—has been predetermined.

Not unlike the Copernican Revolution, which, in the 16th century, dislodged Earth from the center of the universe and threatened rigid social and political conventions, the New Biology dethrones DNA as the center of life, heralding an alternative vision. In this vision, human molecules, cells, tissues, and organs are absorbed in dynamic flux, communication, and feedback. They are capable of constant change, working harmoniously within a networked biosphere that unifies each individual with the whole. Most importantly, the New Biology inaugurates the radical notion that the body can directly access biologically useful energy from the quantum vacuum. In this reenvisioning, biological structures have access to an all-pervading vacuum energy, once described as an ether, and this quantum energy field is operative at subatomic, atomic, molecular, and supramolecular levels.

A particular groundbreaking facet of the New Biology is food's importance as a source of indispensable information, its function reaching far beyond its nutritional composition of varying macronutrients and micronutrients to help epigenetically modify the expression of the majority of our genome.

MASTER MOLECULE OF HEREDITY vs. THE INTERDEPENDENT MODEL OF SYSTEMS

Which human organ do you view as most imperative to life? Some instinctively feel that the brain is the most important organ, because without it cognition would not be possible. Some say it is the heart, which keeps our circulation flowing, or the liver, which stands vigil, filtering the blood. But the answer is *none of the above.* They're all requisite for the intelligent design and operations of our somatic form. These organs are interdependent parts of overlapping systems, superimposed and interwoven into the intricate tapestry of our physiology. Like the notes in a musical composition by Bach, their beauty results from the composite and synergistic way in which they interact.

Consider this: for other domains of science, such as the study of aquatic, marine, and land-based ecosystems, we acknowledge a sophisticated interconnectedness among animal and plant species. Yet this awareness dissipates when we venture more deeply into the human body, down to the level of macromolecules. When it comes to DNA, biologists have abandoned the idea of an interdependent model of systems, embracing instead a hierarchical, linear process to create an origin story of life. In this "central dogma of biology," DNA makes RNA, which makes proteins. DNA, as the supreme biomolecule of life, oversees the genesis of all other biological constituents in a top-down, authoritative fashion. This model traces a one-way trajectory from DNA to RNA to proteins.

However, in truth, a more accurate model would be a bidirectional loop within a web. The New Biology shows us that DNA is not actually at the center of life but is instead one isolated facet of a complex biological economy composed of subsystems, none of which can be ascribed primacy or recognized to exert a privileged level of causation. The New Biology goes even further than that, demonstrating that *there is no center.* Science overwhelmingly shows that life is self-organized, emerging from a network of interpenetrating and interdependent relationships, each with its own niche, specialized in purpose and fundamental to the larger whole. This exquisitely calibrated organization has long been recognized by traditional Eastern philosophies that envisioned all phenomena, from the infinitesimal goings-on of the human body to the macro-level oscillations of the climate, the rhythms of the seasons, and the movements of the planets as a holofractal unity. No one dimension supersedes or holds dominion over another; life operates in an oscillating dance of give-and-take, expansion and contraction, and ebb and flow.

If we utilize a simple linguistic shift from "DNA controls the production of proteins" to "cells use DNA to make proteins," a different narrative emerges.

DNA and Your Health Destiny

This is what the New Biology says about the relationship between DNA, disease, and aging:

- *You*, not your DNA, have control over your health destiny.

- The symptoms of disease are often your body's intelligent response to being exposed to something that is unhealthy or inappropriate. It is always better to look for the disease's root cause than to suppress the symptoms.

- The accelerated decline that we associate with aging is not necessarily predestined by our genes, and it's neither normal nor inevitable.

There is a better way for our bodies to tap into the energy all around us. We need to seek to understand *all* parts of the system in which we live—not just DNA. These include our miraculous microbiome, a sophisticated, life-sustaining microbial reservoir that we are only beginning to learn about.

MicroRNAs for Regeneration

The New Biology contends that what you consume profoundly impacts you in *real time* via the machinery of microRNAs. In fact, noncoding RNAs make up more than 80 percent of transcripts from our genome.[5] RNA is the only biomolecule present in all of life, making it a better candidate for being a universal biomolecule than DNA itself.

RNA can be difficult to study because it can't be extracted easily from cells, being so crucial to their function. Structurally, RNA is similar to DNA. However, it is single- rather than double-stranded, and is therefore much more chemically reactive and unstable. More importantly, it can assume an expanded repertoire of three-dimensional molecular shapes relative to DNA, giving it versatility in structure and function.[6]

RNA and DNA nucleotides are composed of different sugars, ribose in the case of the former and deoxyribose in the case of the latter, and carry slightly different base pairs, with the pyrimidine base uracil (U) found in RNA where thymine (T) occurs in DNA. In most cells, only two chemical modifications to DNA are possible, acetylation and methylation, which are the underlying mechanisms behind epigenetics, which you will remember is the activation or silencing of genes by environmental inputs such as diet and lifestyle. On the other hand, at least 66 chemical modifications can be made to RNA;[7] the roles of these modifications remain largely a mystery.

The explanation underlying these molecular differences between DNA and RNA is that the latter was the first to arrive on the scene, which means that life effectively began with RNA, likely predating the emergence of the first cells. In a transposition of conventional wisdom, then, DNA might have evolved as a specialized form of RNA—adopting chemical inertness and structural rigidity in order to serve as a more reliable warehouse for the safekeeping of heritable information.

For the purposes of this discussion, we will focus in on microRNAs, which are the premier regulators of gene expression and the conduits for free information exchange among the plant, animal, and microbial kingdoms, not unlike cellular phone towers bouncing signals from one seemingly disparate region to the next. MicroRNA, as described by University of Gothenburg professor Jan Lötvall, can zip around from cell to cell inside the bubble-like exosomes—nanoparticle-sized vesicles that are produced when the membranes of cell-sorting compartments bud or pinch off.[8] Exosomes, which contain a mix of proteins, bioactive lipids, and noncoding RNA, may have originally developed as a way for plant cells to talk to one another and to deploy a concerted first-line immune defense when under threat.[9] The exosomes liberated from edible plants when we ingest them may also serve as a portal through which our own digestive tracts can sense and communicate directly with the external environment.

Conventional wisdom holds that cells exchange messages through the secretion of hormones, cytokines, and neurotransmitters, which come from one cell and bind to receptors on neighboring receiving cells to produce physiological effects. But a newly discovered form of exosome-mediated communication suggests that the cargo transported by exosomes can be transferred directly to recipient cells without any intermediaries.[10]

The concept that microRNAs influence the expression of the majority of the human genome[11] and may also serve as a channel for cross-species communication[12] is highly biologically plausible since trillions of digested, plant-derived exosome nanoparticles navigate through our digestive systems on a day-to-day basis, interfacing with the mucosal lining of our gastrointestinal tracts.[13] Previous studies have also highlighted that food-derived microRNAs that piggyback on exosomes have been found to reside in the blood and tissues of animals.[14] MicroRNAs within plants share "molecular homology" with human RNAs, meaning that they look like and can mimic the effects of human RNAs. The significance of these diminutive, noncoding RNAs should not be underestimated. Because they can silence or activate mammalian gene expression, they may influence the course of development, aging, and various disease states.[15]

The animal model brought validity to the concept that exosomes and the microRNAs they contain are instruments of cross-species communication.[16] When administered to mice, exosome-like nanoparticles from grapes penetrated the intestines and triggered enhanced production of intestinal stem cells.[17] This is meaningful because stem cells are a one-way ticket to regeneration. Known as "multipotent progenitor cells," stem cells can differentiate into and replace specialized cell types through a process called mitosis, or cell division, as part of an internal repair system. This ability stands in sharp juxtaposition to terminally differentiated cells of the heart, blood cells of the circulatory system, and neurons of the nervous system, which do not normally proliferate, or multiply— and they also differ from stem cells in that only the latter are capable of long-term self-renewal.

In a study published in the *American Society of Gene and Cell Therapy* journal, researchers issued mice a toxic agent known to cause ulcerative colitis, an autoimmune disease of the colon. They then gave the mice exosome-like particles from grapes. Under ordinary conditions, mice given the toxic substance would have quickly developed colitis. But these mice did not. The mice lived twice as long as the mice that didn't receive the grape substance, suggesting that administration of the grape-derived particles protected them from development of chemically induced ulcerative colitis due to activation of these stem cells. The particles preserved normal histology, or microanatomy of the intestines, in the face of these toxic chemical agents, and they "promoted dramatic proliferation of intestinal stem cells and led to an intense acceleration of mucosal epithelium regeneration and a rapid restoration of the intestinal architecture throughout the entire length of the intestine."[18] The grape particles were also completely safe for the mice, with zero side effects.

The shining gem uncovered by this study is that exosomes, which are present in a variety of plant foods we consume, may exert additive or synergistic effects in course-correcting our own biology, nudging it gently back to the mean or boldly stimulating tissue regeneration by activating our body's own reserve of stem cells. Conversely, one could argue that many acute and chronic diseases could be caused by a lack of dietary exosomes from ancestral foods. Exosomes have been isolated and characterized from an assortment of edible plants, including carrots, grapefruit, and ginger root, all of which have the power to lightly prod deviant biochemical pathways back to the straight and narrow.[19]

For instance, a microRNA derived from broccoli was found to be present in human sera and to inhibit growth of breast cancer through its effect on the gene *TCF7*.[20] Exosome-like nanoparticles from ginger, on the other hand, were found to increase levels of a potent anti-inflammatory signaling molecule, interleukin 10 (IL-10), which tamps down excess immune system reactivity.[21] Flavonoid compounds from berries, known as anthocyanidins, delivered via milk-derived exosomes significantly suppressed both the growth and proliferation of chemotherapy-resistant ovarian cancer cells, suggesting that phytonutrients, or plant chemicals with health benefits, are more effective when carried by exosomes.[22]

While berry anthocyanidins have anticancer properties on their own, their bioavailability, or the proportion ingested that enters systemic circulation and elicits an active effect, is poor, and they are inherently unstable in the absence of attachment to exosomes.[23] Exosomes may therefore be mother nature's delivery service that safeguards healing noncoding RNAs and bioactive plant compounds until they arrive at their final destination.

Exosomes and the microRNAs that they shuttle are some of the reasons why fruits, vegetables, herbs, and spices that come directly from the earth into your kitchen or medicine cabinet set the stage for healing. Because microRNAs can travel horizontally across species—from fruit to mouse, or vegetable to human—they can send messages that tell genes when to express themselves and when to remain quiet. It doesn't take eons to make these changes; they can alter your genes in real time, and these changes can be passed down to your progeny, and from them to their progeny and so forth.

MicroRNAs shuttled about in their environmentally protected extracellular vesicles provide a viable scientific explanation for interspecies cross talk and for the interconnectedness between all the domains of life. Their discovery shows that the systems of the body, like the kingdoms of life and the ecosystems of the planet, all operate on the principles of harmony, symbiosis, balance, and holism. Rather than existential islands unto ourselves, we are united in a grand and awe-inspiring wholeness.

Meet Your Miraculous Microbiome

Since the late 1800s, when Robert Koch and Louis Pasteur tackled the challenge of foodborne infections, microorganisms have been uniformly demonized by the scientific community and pigeon-holed as the singular causative agents behind diseases. Up until recently, the enduring legacy of germ theory, which promulgates the idea that specific germs are the sole cause of specific diseases, is that we have envisioned ourselves to be in a perpetual war against these microorganisms' hostile intrusion. Our conditioning has led us to perceive the microscopic world as the culpable party behind the plagues and pandemics that have snuffed out so much of humanity in singular episodes. Within this conceptual framework, the immune system has been fashioned as the militant armed force against the invasion, and vaccines and antibiotics our only true defense against certain destruction.

The relatively recent discovery of the microbiome, however, is completely redefining the role of microbes in our bodies and shifting the entire frame of reference for our species's self-definition. It turns out that some microbes are hardly the adversary; in fact, they are crucial to protecting us from disease and dysfunction.

A deceptively diminutive term, *the microbiome* refers to our unfathomably complex array of microscopic microbial inhabitants that together weigh only three or four pounds. Yet the microbiome's power is immense, as it contains 99.9 percent of our genetic material. Comprising bacteria, viruses, fungi, and archaea that reside in their respective niches on and inside our bodies, our microbiome is instrumental to digestion and assimilation of nutrients, detoxification of cells and organs, control of the immune system, competitive inhibition of pathogens, reinforcement of the gastrointestinal mucosal barrier, and production of neurotransmitters.[24] Indeed, we relegate life-sustaining functions to these friendly bacteria, including the breakdown of extremely toxic chemicals.[25]

The discovery of the microbiome has radical implications because it undercuts the theory that microbes are a leading cause of disease and death. In fact, mortality from infectious disease—measles, scarlet fever, whooping cough, diphtheria, and polio—had declined precipitously due to improved living conditions, nutrition, hygiene, and sanitation infrastructure even before the use of antibiotics and vaccinations became widespread in the mid-20th century. Magic bullet medical interventions designed to combat germs were credited as being the primary factor in extending the human life-span and putting a discernible dent in the burden of human suffering from communicable disease. These medical interventions conceived from germ theory became the foundation of the allopathic medical paradigm that continues to be exalted as the be-all, end-all of human health.

Yet billions of years have primed our physiology to interface with virtually endless microbial challenges and prepared our body tissues for intimate contact with bacterial, fungal, protozaol, helminth, and viral co-inhabitants. Through our evolutionary past of hunting, foraging, and subsisting off the land, our bodies have undergone millions of years of immunologic evolution with the elements, soil, and fermentation, all of which have attuned us to countless interactions with the microbial world that have served to guide the trajectory of future immune responses, thereby fostering our dependence on microbes as some of our greatest allies.

Our bodies resemble plants in that our susceptibility to pests, or opportunistic infections, escalates when we aren't provided with the proper inputs, such as when our ecosystems are in a state of disharmony, when our microbial soil is depleted, and when our micronutrient status is compromised. The modern pressures of a sedentary lifestyle; pharmaceutical drugs; occupational stress; ultra-processed, nutrient-poor foods; electromagnetic pollution; man-made toxicants; and circadian rhythm–disrupting blue light cause our microbial diversity to suffer, in turn opening the door to sickness.

The ways in which we deviate from our evolutionarily encoded template are the ways in which our microbiomes suffer. When we unnecessarily forgo the fundamental inoculation of microbes that comes with vaginal birth in favor of Cesarean section, for instance, we are sacrificing the postnatal transmission of maternal flora that seeds the baby's microbiome—one of the most critical exposures in molding the composition of the infant's microbial ecosystem. When we opt for bottle-feeding our babies instead of providing them with the gut-mammary transfer of mom-derived bacteria, gene-regulatory microRNAs, and prebiotic sugars designed to encourage bacterial growth in the infant, we set the stage for the bacterial imbalance known as dysbiosis, the precursor to a dysfunctional immune system, which is a breeding ground for infectious challenges. Breast milk contains special sugars known as oligosaccharides, including lactose and 1,000 other distinct nondigestible molecules that provide a substrate for bacterial fermentation[26]—in other words, one of the explicit purposes of breast milk is to allow our microbiomes to flourish. Babies with microbiota underdevelopment are at an increased risk of autoimmunity, allergies, asthma, allergic rhinitis, late-onset sepsis, coronary artery disease,[27] and obesity. The pattern of early seeding of the microbiome can even predispose babies to vaccine injury, with certain signatures of dysbiosis—absence of bifidobacteria in particular—leading to systemic inflammation and a greater likelihood that vaccines will cause adverse effects.[28]

Although how we are born and our initial feeding methods are not under the realm of our control—in some cases, Cesarean birth is the only option and breast milk is unavailable—other variables that either impede or cultivate microbial diversity fall well within our purview. These include avoiding gut-disrupting antibiotics, eating organic fruits and vegetables, managing stress, and minimizing exposure to toxicants in our home environment.

When we malign all bacteria as microorganisms to be feared and eradicated, we indiscriminately target commensal and virulent microbes alike. We do so with antibiotics, hand sanitizers, chemical cleaning agents, triclosan-laden antibacterial soaps, and gut-disrupting pharmaceuticals like acid-blocking drugs and over-the-counter pain relievers. While they are purportedly designed to heal, these prescriptions inevitably destroy the system that has evolved to protect us.

Being stalwart guardians of our microbiomes is of utmost importance if we are making the health of our future generations, which is perhaps the most fundamental evolutionary imperative we have, a priority. Because our microflora consists of a selective array of commensal microorganisms that ultimately originated from the environment—the air we breathe, the soil we interact with, and the water and food that we ingest—our mission must encompass a wider breadth and a more far-reaching scope if we are to save our microbiomes from certain demise.

The Microbiome as a Key to Evolutionary Survival

A growing body of microbiome research is challenging the prevailing genome-centric story of human evolution, namely that extremely gradual changes in the protein-coding nucleotide sequences of our DNA are primarily responsible for the survival of our species over the ages. This is exemplified by a study published in the journal *Nature* that found that Japanese subjects had a strain of bacteria in their gut that were loaded with both the genes and enzymes required to digest the polysaccharides found in sea vegetation, which are normally indigestible to humans.[29] Absent from the human genome, these genes were found to originate from a strain of the marine bacteria *Bacteroidetes*, *Zobellia galactanivorans*, which naturally lives on the red marine algae commonly consumed in East Asia as nori—the dried and roasted sea vegetable that is formed into a sheet and used as the green wrapper of a sushi roll. These bacterium-derived genes fall outside the bounds of the human genome and are not found in the gut bacteria of North Americans.

The human genome contains an informational blueprint capable of producing a mere 17 carbohydrate-active enzymes (CAzymes),[30] a small armament developed over millions of years to help us digest terrestrial plants. The average human microbiome far outpaces our own carbohydrate-digesting ability, containing as many as 16,000 different CAzymes. In other words, our micro-biome is a treasure trove of carbohydrate-digesting enzymes, allowing us additional biosynthetic pathways to process new food supplies.

The astounding diversity of CAzymes found within strains like the human gut symbiont *Bacteroides thetaiotaomicron*, which alone contains 261 carbohydrate-digesting enzymes known as glycoside hydrolases and polysaccharide lyases, begs the question of how this immense diversity evolved. The *Nature* study provides a novel explanation: human gut flora acquiring new genes from microbes living *outside* the gut, presumably through the phenomenon of horizontal gene transfer. In particular, the researchers showed that genes coding for porphyranases, agarases, and associated pro-teins needed to degrade marine vegetation were transferred to the gut bacterium isolated from Japanese individuals.

The implication is that when a population eats a food like nori for long enough, the useful genes from marine bacteria residing on nori can be shunted into already-existing bacterial strains in their guts. Bacteria in our guts can therefore enlarge, elaborate upon, and compensate for deficits in our "hardwired" genetic capabilities. Through shifts in our microbiome, our entire physiol-ogy can adapt to changes and challenges in our environment and nutritional milieu. The immense plasticity of our microbiome, therefore, improves our ability to survive and remain in harmony with our natural environment.

Another example centers around the ability of our commensal flora to mitigate some of the ill effects of consuming gluten-containing grains. One reason these popular Western foods are so problematic is that they contain what is colloquially referred to as "gluten," a mixture of addictive, hard-to-digest, and immunologically problematic proteins rich in proline also found in rye, spelt, and barley.[31] The primary issue with them is implicit in the word *gluten*, which means "glue" in Latin. The words *pastry* and *pasta*, in fact, derive from "wheat paste," the original concoction of wheat flour and water that made such good plaster in ancient times. Gluten's adhesive and difficult-to-digest qualities come from the high levels of disulfide bonds it contains. These sturdy sulfur-based bonds, also found in human hair and vulcanized rubber, resist digestion and decomposition and give off a sulfurous odor when burned.

Wheat is a hexaploid species, the by-product of three ancestral plants becoming one, containing no less than six sets of chromosomes and 6.5 times the number of genes found in the human genome. Thus, it is capable of producing no less than 23,788 different proteins.[32] Clearly the monolithic term "gluten" is misleading, as any one of these proteins is capable of inciting an antigenic response, wherein the immune system identifies the protein as other and launches an innate or adaptive immune response, sometimes attacking self-structures in a case of friendly fire.

One saving grace that has ameliorated some of the effects of wheat consumption is our gut bacteria. Research reveals that a wide range of bacteria in the guts of Westerners are capable of degrading thousands of difficult, if not impossible to digest, proteins in modern wheat.[33] Indeed, without the help of these gluten peptide–degrading microbes, the sudden Neolithic introduction of gluten-containing grains into the human diet may have had even more catastrophic health consequences.

Tending to Your Microbiome

Cultivating practices that protect and nourish our microbiome are just as important as our efforts to reduce exposures to genotoxic chemicals and radiation that damage our genetic material. It is also incumbent upon us to understand that antibiotics, literally translating to "against life," in the form of both pharmaceutical prescription drugs and the thousands of pervasive, man-made chemicals that kill microbial life, have devastating and perhaps irreparable consequences to beneficial microbes when used indiscriminately or unconsciously—such as with the fluoridation and chlorination of city water or the bacteria-destroying use of the broad-spectrum, glyphosate-based herbicide Roundup on a mass scale.

Each of us is eating for one hundred trillion microorganisms with every bite we take.[34] Especially important is the incorporation of dietary fiber in the form of microbiota-accessible carbohydrates or prebiotics, which can be readily found in foods such as Jerusalem artichokes, onions, garlic, leeks, asparagus, green bananas, cocoa, jicama, almonds, blueberries, carrots, cassava, pumpkin, and taro.[35] Prebiotics are a special class of fiber that resists hydrolysis by gastric acidity and mammalian enzymes and is instead selectively fermented by the intestinal flora, augmenting the growth or activity of flora that confers a health benefit to the body.[36] Also important is the avoidance of microbiome-disrupting foods such as synthetic additives, colorants, and flavorings; artificial sugars; grain-fed meats; oxidized and genetically engineered vegetable oils; hybridized wheat; glyphosate-laden food crops; and processed dairy, the consumption of which has increased in parallel with the escalating prevalence of "diseases of affluence," including metabolic syndrome, coronary artery disease, osteoporosis, and cancer.

When considered as a whole, microbiome research peels back the layers of our very essence and lays bare one gleaming, iridescent fact: we must make a conscious effort to get out of our own way to preserve and leverage our relationship with the natural world. We are not separate or superior to the environment, nor are we detached from the ecology of it. Our genetic potential is optimized in the presence of biologically appropriate nutriment that supports our mutualistic and indivisible interdependence with all the plants, animals, and microbes on Earth.

The seemingly supra-human genetic capabilities of our gut microbiome may have been the primary determinant in our species's survivability because they allowed our species to adapt quickly to changing environments and available diets. Research is only just beginning to bring to light how profoundly the microbiome can and does extend our genetic capabilities.

The Connection between Mother and Newborn

The latest research into the role of the microbiome in sustaining physiological resilience undermines germ theory *and* presents a challenge to traditional gender dynamics.

We've long known that both men and women pass on nuclear DNA in the form of chromosomes. Yet only women can pass on the DNA that is found within mitochondria, the organelles traditionally considered the energy factories of the cells.

Because we are all designed to gestate in the womb and enter the world through the birth canal, from which the neonate's microbiome is derived and established, it follows that most of our genetic information is maternal in origin. Even when the original colonization eventually changes and is superseded by environmentally acquired microbial strains in infancy, childhood, adolescence, and adulthood, the original composition and subsequent trajectory of microbial changes is a direct by-product of the mother's terrain. Like a gardener planting the seeds, tending to her plot, and provisioning the conditions for growth, the mother is the guiding force for which foliage and greenery will flourish and thrive within the baby. As such, the microbiome of the mother is the bedrock of the baby's microbiome.

The conditions surrounding gestation, therefore, are important because the maternal-to-fetal microbiome trafficking in utero, maternal diet, and mode of birth take on vastly greater importance than previously imagined.

Honey, Please Pass the Genome

With scientific advances, we have reached a critical juncture where certain long-buried pearls about our physiology are being revealed, unfolding in shimmering opalescence before our eyes. The central tenet—and the one that may be most shocking—is that we are more microbe than human. Not only are we meta-organisms, with the vast majority of our genetic information being microbial in nature, but when we peel back the curtain on the "private" genetic contribution of our own cells, we find that the human genome itself is almost one-tenth retroviral in origin.[37]

Even our mitochondria, popularized in high school classes everywhere as the "energy powerhouses" of the cell, are alien in origin. According to the endosymbiotic theory, mitochondria were once ancient, free-floating proteobacteria that surrendered their independence by becoming subcellular organelles, leading to the evolution of eukaryotic cells that presently make up our bodies.

The distant past, therefore, is embedded within the present; our cells are enriched with billions of years of biological information, and depending on what we eat or do not eat, the information either remains latent or is activated in an expertly executed schematic. Each cell in our bodies, along with all the cells in all living creatures on the planet today, derives from a last universal common ancestor (LUCA) estimated to have lived some 3.5 to 3.8 billion years ago in the primordial ocean. This was echoed by Charles Darwin, the father of evolution, who said that "probably all the organic beings which have ever lived on this earth have descended from some one primordial form, into which life was first breathed." Thích Nhất Hạnh, a Vietnamese Buddhist monk, peace activist, and global spiritual leader, articulated the same insight when he wrote these words: "If you look deeply into the palm of your hand, you will see your parents and all generations of your ancestors. All of them are alive in this moment. Each is present in your body. You are the continuation of each of these people."[38]

Our degree of reconciliation with our evolutionary past—and hence our level of alignment with the molecular and energetic fabric that is the essence of who we really are—will determine our ability to cultivate health and resist illness. One of the pillars of stepping back into alliance with our authentic selves is eating the food our body expects to encounter, the sustenance it has been conditioned over the millennia to use as fuel. Hippocrates's proclamation that "we are what we eat" was true not only in physical terms—the food we eat produces molecular building blocks from which our bodies are constructed—but also in microbial terms.

The billion-dollar question, of course, is this: What did our ancestors eat? The stereotype of the caveman revolves around a meat-heavy dietary template. Animal products were indeed important in our evolutionary past, but not in the way that you might think. A turning point in evolution for our hominid predecessors was the inclusion of high-quality, easily digestible nutrition from coastal and inland freshwater seafood, which dovetailed with the rapid expansion of gray matter in the cerebral cortex of the brain. A staple of the mid–Upper Paleolithic period, freshwater or marine sources of protein made up between 10 and 50 percent of the diet early modern humans consumed. The inclusion of this protein and fat was concurrent with the development of many hallmarks of abstract thought, such as pottery figurines, knotted textiles, burial decorations, and personal ornamentation.[39] Our large human brains, especially their frontal lobes, expressed capacity for executive thought, critical thinking, problem-solving, memory retention, toolmaking, language, and learning. All this may be directly attributable to the easily assimilated long-chain fatty acid in seafood known as docosahexaenoic acid (DHA), which is important for membrane-rich brain tissue.

But Paleolithic humans ate a variety of other forageable foods, too, including honey. According to Alyssa Crittenden, a behavioral ecologist and nutritional anthropologist at the University of Nevada, Las Vegas, honey was a central food for early humans. Excavated rock wall art from around the world displays likenesses of early humans climbing ladders to smoke out and collect honey from honeycomb-filled hives. Crittenden also notes that traditional hunter-gatherer populations in Africa, Australia, Asia, and Latin America incorporate honey and bee larvae as integral parts of their diets.

The idea that honey may be a cornerstone for our species's microbial health is substantiated by a study published in the journal *PLOS ONE*, which discovered the presence of lactobacillus species in honeybees, suggesting an 80-million-year or older history of association.[40] In our fostering of an ancient co-evolutionary relationship with honey, it has become an integral facet of our microbial identity, where our own immune systems and microbial populations may share dependency on honey-based microbes.

Honey contains a range of beneficial microbial life-forms contributed by bees and the plants they forage, including the lactic acid–producing bacteria lactobacilli, which support the immune systems and behavioral patterns of individual bees and the hive as a whole. When eaten raw, honey may contribute health-promoting bacterial strains to our bodies. Strains of lactic acid bacteria, for instance, can improve chronic constipation,[41] reduce childhood dental caries[42] and eczema,[43] reduce nosocomial (hospital-acquired) infections,[44] reduce infectious complications in elective liver donors,[45] decrease the duration of respiratory infections in the elderly,[46] alleviate symptoms of irritable bowel syndrome,[47] and reduce the incidence and severity of the life-threatening condition necrotizing enterocolitis in very low-birth-weight infants.[48]

Honey has also been shown to heal wounds[49] and burns,[50] reduce radiation-associated pain in cancer patients, improve cholesterol profiles,[51] and enhance DNA repair in residential populations chronically exposed to pesticides.[52] One of nature's ultimate medicinal substances, it is as effective as the mouthwash chlorhexidine in reducing plaque formation,[53] treats nocturnal cough better than the over-the-counter cough suppressant dextromethorphan,[54] has superior efficacy to standard hydrogel therapy in the treatment of venous ulcers,[55] and has efficacy against urinary tract infections.[56] It can even help address the antibiotic-resistant infection known as methicillin-resistant *Staphylococcus aureus* (MRSA).[57]

Since Paleolithic times, the topography of our inner microbial soil has become completely ravaged. Most recently, the daily barrage of synthetic dietary inputs and battery of antimicrobial toxicants has plunged us into a post-industrial chemical soup. It is plausible, however, that honey could help heal these wounds and that ancestral foods infused with equally ancient symbiotic bacteria could help us recover and "travel back" in biological time to a far more stable state of health. Consuming honey and other real, microbiota-impregnated foods may be absolutely necessary for the continued healthy expression of our DNA, establishing vital anchors for the informational integrity of our species identity.

The Life Bridge: Our Bodies Are Connected to Earth through Microbes

The American herbalist Paul Schulick aptly named the interstitial layer of microbial communities within the soil and our guts a "life bridge," which can be visualized as a bridge that connects our bodies via microbes directly to the Earth, as well as between the ancient past and the present, forming an inseparable whole. Think about ancient farming practices that use wild soil from old growth systems as a microbial inoculant in newer farming land to produce vitally nourishing food. These old-growth microbial communities, perhaps a by-product of millions of years of co-evolution, could contribute a wide range of biotransformed soil metabolites for a plant's nutritional needs, as well as infuse the edible plants themselves with strains of bacteria, fungi, and viruses important to our own health.

When we allow our evolutionary compass to guide us home to ourselves, we naturally gravitate toward certain foods and avoid others. In the next chapter, we will explore some of the frontiers in the science of food and energy and learn how to assess new inventions, sidestep those that make us sick, and navigate toward the inputs that best align with what our bodies need and crave at a cellular level.

CHAPTER THREE

THE NEW BIOPHYSICS OF ENERGY SYNTHESIS

How the Body Harvests Nature's Alternative Energy Sources to Power Cellular Pathways, Build Resilience, and Promote Our Evolutionary Edge

Food is an important energy source, but it is not the only one that powers your body. Until recently, we have regarded the body as a mostly glucose-burning or glucose-fermenting biomachine, with a convenient backup system for fat burning. Most people believed that the majority of our body's energy is stored and transferred by mitochondria in the form of ATP (adenosine triphosphate) and that ultimately all our energy needs can be met by our food. The New Biology, however, is revealing that sunlight, melanin, water, and chlorophyll all provide alternative sources of energy. Like plants, humans can capture energy through the direct transformation of environmental energy into metabolic energy. There is also exciting evidence indicating that the human body can access zero-point energy directly from the quantum vacuum. In this chapter, I'll also explain how certain dietary and lifestyle choices can make it easier for our bodies to access these alternative forms of energy.

WATER: YOUR BODY'S MOLECULAR BATTERY

We know that cells can regenerate, microRNAs can communicate genetic information from food to your body, and the microbiome extends and complements our cells' genetic capabilities. We know that our bodies are innately intelligent and that most disease symptoms are compensatory adaptations seeking to re-establish equilibrium. Water plays a critical role in this paradigm.

Water makes up two-thirds of the human body by weight and 99 percent of our bodies' molecules by number. Although essential to life and a variety of biological functions such as enzymatic activities, protein-folding dynamics, and myriad cellular responses, water is often thought of as inanimate background material relative to nucleic acids and proteins, the latter of which are considered the most valuable players in the central dogma of biology. Scientists have been limited by the assumption that the phenomenology of water can be explained through the principles of surface tension, capillary action, condensation, evaporation, sublimation, and Brownian motion (the erratic motion of particles suspended in a fluid that occurs due to collision with molecules in the surrounding medium). But we have yet to explain some of the vagaries and mysteries of water's behavior, such as how the so-called Jesus lizard walks on water's surface, how electrodes inserted into two adjacent beakers of water cause a bridge of water to form between them that can be sustained indefinitely (even when the beakers are separated by a few centimeters), or the Mpemba Effect, a process through which hot water can occasionally freeze faster than cold.

By envisaging water molecules through the lens of reductionism and focusing myopically on the molecular structure of H_2O, we have overlooked the collective behavior of water molecules— how they interact, share information, and work together. Every schoolchild can mindlessly recite the three phases of water: solid, liquid, and gas. Around a century ago, however, chemist Sir William Hardy, as well as Martin H. Fischer, M.D., and Gertrude Moore,[1] suggested that there might be a fourth phase of water that is liquid crystalline–like in form. In the 21st century, Dr. Gerald Pollack, a professor of bioengineering at the University of Washington, took interest in this idea. When he placed a gel-like hydrophilic or "water-loving" material next to liquid water and added particles to the water, the water took on a different set of characteristics. The particles migrated away from the place where the gel met the water, to a distance approximately the width of a human hair away from the interface, leaving the water close to the gel in a purified state, devoid of suspended particles and solutes. Pollack continued to study the properties of this negatively charged and purified zone between the gel and the water, which he aptly named exclusion-zone, or EZ, water, because everything was progressively excluded, including the minerals that can appear in regular bulk water.[2]

This fourth phase of water, also known as "ordered" or "structured" water, is ubiquitous in both nature and the human body. The crucial factor here is that the separation of positive and negative charges that occurs with EZ water creates a battery, or a repository of energy that can be freely extracted. We can acquire biologically useable energy from water.

Pollack and his team were perplexed as to what provided the energy to create charge separation. The surprising answer came in the form of a student walking through the lab with a lamp, which was observed to dramatically increase the quantity of EZ water. This effect was caused by the flashlight's electromagnetic radiation enhancing the EZ zone, charging the water like a battery. Although any spectrum of radiant energy may have a charging effect on water, infrared light—light invisible to our eyes but that we feel as heat—appears to be the most potent. The reality is that infrared energy is found throughout our environment and is constantly being emitted by our bodies. This is largely due to the fact that more than half of the near-thermal-spectrum radiation given off by the sun is in the infrared bands. As the water in our bodies collects the energy of the sun, it naturally splits positive and negative moieties, the latter of which builds the EZ layer. The ultimate result is that our body's energy supply is enhanced in a powerful way.

Because 50 to 75 percent of body mass is water, two-thirds of which resides in the intracellular compartment,[3] the implications of EZ water for human health and as an energy source are boundless. Whereas conventional thinking about how the body gets most of its energy is focused on ATP, the EZ-structured water molecules in our bodies take in massive amounts of incident electromagnetic radiation from the environment. Because all elements within our cells are bathed in EZ water, each biomolecule serves as a nucleating site upon which structured water can be built, creating shells of EZ water, available to power cellular reactions, including providing ample power for the trillions of mitochondria within our body. EZ water spontaneously absorbs ultraviolet, visible, and infrared wavelengths and converts them into charge separation that can be used as power, including driving red blood cells through capillaries or vascular flow in plants.

This process has an uncanny symmetry with photosynthesis, which is premised upon the harnessing of solar energy by light-harvesting, plant-based antenna structures such as bilins, chlorophyll, and carotenoids—chromophores that convert the energy of the sun into charge segregation with expedient efficiency.[4]

If you take a hollow tube made from hydrophilic material, submerge it in water, and shine a light on it, positive and negative charges separate, causing a constant flow of water to run through the tube for as long as the light shines.[5] This explains, then, how red blood cells, which are actually too big to fit comfortably through our narrow capillaries, can navigate through the circulatory system. The radiant energy–driven flow overcomes the need for high-driving pressure gradients that would otherwise be required to propel red blood cells through capillaries with even smaller diameters. As Pollack suggests, perhaps it's not the heart alone that creates the pumping energy; perhaps it's light-powered water. Pollack's pioneering work casts doubt on our former assumptions about water as a mere background carrier for more important molecules, as structured water has been found to encase every macromolecule and to be intrinsic to the execution of our cellular processes.[6]

EZ water could also help explain the legendary healing powers of certain waters, such as the Lourdes spring and the Ganges river, and especially those that emanate from glacial melt or underground springs. Because the pressure on these springs is known to restructure bulk water into EZ water, these springs could be abundant sources of naturally purified EZ water, potentially explaining why people have turned to them for millennia as sources of healing.

PLANT INTELLIGENCE: BRIDGING THE DIVIDE BETWEEN PLANTS AND ANIMALS

The emerging theories about water, light, and energy echo the research on exosomes as cross-kingdom messengers, providing a plausible mechanism for how the Earth's inhabitants—plant, fungal, bacterial, and animal—are linked together in an open-access, information-sharing network. Provocative new research published in *Plant Signaling & Behavior* proposes that plants, incapable of escaping environmental stresses in the manner of animals, have developed advanced, sophisticated forms of biological quantum computing and cellular light memory, processing information encrypted in both the energy and intensity of light in what could only be described as a form of plant intelligence.

According to the study, plants can gather, store, and memorize information in the form of the spectral composition of light so that they can predict environmental changes. They also appear to exercise agency or "choice" vis-à-vis different scenarios, such as "what to do" in varying light, temperature, and relative humidity conditions.[7] Furthermore, the study hypothesizes that plants may absorb more light energy than is needed for photosynthesis alone. This may be done for the purpose of training via light for young, naïve leaves in light acclimatory and immune defenses, wherein older, more experienced leaves instruct emerging young leaves with photoelectrophysiological signaling and cellular light memory mechanisms. Attributes previously assigned to the lexicon of human traits, then, such as learning, memory, thinking, and anticipation of future events, are ubiquitous in the plant kingdom.

Despite being immobile, plants have evolved their own highly skilled ways of acquiring energy, defending themselves, reproducing, and contending with their environments, many of which resemble the collective and unifying intelligence that emerges in insect colonies, which is based upon the science of networking, distributed intelligence, and the dynamics of swarm behavior. The modular design of plants, for example, with built-in redundancy and decentralization, means that they can lose limb without losing life. Their sessile lifestyle, which renders them firmly affixed to the ground, has led to their development of exquisitely sensitive apparatuses that allow them to respond to environmental cues and stimuli and to gain a nuanced understanding of their immediate surroundings.

In addition to analogs of our five senses, plants can sense light, pressure, gravity, hardness, volume, moisture, salt and other minerals, microbes, and chemical signals emitted by neighboring plants. They make complex decisions regarding allocation of resources, growth away from competitors, and deployment of a stockpile of molecular munitions that can entice pollinators, enlist the service of animals, and deter predators. The nascent field of plant neurobiology increasingly illuminates the intelligence of plants—how they communicate in the invisible molecular vocabulary of chemical signals, employ rudimentary forms of memory, assimilate information from both biotic and abiotic stimuli to "make decisions," and produce anesthetics in response to injury or stress. These discoveries reframe our ideas around self-consciousness, free will, and intentionality, all of which we have previously associated exclusively with the animal kingdom.

LIGHT, ENERGY, AND MITOCHONDRIA

Just as plants exhibit sensorial qualities we once believed to be the sole province of animal life, new research indicates that humans exhibit capabilities we once thought solely possessed by chlorophyll-containing life forms. It turns out that humans may be able to directly convert sunlight into biological energy,[8] upsetting the basis for our elegant taxonomic subdivision between the plant and animal kingdoms.

Traditional taxonomic divisions differentiate plants as autotrophs (which produce their own food) from animals as heterotrophs (which eat other living things for food). While generally these two zoological classifications are considered nonoverlapping, important exceptions have been acknowledged. For instance, photoheterotrophs—hybrids between autotroph and heterotroph—can use light for energy but cannot use carbon dioxide, as plants typically do, as their sole carbon source, so they must "eat" other things. Some classical examples of photoheterotrophs include green and purple nonsulfur bacteria, heliobacteria, and a special kind of pea aphid that has borrowed genes from fungi to produce its own plantlike carotenoids to harness light energy and supplement its energy needs.[9]

Examples of photoheterotrophy can also be found in worms, rodents, and pigs (one of the closest animals to humans physiologically), which have been found to be capable of taking up chlorophyll metabolites into their mitochondria, enabling them to use sunlight energy to supercharge the rate (up to 35 percent faster) and quantity (up to 16-fold increases) of adenosine triphosphate (ATP) production within their mitochondria. This truly groundbreaking discovery from Columbia University Medical Center researchers, published in the *Journal of Cell Science*, completely overturns the classical definition of animals and humans as solely heterotrophic creatures.[10]

This feat is made possible by a metabolic by-product of chlorophyll named pyropheophorbide a (or Ppa for short), which is taken into animal mitochondria. In the presence of the chlorophyll metabolite and light, researchers observed a striking increase in the amount of ATP that mitochondria produced. Animals that were given Ppa but not exposed to light did not show this effect, nor did a control group that was not given Ppa at all. In accordance with well-known mechanisms that link improved mitochondria function to increased cellular longevity, feeding the same metabolite to the roundworm Caenorhabditis elegans with concomitant light exposure significantly increased its life-span, though sunlight was deadly in the worms that did not receive chlorophyll. Thus it is reasonable to wonder whether consuming plant blood is protective for us humans, too.

This study likewise raises questions regarding the increased public ambivalence concerning sunlight exposure, where the sun has been increasingly viewed as a vector of lethality in skin cancer causation and humans have adopted the practice of slathering on petrochemical-based sunscreen as a precautionary measure. However, one crucial question that remains unexplored is whether sunlight is only toxic when chlorophyll is absent from our diet and tissues or if it is healthy when it appears in optimal doses alongside appropriate chlorophyll consumption.

The biological imperative of sunlight exposure, then, extends well beyond the immunomodulatory, anti-inflammatory, gut barrier–reinforcing effects of vitamin D—and even beyond the ability of sunlight to generate structured water in our bodies. The study points out that both sun exposure and consumption of green vegetables are correlated with better health outcomes, which are often chalked up to vitamin D or antioxidants, respectively. But, according to the study, these simplistic accounts may be incomplete, since we evolved in the sun, with organs that were literally bathed in its photonic energy. The study concludes that given the intimate evolutionary history between *Homo sapiens* and the sun, it is not inconceivable that we have also evolved to exploit this source of energy, oscillating between glucose- and sunlight-dependent processes for derivation of our cellular energy currency.

The implications of this study are profound. If animal cells have evolved to be able to harvest sunlight through the help of the "blood" of our plant allies, it might be reasonable to presume that we could optimize our biological potential through the use of a certain amount of chlorophyll and take full advantage of the sunlight to meet our metabolic energy needs. As such, there could be a clear survival advantage conferred by regular consumption of chlorophyll-rich plant material. The paleo-oriented diet communities, therefore, should perhaps be compelled toward placing more emphasis on chlorophyll-rich foods as centerpieces of a truly ancestral diet.

Noteworthy properties of sunlight exposure, including its analgesic effects and ability to improve alertness and regulate lifespan, make more sense in the context of this research. For example, a prospective study of patients undergoing spinal surgery explored the difference in the experience of those who stayed on the bright side of the hospital as opposed to those who didn't. Patients who were exposed to a 46 percent higher intensity of natural sunlight on average during their hospital recovery period experienced less perceived stress, marginally less pain, and required use of fewer analgesic medications.[11] In terms of cognitive benefits, a study published in the journal *Behavioral Neuroscience* found that subjects who were exposed to six hours of sunlight felt significantly more alert at the beginning of the evening and less sleepy at the end of the evening compared with those who were exposed to artificial light.[12]

That our health may be directly married to the solar cycles, a tenet to which Eastern philosophies have long given credence to, was explored by a study from the journal *Medical Hypotheses*, which reviewed the possibility that sunlight directly affects the human genome. The study suggests that when solar cycles are experienced during the critical developmental periods of conception or early gestation, genetic changes that directly modulate the expression of disease and affect the length of our lives may be accelerated.[13]

Research suggests an intimate evolutionary relationship between our physiology and the consumption of green vegetables, which provide antioxidants, nutrients, and fiber, as well as supply the mitochondrial co-factors that, when mixed with sunlight, can suffuse our bodies with energy for health and longevity. The potential for increased ATP production without an accompanying increase in free radicals[14] means that these dietary sources of chlorophyll can even slow the aging process at the cellular level. From a practical standpoint, this means we would all be better served by crossing the nutritional bridge to become more photoheterotrophic organisms by drinking more green juices and consuming more green foods.

But chlorophyll in isolation, no matter how you get it, isn't enough. We concurrently need sunlight in order to obtain the full range of its life-imbuing, health-imparting wavelengths. That means engaging in outdoor activities, with an emphasis on early-morning sunlight exposure for the added benefits to our circadian rhythm.

In what might be one of the most phenomenal discoveries of our time, these findings point to the animal kingdom's ability to derive energy directly from the sun—a constant, daily, guaranteed source of energy. It sheds a spotlight on the newly discovered capacity of mammals, humans included, to borrow the light-harvesting capabilities of "plant blood"—chlorophyll and its metabolites—and to utilize them to photo-energize mitochondrial ATP production. And it dethrones the widely held belief of the scientific community that humans are simply glucose-, fat-, and protein-dependent biofurnaces.

Melanin, Radiation, and the Conversion of Light to Metabolic Energy

Melanin, the central pigment within our skin, and distributed throughout our bodies, is one of the most interesting biomolecules identified thus far. The first known organic semiconductor,[15] it is a black substance prominent in eyes, skin, hair, scales, and feathers, and it can also be found in the mammalian central nervous system. From the ink of the octopus to the protective colorings of bacteria and fungi, melanin offers protection against a variety of biochemical and predatory threats and chemical stressors, and, most famously, acts as a photoprotective factor against ultraviolet radiation. It absorbs all visible wavelengths of the electromagnetic spectrum, hence its dark coloration, and, most notably, converts and dissipates potentially harmful ultraviolet radiation into heat. It serves a wide range of additional physiological roles, including free radical scavenging, charge transfer, toxicant chelation, endocrine functions,[16] and gene protection. Melanin's proposed ability to convert sunlight into metabolic energy—akin to the way chlorophyll harvests sunlight in plants—means that our species should be reclassified from heterotrophic to photoheterotrophic, and, even more significantly, may raise the prospect that melanin offers protection against ionizing radiation *while* transforming it into metabolically useful energy.

As the molecule that is crucial in determining skin color, melanin has fundamentally shaped the way we humans perceive ethnic and racial differences and tribal affiliation. Given its function as an evolutionarily encoded heuristic that has allowed the human brain to rapidly identify in-group versus out-group dynamics, it has played a role in genocide, slavery, and the rise and fall of civilizations, all of which have been at least partly due to misperceptions about what it means to have more or less melanin in the skin.

The variation in human skin from dark, melanin-saturated African skin to light, relatively melanin-depigmented Caucasian skin may merely be a direct by-product of our last common ancestor from Africa migrating toward sunlight-impoverished higher latitudes 60,000 years ago. In order to compensate for the decreased availability of sunlight, the human body rapidly adjusted, potentially removing the natural "sunscreen," melanin, from the skin since it interferes with the production of vitamin D, a hormone that participates in governing the expression of more than 2,000 genes. Without adequate vitamin D, our genome would completely destabilize, and immune balance would become disturbed, so the reduction of melanin to augment vitamin D status likely saved the lives of humans who migrated to cooler climates. But this evolutionary adjustment may have come at a significant cost. Humans with lighter skin tones may have gained vitamin D accessibility at the expense of the ability to convert sunlight into metabolic energy.

The resolution to this energy paradox might be found in the discovery that melanin has the intrinsic ability to transform light energy into chemical energy through the hydrolysis of the water molecule, a function formerly consigned to the domain of the plant kingdom. The chemical energy liberated via the dissociation and subsequent charge separation of the water molecule by melanin, in fact, has been estimated to meet over 90 percent of cellular energy needs.[17]

Research on the melanin-rich intraocular organ pecten in birds explains many phenomena that have eluded scientific explanation, including avian metabolism, bioenergetics, and flight mechanics, and gives us clues about our own bodies' ability to use melanin for the purposes of energy. The albatross, for instance, is capable of traveling 10,000 miles in a single flight, a bioenergetic feat that has long baffled the scientific community. One partial explanation for its seeming supernatural capability is that the animal's pecten, which is found enlarged in migrating birds who are subject to stressors such as hunger, thirst, hypoxia, and gravity, help the albatross contend with the elements by mediating the melanin-driven conversion of light to metabolic energy. This is one example among several that challenge the widely held assumption that animals are incapable of directly utilizing light energy.[18]

HAIRLESSNESS, SUNLIGHT, AND PALEO-DEFICIT DISORDER

Melanin may also explain another curious fact: that humans are the only species among hundreds of different primates who are almost completely hairless, which is why we are known in biology as the "naked ape." Approximately 6 million years ago, the mutation for human hairlessness was introduced into the genome, causing us to diverge from hairy chimpanzee lineages. The evolutionary reason, however, is hard to pin down. Being hairless left us vulnerable to fluctuations in weather since, in comparison to other primates, we must expend significant extra energy to produce body heat to stay warm. We are also more exposed to ultraviolet light, which degrades folate in the human body, leaving fetuses more likely to develop neural tube defects. What advantages, then, could hairlessness impart?

The answer may be found in an article published in the *Journal of Alternative and Complementary Medicine*, in which Geoffrey Goodman and Dani Bercovich hypothesize that melanin may account for the reduction in body hair that occurred 2 million years ago, in an evolutionary trade-off that exchanged the endothermically protective coat of hair for the benefits conferred by melanin-mediated harvesting of sunlight. Human hairlessness occurred concurrently with an augmentation in the melanin content of the skin, paving the way for a process called photomelanometabolism.[19] In what is known as "ultrafast internal conversion," melanin can convert 99.9 percent of potentially gene-damaging ultraviolet light into harmless heat, fulfilling both sun blocking and energy-generating functions.[20]

As explained in a paper published in *Medical Hypotheses* by retired medical practitioner Iain Mathewson, new research on low-level light therapy, also known as photobiomodulation, may explain the immediate benefit conferred by hairlessness, as it shows that exposure to the red and near-infrared radiation found at sunset increases mitochondrial respiratory chain activity and results in extra synthesis of ATP in all superficial tissue sites, including those of the brain.[21] Under Mathewson's hypothesis, a random mutation for hairlessness occurring in one of our African forebearers millions of years ago would have conferred an immediate survival advantage over her hairy relatives by enabling her body, especially her brain, to access the red and near-infrared wavelengths generated by ancient sunsets.

The rapid expansion of our species's brain volume, known as encephalization, occurred at the same time as the adaptive event of human hair loss, around 2 million years ago. Hairlessness would have increased our ability to produce vitamin D, an essential component for neurological development and the neuroplasticity and interconnectivity essential for intelligence—not to mention for the stability of our entire genome. This could have further increased brain development in the sheer size and complexity of neural circuits. Most significant, however, is the resulting necessity for the increased production of melanin, first as a sun protectant but secondarily as a means to endow humans with the ability to harness electromagnetic radiation for metabolic energy in a fashion similar to chlorophyll.

The ability to use melanin to absorb electromagnetic radiation and utilize its energy to dissociate the water molecules in our bodies (producing what Gerald Pollack says "amounts to a light-energy driven proton pump")[22] may have reduced the energy expenditure required for hunting and foraging food. In other words, the energy freed up by using melanin in this novel way may have enabled the expansion of energetically intensive brain tissues such as the cerebral cortex, which is responsible for the higher thought processes of speech, information processing, impulse control, and decision making.[23]

The development of these higher cognitive processes allowed for the materialization of sophisticated technologies, the agrarian revolution, hierarchical social structure, and advanced human civilizations. This turning point—first the hairlessness, then the expansion of the brain—may be directly traced back to melanin, exemplifying how paramount it is to our species's resilience and survival.

MELANIN AND THE HOLY GRAIL
OF RADIOPROTECTIVE FOODS

Not only can melanin convert light into heat, but new research raises the possibility that it can also transform other forms of radiation into metabolically useful forms of energy. Hints at this phenomenon arose when scientists noticed that a group of fungi had colonized within the walls of the still-hot site of the Chernobyl nuclear meltdown.[24] Fungi were also found at a nuclear test site in Nevada in the 1960s, where they had survived radiation doses of up 6,400 grays, around 2,000 times the dose that is lethal for humans,[25] suggesting that certain kinds fungi are not deterred by radiation but, on the contrary, seem to thrive on it. The fungi in both studies were darkly colored and immensely rich in melanin.

Taken alongside evidence that bacteria that produce pyomelanin, a cousin to melanin, thrive in soil contaminated with uranium,[26] and the findings that exposure to ionizing radiation actually promotes the growth of certain melanized fungal species inhabiting nuclear reactors, space stations, and the Antarctic mountains, it seems plausible that melanin allows certain organisms to "eat" radiation.[27] A study published in *PLOS ONE* revealed that melanin-containing fungal cells saw increased growth relative to nonmelanized cells after exposure to ionizing radiation and that the irradiated melanin from these fungi also changed its electronic properties, which the study noted raised "intriguing questions about a potential role for melanin in energy capture and utilization."[28]

Collectively, this research suggests that, more than surviving radiation exposure that is normally lethal to most forms of life, fungi may be using melanin to feast on the free lunch of anthropogenic radioactivity. Therefore it is logical to ask whether the consumption of melanin from fungi might protect those higher on the food chain—like humans—from radiation exposure.

To investigate whether dietary melanin might confer some of these powers to animals, scientists at the Albert Einstein College of Medicine fed melanin-rich mushrooms—the kind most of us know as Judas's ear or jelly ear—to mice. A second group of mice was fed white, melanin-poor porcini mushrooms, a third group ate white porcini mushrooms that were supplemented with melanin, and a final control group received no mushrooms or melanin at all. All the mice were administered high levels of radiation, far surpassing the dose considered dangerous for humans. After 13 days, all the mice in the control group had died, and the mice that ate the nonmelaninized porcini mushrooms died almost as fast as the controls. Impressively, however, 90 percent of the mice that had been given melanin-rich mushrooms or white mushrooms supplemented with melanin survived.[29]

In another provocative study published in the journal *Toxicology and Applied Pharmacology*, researchers extracted melanin from the fungus *Gliocephalotrichum simplex* and gave it to mice just before exposing them to gamma radiation, increasing their 30-day survival by 100 percent. The probable mechanism of action was suggested by a study published in *Bioelectrochemistry*,[30] in which ionizing radiation was found to alter melanin's oxidation-reduction potential. Whereas most other biomolecules experience a destructive form of oxidative damage as a result of radiation exposure, melanin remained structurally and functionally intact, appearing capable of producing a continuous electric current that could theoretically be used to produce metabolic energy in living systems. This would explain the increased growth rate, even under low nutrient conditions, in certain kinds of gamma-irradiated fungi.

In an eye-opening statement, researchers noted that these effects need to be studied in humans but that in nuclear emergencies, "diets rich in melanin may be beneficial to overcome radiation toxicity in humans."[31]

Rectifying the Root of Illness: Paleo-Deficit Disorder, Sunlight, and Grounding

Sunlight once determined the highly orchestrated sleep and wake cycles of humans, as the near-red and infrared wavelengths of the sunrise synchronized the circadian oscillator of a brain region called the suprachiasmatic nucleus (SCN), regulating "clock genes" that rely upon light input to align their expression with solar time. This SCN, the central pacemaker of the brain, is photo-entrained by way of sunlight entering light-sensitive retinal ganglion cells in the eye, which in turn oversees diverse aspects of human biology including cellular bioenergetics, immune and endocrine function, as well as body temperature, sleep, and feeding. The circadian rhythm perfectly epitomizes the intelligence of the human form, as it optimizes allocation of cellular energy and allows for flexible adaptation to the unpredictable and fluctuating environments of life on earth. It's no surprise, then, that disturbance of the circadian rhythm is linked to neurodegenerative disease, cancer, obesity, cardio metabolic disease, neuropsychiatric disorders, and decreased life-span.[32] One of the primary culprits for circadian rhythm disruption is lack of sunshine, and the other is our reliance upon man-made technology along with its artificial light.

Today, a central feature of modern society is a career spent in a cubicle, bombarded by blue light–containing artificial wavelengths of light that are highly destructive to our circadian rhythm. In fact, it's been estimated that 60 percent of people spend more than six hours a day in front of a digital device, besieged by blue light emitted from electronics. Blue-containing LED screens disrupt restorative sleep, a critical period for detoxification, by interfering with the production of melatonin and overriding our body's instinct to sleep and wake according to the solar day. They also interfere with our ability to track seasonal changes and our capacity to express genes in the most advantageous manner.

This lack of sunlight is the primary driving factor in creating what researchers Alan C. Logan, Martin A. Katzman, and Vicent

Balanzá-Martínez have called paleo-deficit disorder,[33] which describes the myriad ways in which we have strayed from the evolutionarily appropriate inputs our genes expect. What this means is that our bodies have evolved with an instrumental requirement for sun exposure. Without it, we're more vulnerable to a host of diseases, including the autoimmune thyroid disorder Hashimoto's thyroiditis, multiple sclerosis, inflammatory bowel disease, rheumatoid arthritis, systemic lupus erythematosus, cardiovascular disease, and 25 types of cancer (including cancers of the breast, bladder, cervix, colon, and lung), as well as skin conditions such as acne, rosacea, eczema, psoriasis, and dermatitis.

The prevailing cultural zeitgeist is to cover up, find the shade, slather our bodies in sunscreen, and avoid midday sun exposure. This flies in the face of the results of a prospective study following 38,000 Swedish women for 15 years, in which sun exposure was found to be associated with a significant reduction in all-cause mortality (death from any cause), as well as significant reductions in cardiovascular mortality (death from heart attacks, stroke, and coronary artery disease).[34] Furthermore, whereas intermittent sun exposure was correlated with a 60 percent increased risk of melanoma, chronic sun exposure was actually protective against this most fatal form of skin cancer.

Although burning should always be avoided, habitual insulation from the sun is also detrimental. The solution, then, is twofold: first, we should minimize or entirely eliminate contact with electronics after dusk or, failing that, wear blue-blocking eyewear to shield against light pollution from self-luminous devices used at night, which has been shown to improve sleep efficacy, sleep latency, and melatonin production.[35] Secondly, we should commit to spending at least one day a week exposing our bodies to the whole spectrum of light from sunrise to sunset, practicing natural photobiomodulation unencumbered by sunscreen, extensive clothing, or sunglasses for maximal exposure.

To further mend the evolutionary mismatch, we should firmly root our bare feet on the ground while we receive this life-giving sun exposure, practicing what is known as grounding or earthing. Throughout evolutionary history, human beings have gone shoeless, or worn footwear fashioned from animal hides that allowed equilibration with the electrical potential of the earth. These practices have been discarded with what is perceived as the linear trajectory of mankind toward advancement. Sadly, however, our divorce from the earth is in fact a fatal regression, leading to the loss of that pivotal energetic transfer and free radical neutralization from the ground to our bodies.[36]

The advent of plastic- or rubber-soled shoes, elevated beds, and high-rise buildings has insulated our bodies from the electrical field of the earth, which has coincided with unparalleled increases in the incidence of chronic illness. Furthermore, our departure from the ground has decimated our defenses against electromagnetic pollution, as studies have demonstrated that grounding reduces the voltage induced on the body by a factor of 70 upon exposure to alternating current (AC) electric potential.[37] This transfer of electrons from the earth to the body prevents the electromagnetic frequencies from interfering with the electric charges and activities of our bodies' molecules, which is not insignificant given that, according to a paper in the *Journal of Environmental and Public Health*, "there is no question that the body reacts to the presence of environmental electric fields."[38]

This means that the ground represents a reservoir of free and mobile electrons, negative charges that have the potential to neutralize the positively charged free radicals, or reactive oxygen species (ROS), that can damage cell constituents and lead to disease and degeneration. Because ROS is a direct link to inflammation, and inflammation leads to disease, it is incumbent upon us to fight it with an evolutionarily compatible toolbox at every turn. Inflammation is positively charged, and the earth is negatively charged, so putting our bare feet on the ground may elicit an antioxidant effect, scavenging free radicals and mitigating their harm.[39]

In the absence of contact with the earth, distorted electrical gradients can accumulate due to uneven distribution of charges, which can in turn affect the functioning of enzymes. This may explain why studies have shown grounding to have therapeutic benefits that include normalization of the circadian rhythm and improved sleep,[40] relief from chronic joint and muscle pain,[41] better glycemic control, rapid resolution of inflammation,[42] and reduced blood clotting.[43] Grounding has even been shown to shift the autonomic nervous system from sympathetic fight-or-flight to parasympathetic rest-and-digest, also known as breed-and-feed. In fact, participants in a grounding condition exhibited immediate deactivation of the former and concomitant activation of the latter.[44]

Grounding has been transplanted from the realm of alternative medicine folklore to the domain of a scientifically substantiated therapy for ailments of many kinds, including aging, since aging is inextricably linked to inflammatory burden.[45] Grounding has shown preliminary evidence of improving autoimmune conditions and may also elicit improvements in cardiovascular arrhythmias, hypertension, osteoporosis, asthma and other respiratory conditions, sleep apnea, and premenstrual syndrome (PMS).[46] The applications of grounding are truly limitless. Similar to the effects of chlorophyll, electrons from grounding supercharge the electron transport chain of the mitochondria, suggesting that grounding can contribute to the energy-intensive processes of repair and regeneration that are required for healing from disease.

What is truly remarkable, however, is the possibility explored in a recent review in the *Journal of Inflammation Research*, which proposed that innovations in biophysics and cellular biology show "the human body is equipped with a system-wide collagenous, liquid-crystalline semiconductor network known as the living matrix,"[47] which is capable of directing electrons to any bodily location in the event of injury or disease in order to confer protection at the cellular, tissue, and organ level. In fact, this vast whole-body redox network is considered the primary antioxidant system of the body in some research circles.

The surface of the earth, therefore, represents an untapped and indispensable therapeutic resource with the potential to improve a myriad of inflammatory maladies. Failing to recharge our bodies with regular contact with the earth is a certain recipe for degeneration and debility—and one of the foremost ingredients for paleo-deficit disorder.

The New Biophysics: A Deep Dive into the Quantum Rabbit Hole of Esoteric Physiology

The energy needs of the human body have long been envisioned as dependent upon physical "fuel" being fed to the glucose-burning furnaces within the mitochondria of our cells. Indeed, our fixation on the caloric content of food reflects this outdated and fundamentally inaccurate concept. Calories are simply a measurement of the amount of heat given off when we internally incinerate food, which is a crude metric when we consider the complexity, elegance, and mystery of human metabolism.

Our bodies, in addition to utilizing ATP-based mechanisms of energy transfer, are capable of harnessing "free" energy directly from the sun through a variety of means, including water-, melanin-, and chlorophyll-mediated processes. No doubt, there are many other energy-generating processes at play yet to be discovered. But while examples of alternative energy sources based on EZ water or melanin may seem like a radical departure from conventional theories of cellular bioenergetics, they actually still aren't radical enough to account for what is really going on.

The truth is that our bodies can access, accumulate, and put to work immense quantities of free energy, or energy that does not need to be extracted from physical substances such as food. The body has an even more direct, limitless source of energy that it can, and does, continually access—one that may finally explain accounts of humans living without food or water for prolonged periods of time. Recent experiments reveal that, despite long-standing assumptions that cytosol, the aqueous part of a cell's cytoplasm, has zero electric fields, it actually contains an electric field strength as high as 15 million volts per meter.[48] (For comparison, high-voltage power lines typically operate at 155,000 to 765,000 volts per meter.) Even more astounding is the fact that the inner membrane of a single mitochondrion has an electric field strength of 30 million volts,[49] which is comparable to the electrical field generated by the flares coming off the surface of the sun or a thunderbolt.

But where does this immense energy come from? In order to answer this question, we'll have to explore some of the most foundational discoveries of quantum physics. After all, all our bodies' molecules are composed of atoms, whose fundamental structure lies at the sub-sub-sub-atomic level of the quantum of action, which means understanding human physiology and cellular bioenergetics will require at least a basic understanding of quantum physics.

In the New Biophysics, space is described as the quantum vacuum, unlike its more passive precursor of classical physics, where it is visualized as an empty and invisible container for physical things. The quantum vacuum is not a void but is instead teeming with zero-point energy, that is, the vibrational energy at baseline or ground state that remains present even when the system being observed from a classical perspective is at absolute zero and appears completely empty and motionless. In quantum field theory, estimates of the vacuum energy density within "empty space" range from infinity to the mass density of about 10^{96} kilograms per cubic meter (that's a 10 with 96 zeros behind it!), which in practical terms *is infinite*. This is the reason American physicist Richard Feynman remarked that "one teacup of empty space contains enough energy to boil all the world's oceans." Similarly, Swiss physicist Nassim Haramein predicts that the zero-point vacuum energy contained within the volume of a single proton is equal to the mass of all protons in the observable universe.

Within this understanding of empty space, matter (in the form of virtual particles) is constantly popping in and out of existence within the quantum vacuum, similar to a foam coalescing and disappearing at the bottom of an immense waterfall of energy.

The version of reality described by quantum field theory physics seemingly violates basic laws of thermodynamics, with its conservation of energy and matter, and completely contradicts the classic Newtonian, macroscopic experience of space and objects within which we live. Yet it is the best explanation for how forces and particles behave, with a wide range of modern technologies like laser systems, MRIs, and semiconductor devices owing their existence to it.

So, how does this relate to the New Biology? If quantum field theory is accurate, and a practically infinite source of energy is available to biological systems at any point in space, everything we have learned about how the cell works and what our bodies need to survive would need to be revised. Indeed, an entirely new field called quantum biology has sprung up in order to understand how these discoveries at the level of the quantum of action affect biological systems, from the most basic molecular building blocks of the cell all the way up to human physiology and the origin and nature of consciousness itself.

A concrete example of a biological system that harnesses energy from the quantum vacuum can be found in the wall-crawling gecko lizard, which can hang from ceilings and scale smooth surfaces like glass, seemingly boldly defying basic physical laws of gravity.

In quantum physics, there is a phenomenon known as the Casimir effect.[50] By placing two uncharged metallic plates extremely close together (a few micrometers apart), without any external electromagnetic field present, the quantum vacuum energy draws the plates together from the wide range of electromagnetic frequencies in the energy density of the vacuum of space. The longer wavelengths are excluded from within the small opening between the plates, hence pushing the plates together from the outside in, proving the vacuum is full of "real" energy and can affect the objects in "real space."

The gecko, it turns out, has extremely small Casimir-like plate structures at the end of its bulbous feet in the form of millions of microscopic hairs. When applied to a flat surface, these hairs harness the Casimir effect to help keep the gecko stuck to the wall. While there are other proposed contributing factors, such as electrostatic effects, the Casimir effect is believed to be a primary cause.

Using engineering principles of biomimicry, researchers at Stanford have harnessed the Casimir effect to create a "Spider-Man" suit that allows humans to crawl up buildings.[51] The suit's "gecko gloves," capable of forming a strong bond with smooth surfaces and distributing large loads like the weight of the human body evenly, comprise a pad of 24 independent tiles with progressive and degressive load-sharing elements, covered in synthetic adhesives that contain sawtooth-shaped polymer structures approximately the width of a human hair.[52] So promising is this technology that applications of these pads are being explored on the robotic arms of spacecrafts in NASA's Jet Propulsion Laboratory.

The unusual, quantum-mechanical origin of the gecko's super-power even makes sense from a conventionally minded evolutionary perspective. Should we really be surprised that after billions of years of trial and error, where even the slightest advantage has life-and-death consequences, living things would eschew a quantum free lunch? Indeed, the Casimir effect and other zero-point energy–harnessing processes are operative at the most fundamental building blocks of our biological architecture.

BIOLOGICAL ZERO-POINT ENERGY

Of all the areas of exploration at the interface between quantum physics and biology, most relevant to our body's ability to sustain and regenerate itself even when up against incredible forces of adversity and scarcity is an understanding of where the body gets its energy.

Zero-point energy–harvesting processes within the human body are believed to be concentrated most intensely where conventional thinking on the matter expects them to be: within our cells' mitochondria. The primary reason why eukaryotes (plants, fungi, animals) are so complex versus single-celled organisms is because of the exceptional bioenergetics afforded to them through the endosymbiotic event estimated to have occurred about 1.8 billion years ago that created our mitochondria. Since protein synthesis uses about 75 percent of the cell's energy and mitochondria provide eukaryotes with 200,000 times more energy than a prokaryotic cell, they are able to support a genome that is 200,000 times larger.[53] This has afforded eukaryotes their immense evolutionary diversity and complexity relative to the simpler prokaryotes.

According to Douglas Wallace, Ph.D., one of the world's preeminent researchers in the biology of mitochondria, each mitochondrion stores energy within an electrical field with 180 millivolts of potential energy. There are 10^{17} mitochondria in your body (100 quadrillion).[54] Taken together, that sums up to about the potential energy of a lightning bolt stored in each human body!

While the discovery that your body has a lightning bolt of electrical potential within the totality of its mitochondria is amazing, it turns out that *each mitochondrion within each cell of your body has a magnetic field strength of 30 million volts per meter.* That electrical potential equates to as much energy as is found in a lightning bolt *in each mitochondrion.* With up to 5,000 mitochondria per heart muscle cell, an even greater density of 100,000–600,000 mitochondria per oocyte (mature egg cell), and trillions of cells in the human body, there's a near-infinite amount of potential energy available to the cells of your body at any given moment, which is inconceivably vast in contrast to the conventional explanation for the origin of cell energy.

If there is enough energy in a teacup of empty space to convert all the world's oceans to steam, it doesn't seem so outrageous that the mitochondria within our bodies are capable of harnessing trillions upon trillions of volts of potential energy from the quantum vacuum, transforming it into matter and transmuting elements. If such is the case, the entire framework of present-day biology, including the conventional body of knowledge concerning human physiology and nutrition, stands to be revised. As we dive deeper into the implications of the New Biology, we will find that conventionally accepted truths about human physiology are still a Wild West of assumptions and myths yet to be fully examined and explored.

Biotransformation of Elements

If the invisible space within and all around us is *not nothing* but a very energetically and informationally packed *something*, constantly giving rise to other somethings (e.g., virtual particles and antiparticles), should we be surprised if biological systems are capable of similar transformative and *de novo* feats of creativity? Consider as an example how widespread the belief in a cosmological big bang is, with hundreds of millions of adherents worldwide. The unequivocal faith in the big bang as the process that manifested the universe into material existence is basically the belief that out of *nothing* you can have a *very big* something. Yet conventional scientific thinking forbids this kind of radical creativity exist anywhere else, and certainly not within biological systems.

Regardless of immense resistance to this idea, the medieval precursor to modern chemistry, alchemy, with its long-sought-after transformation of baser elements like lead into gold, represented more than merely dabbling in metaphor and indulging in magical thinking. In retrospect, we, in the postnuclear age, are intimately familiar with powerful exceptions to the strict laws of conservation of energy and mass through technologies like particle accelerators and the phenomenon of radioactive decay—two instances where elements can and do change into one another. Physicists even managed to synthesize gold from mercury in a nuclear reactor back in 1941,[55] albeit in infinitesimal quantities and as a radioactive isotope.

Conventional thinking would have us believe that these exceptions only occur when exceptionally high pressures and temperatures are involved and not in the relatively cold, wet "reactors" of living things such as human cells. Yet the body is indeed capable of transmuting the elements of calcium, magnesium, potassium, copper, and iron into one another, nonradioactively, at our body's normal temperature ranges, a phenomenon that has been studied by scientists for over 200 years.

It was the celebrated French chemist Nicolas-Louis Vauquelin (1763–1829) who first discovered the phenomenon of biotransformation when he observed that chickens produce far more calcium in their eggshells than they ingested, leading him to write: "Having calculated all the lime in oats fed to a hen, found still more in the shells of its eggs. Therefore, there is a creation of matter. In that way, no one knows."[56] This finding violated the dictum of Vauquelin's contemporary, Antoine-Laurent Lavoisier (1743–1794), the "father of modern chemistry," who posited that while the combination of elements could be changed, elements themselves were unchanging, and therefore nothing was created. Henceforward, Vauquelin's findings would be mostly ignored. Despite that, other scientists would follow who confirmed Vauqelin's discovery:

1. **William Prout** (1785–1850): Studied incubating chickens and found that hatched chicks had more lime (calcium) in their bodies than originally present in the egg, which was not contributed from the shell.

2. **Albrecht von Herzeele** (1821–?): In 1873 von Herzeele published *The Origin of Inorganic Substances*, in which he presented research proving that plants continuously transmute material elements into one another.

3. **Vogel** (?–?): In 1844, Vogel studied watercress seeds and found that after germinating and growing them with distilled water, the resulting plants contained more sulfur than was present in the seeds.[57]

4. **John Bennet Lawes** (1814–1900) and **Joseph Henry Gilbert** (1817–1901): During 1856 to 1873, these

two British scientists found plants "extracted" more elements from the soil than the soil itself contained.[58]

5. **Henri Spindler** (?–?): During 1946 and 1947, Spindler discovered that two species of *Laminaria*, a marine algae, created iodine.

6. **Rudolf Hauschka** (1891–1969): In experiments conducted between 1934 and 1940, Hauschka discovered that weighed cress seeds, sealed in glass containers, increased in weight during the full moon and decreased in weight during the new moon.

7. **Pierre Baranger** (1900–1970): In thousands of experiments conducted between 1950 and 1970, Baranger saw the transmutation of various elements when comparing seeds before and after germination.

Despite these early examples, it was not until the 1960s that the French researcher C. Louis Kervran, who also held an academic position as a member of the New York Academy of Sciences, brought mainstream attention to the phenomenon. Not only was he the first scientist to do so in the postnuclear era, but he was also nominated in 1975 for a Nobel Prize in Physiology or Medicine for his compelling body of research on biotransmutation. Kervran's meticulous observations from the experiments he conducted showed conclusively that living organisms transform elements into one another.

Several famous examples include his observations in 1959 of Sahara oilfield workers who worked intensely under extreme temperatures (over 130°F) and excreted a very high percentage of potassium after taking sodium-containing salt tablets. Kervran concluded that the sodium was converted into potassium in an endothermic reaction that brought down the workers' temperatures. Another famous observation he made is that hens in France's northwesternmost region, Brittany, where the soil is notoriously low in calcium, lay perfectly normal calcium-replete eggs daily. He discovered the hens consumed potassium-rich mica from the soil, which they then converted into calcium. Kervran would later do extensive experiments with seeds, which substantiated his finding that biotransmutation of elements is constantly occurring. But while his work and observations were truly groundbreaking, upsetting the prevailing dogmas of chemistry and physics, he was not able to provide an explanation for how these bionuclear reactions were being facilitated at the atomic level. Nor was he able to prove the phenomenon's occurrence within quantitatively controlled conditions, such as in the context of a single-cell experiment.

That empirical evidence and physical explanation would come with the work of a Ukrainian scientist, Vladimir Vysotskii, who started working on biological transmutations in the 1990s. Vysotskii was the first to show that specific strains of bacteria, such as *Bacillus subtilis* GSY 228, *Escherichia coli* K-1, and *Deinococcus radiodurans* M-1, and a strain of yeast known as *Saccharomyces cerevisiae* T8, are able to transmute metals (such as manganese into iron) and accelerate the decay of the radioisotope radioactive cesium (Cs-137), which has a half-life of 30 years, transforming it into a form of barium (Ba-138), with a half-life of only 310 days. In 2015, Japanese researcher Hideo Kozima reexamined data from Vysotskii's experiments and provided a unified explanation, called the Trapped Neutron Cold Fusion (TNCF) model, of both the cold fusion and biotransmutation phenomena.[59] Vysotskii's findings are detailed in his book *Nuclear Transmutation of Stable and Radioactive Isotopes in Biological Systems* (2009).

Vysotskii's groundbreaking work is extremely compelling and relevant to human health, especially when we consider that the human microbiome is made up primarily of bacteria and that *we are composed mostly of our microbiome*. We've already seen how the microbiome is capable of extending our genetic capabilities far beyond what our hard-coded eukaryotic genome provides. It is therefore not outside the scope of possibility that these bacteria could also be responsible for the transmutation of elements.

This possibility has revolutionary implications for revealing the truly immense power and resilience inherent to our microbiome-based physiology. Our body has at least as many bacteria as cells, and each cell contains within it mitochondria that look and behave very much like bacteria due to their genetic and structural homologies.[60]

Could our microbiome also facilitate the mitigation of radio-isotope exposure from our environment? If so, we may have a deeper level of human resilience and regenerative potential than previously conceived, which may be necessary for our species's very survival in this postnuclear era.

MITOCHONDRIA: TURNING ENERGY INTO MATTER

One of the most revolutionary discoveries of our time is that mitochondria are capable of profound feats of alchemical transformation. This includes transforming the immense energy available to them into matter.

In 1978, Army research scientist Solomon Goldfein performed a series of experiments with mitochondria in order to evaluate the veracity of C. Louis Kervran's claims of transmutation of elements within biological systems. Goldfein's experiments proved Kervran correct, and moreover, they uncovered something truly paradigm-shifting about the creative power of our mitochondria. In his report, "Energy Development from Elemental Transmutations in Biological Systems,"[61] Goldfein revealed two remarkable phenomena. First, mitochondria are capable of producing more energy than would be expected according to classical laws of physics and biochemistry (an implication of which is that they are accessing free energy from the quantum vacuum), and second, mitochondria act like microscopic particle accelerators, with the resultant energy generated enabling the cell to transform elements into one another. Goldfein was able to identify six ways that each requirement for a cyclotron particle accelerator is met on a molecular scale. While it is also an essential part of our cellular bioenergetics, the biologically active form of magnesium ion–bound ATP (Mg-ATP) serves an entirely new role as a nanoparticle accelerator, its helical structure enabling the acceleration of the hydrogen ion (H⁺) to the relativistic speeds sufficient to transform target atoms into other elements, such as sodium to magnesium, potassium to calcium, manganese to iron, and so on and so forth. Goldfein's discovery overturns the conventional view that ATP's primary role is to function as a carrier molecule for the energy needed to sustain life. Indeed, if Goldfein's findings are accurate, the Mg-ATP chelate functions as a particle accelerator with immense creative and biotransformative potential.

The only other researcher since then who has visualized mitochondria as capable of functioning like a particle accelerator is Dr. Jack Kruse, who has written extensively on the topic of quantum biology. He has applied the most famous formula in physics, Einstein's mass-energy equivalence equation ($E=mc^2$), to quantum biology. What's more, he points out its reversibility: not only does matter convert to energy/light, but energy/light can transform into programmable matter.

WATER: THE PHILOSOPHER'S STONE OF THE NEW BIOPHYSICS

Water cavitation occurs naturally and can also be induced in experimental settings. It involves the formation of a vapor-filled cavity in a liquid such as water in places where the pressure is low. When high pressures are applied, these cavities, also called voids or bubbles, collapse into themselves, generating a shockwave of extremely high levels of heat, sound, and light in a phenomenon known as sonoluminescence. An acoustical wave or laser passed through water is capable of inducing a water cavitation bubble that produces millions of times more energy than induced it. The energy is so intense that temperatures equal to that of the sun have been measured off these tiny collapsing water bubbles.[62]

The science of water cavitation has been studied for decades, due in large part to sheer necessity, because it is highly destructive to man-made machines. Propeller blades on ships, for instance, often undergo great wear and tear due to the natural formation of water bubbles in their operation. Only recently has the science advanced to the point where the phenomenon's immense power could be harnessed and directed for specific technological applications.

Mark LeClair, a scientist specializing in harnessing water cavitation for nanotechnological applications, came upon a revolutionary discovery when he performed a series of grant-funded experiments using a laser to induce cavitation bubbles. An unexpected result of the experiment was the production of excessive energy (evidence of zero-point energy harnessing), with 840 watts powering the pump and 2,900 watts produced. This result alone has huge implications for the development of clean, sustainable alternatives to fossil and nuclear fuels. But what was even more remarkable was that the cavitation event revealed both the transmutation and de novo synthesis of elements, during which water was transformed into energy and matter. Incredibly, the elemental distribution of the transmuted material was a near-perfect match for supernovas (thought to be the origin of all the elements on the planet) and the ratio of elements found in the earth's crust, with strong corroborating evidence of micro black hole formation preceding the creation of elements.

This experiment appeared to show that a nucleosynthesis event, similar to stellar nucleosynthesis, can be induced in water, a finding that completely rewrites our understanding of where the elements found on the earth, and even those of the sun, originated.[63]

LeClair's cavitation experiments also revealed a hitherto unknown crystalline form of water, twice as strong as diamond and up to 5.5 times denser than ordinary water. The formation of the water crystal induced a shockwave observed to reach the relativistic speeds and energies required to trigger intense nuclear fusion, fission, and transmutation. One way to explain this cavitation-induced sonoluminescence and nucleosynthesis is the concept that the immense energies that are released come from the quantum vacuum. Dr. Claudia Eberlein's pioneering paper "Sonoluminescence as Quantum Vacuum Radiation" speaks to that point; Eberlein points out that only the zero-point energy spectrum matches the light emission spectrum of sonoluminescence.[64]

These discoveries also have profound implications for our understanding of the origin of life. LeClair's water crystal was observed forming linear or helical strands with large, icosahedral-hexagonal heads and long, narrow whip tails forming coils that can supercoil, similar to DNA. As LeClair observed, the discovery of the crystal and its effects will have a dramatic impact on the physics, chemistry, and biology of water. Furthermore, this discovery indicates that water cavitation may be at the root of the origin of life itself by providing the geometric template for self-replicating information-storage molecules. When we consider that the origin of life is believed to have occurred in hydrothermal vents deep on the primordial ocean floor, where one would find a proton gradient, prebiotic building blocks, and water cavitation bubbles, LeClair's work adds a missing piece to the ancient puzzle of how and where life on this planet originated.

Water cavitation provides us with a powerful example of both the extraordinary energies available within the elements of which we are composed and our creative potential. But do we have the biological systems to harness it?

Two very special species of shrimp point to the affirmative. The first, known as the mantis shrimp (typically four inches long), possesses a claw strike so powerful that divers who had had the misfortune of being struck by one named them "thumb splitter." Their strike can carry up to 200 pounds of force, enough to break through aquarium glass, and is as powerful and fast as a .22-caliber bullet.

The second, smaller pistol shrimp (1.2–2 inches long) is aptly named for its disproportionately large claw comprising two-part pistol-like features: a "hammer" that moves backward into a right-angled position cocked in its joint, and a receiving part the hammer is released into. The wave of bubbles it emits is powerful enough to break glass jars and stun its prey. Acoustically, the snap of its claw produces a cavitation bubble moving at a speed of 100 km/h (62 mph) that generates a sound reaching as high as 218 decibels. (For perspective, a thunderclap is 120 decibels, and a jet taking off 80 feet away will generate 150 decibels, which is loud enough to rupture your eardrum.) The pistol shrimp's click only lasts one millisecond. But in that millisecond the collapsing cavitation bubble produces heat of over 5,000 K (4,700°C). In comparison, the surface temperature of the sun is estimated to be around 5,800 K (5,500°C). The sound wave also produces a burst of light through sonoluminescence, which is believed to cause temperatures four times that of the sun (around 20,000 Kelvin) within the core of the collapsing bubble.

The way in which these species of shrimp generate enough power to accomplish these feats penetrates to one of the key realizations of this book, namely, that there are sources of energy available to living things that far exceed any conventional estimates or mechanisms commonly accepted today. If organisms as diminutive as shrimp are capable of harnessing enough zero-point energy to produce temperatures as hot as the sun, and the mitochondria within our bodies are capable of harnessing trillions upon trillions of volts of potential energy and transforming it into matter, only time will tell what we are truly capable of achieving.

When it comes to the New Biology, the convergence of quantum biology, epigenetics, mind-body and narrative medicine, and spirituality has never been more compelling and exciting than it is today. Within the nexus of these disciplines, we can now arrive at plausible explanations for phenomena that, for many decades and in some cases centuries, have often seemed fantastical, perplexing, and downright heretical.

PART TWO

RETHINKING CHRONIC DISEASE, PREVENTION, AND HEALING

THE ROLE OF STEM CELLS IN REGENERATION

CHAPTER FOUR

BEYOND GENE MUTATION

Cancer's Origin, Prevention, Treatment, and Lifesaving Patient Empowerment and Resilience Strategies

On Friday, December 23, 1971, President Richard Nixon signed the National Cancer Act, which allocated $1.4 billion over three years to fight the "war on cancer," which, at the time, was the second-leading cause of death in the United States.[1] This powerfully evocative Vietnam War–era metaphor suggested that cancer is an insidious adversary to be conquered and subjugated by sheer force. The consequence of this battlefield zeitgeist was that the war was waged with the conventional weapons of surgery and chemotherapy, designed to strike the enemy and decimate its defenses. The war even went nuclear with radiation therapy. But despite a concerted campaign by bureaucratic agencies, academic research institutions, nonprofit organizations, and pharmaceutical corporations, the battle may have been waged blindfolded.

At the 2012 World Oncology Forum held in Lugano, Switzerland, a group of thought leaders from across cancer research and treatment concluded that "enduring disease-free responses are rare, and cures even rarer."[2] In the journal *Frontiers in Oncology*, Bryan Oronsky and his colleagues explicitly said that the conventional tools we wield to target treatment-resistant cancer cells inadvertently amplify their power:

> Chemotherapy and radiation are the ultimate stress test for cancer cells, leading to an unintended "survival of the fittest" response in which the most sensitive cells are culled from the treatment-resistant herd; inevitably the price of this selection pressure is the emergence of acquired resistance and therapeutic failure, making aggressive therapy a self-defeating process. Nature abhors a vacuum and fills it up with resistant tumor cells, which ultimately dooms the outcome to failure.[3]

As of 2015, patients worldwide were spending $100 billion per year on cancer treatments, including surgery, chemotherapy, and radiation, while cancer diagnosis rates and deaths from cancer continue to grow unchecked. One quarter of the population still falls prey to an "enemy" that is universally feared but remains poorly understood at a fundamental level.[4] According to the International Agency for Research on Cancer, in 2012 there were 14.1 million new cancer diagnoses,[5] and according to the CDC in 2016, cancer was fast approaching heart disease as the number one reason we die.[6] Toxic and invasive therapies are being used liberally and inappropriately for patients with indolent or slow-growing diseases such as chronic lymphocytic leukemia, follicular low-grade non-Hodgkin lymphoma, and prostate cancer,[7] as well as for solid cancers (abnormal masses of tissue that usually do not contain cysts or liquid areas), for which there is no empirically demonstrated benefit to either survival or quality of life from using maximum tolerated doses.[8]

The language we use to describe cancer often creates the impression that it is a predetermined time bomb produced by defective genes. In this model, malignancy represents a cell gone rogue due to the accumulation of point mutations—where one nucleotide is substituted for another in a gene sequence—in the genes controlling the cell cycle and proliferation. As a result, we have characterized tens of thousands of candidate genetic alterations in tumor cells, premised upon the assumption that identification of the cancer genome will lead to a suite of targeted therapies and a comprehensive elucidation of cancer biology.[9] The tenet we have been led to believe is this: if we can isolate the genes responsible, we can find a cure.

While exposure to mutagenic substances contributes to the initiation and promotion of cancer, it is not a complete explanation for the origin of neoplasms. There is much more to cancer than the pat story of our arbitrary genetic inheritance or mutation events putting us on a collision course with death. Yet this model has led cancer patients to abdicate their autonomy and leaves them with the impression that they are merely bystanders in an arms race waged between their cancer cells and the tools at the disposal of their oncologists. Cancer patients then may surrender their fate to medical professionals without even considering alternatives, including proven, lifesaving, and life-enhancing holistic approaches.

It's time to reframe our approach to the challenge of cancer. The all-or-nothing extremism of the medical monolith must be removed in favor of a more nuanced perspective on oncogenesis. In this newfound paradigm, cancer should be regarded as a dynamic process, a spectrum of deviation from the norm, and an adaptive response to a radically divergent environment from the one in which we evolved.

FEAR FUELS CANCER

We can't talk about cancer without talking about fear. The fear surrounding cancer has burrowed itself into the deepest recesses and darkest crevices of our being and extinguished all hope. This primal fear has become the lens through which we envision cancer, coloring and clouding our judgment. It has latched on to our fight-or-flight psychology and activated our most primal, black-and-white thinking. Cancer is the aggressor. Fear is the reason we believe we have to fight for our lives and engage in outright war with our own bodies.

This expectation of deadly effects on our physiology, then, becomes a self-fulfilling prophecy. Research published in the journal *Cancer Genetics and Cytogenetics* has found that cancer cells express receptors for adrenaline known as adrenergic receptors, which respond to the outpouring of catecholamine hormones—dopamine, epinephrine (adrenaline), and norepinephrine (noradrenaline)—that occurs with psychological stress. The ensuing hormonal release leads to the poor response of tumors to chemotherapy and is also considered a risk factor for poor prognosis. For example, in patients with colorectal cancer, adrenaline leads to increased expression of an oncogene called *ABCB1*, which encodes P-glycoprotein.[10] P-glycoprotein transports xenobiotic (foreign) substances, including chemotherapy drugs, out of the cell through efflux pumps, thereby shielding cancer cells from the anticancer effects of conventional treatments. The effects of stress are also associated with increased activity in the mitogen-activated protein kinase (MAPK) pathway, a cascade that increases cancer cell survival, dissemination, and resistance to drug therapy.[11] Stress, then, through the synchronous release of multiple hormones, amplifies the cancer process.

The allopathic model, with its misplaced emphasis on "objective" signs and verifiable biomarkers at the expense of patient beliefs, perceptions, and attitudes, is another relic of metaphysician René Descartes, who severed body from mind in his philosophy of dualism five centuries ago. The legacy of the "ghost in the machine" can be found in the mind-set of a cancer patient, which has been shown to affect prognosis within conventional oncology. A prospective, longitudinal study conducted jointly in Malaysia and Boston found that one-fifth of recently diagnosed cancer patients develop post-traumatic stress disorder (PTSD), and more than one-third continue to exhibit PTSD symptoms four years later.[12]

Studies have shown that the psychological toll of cancer diagnosis affects the risk of death.[13] According to nationwide health registries in Sweden, the risk of suicide during the first 12 weeks following cancer diagnosis was elevated 4.8-fold and remained elevated beyond the first year after diagnosis for all cancers, including esophagus, liver, pancreas, and lung. The study found that cancer patients were 5.6 times more likely to die from heart-related causes, such as heart attack, in the days after receiving a positive cancer diagnosis—not from the cancer but from the heartbreak and devastation wrought by the news. Furthermore, the increased rate of suicide following cancer diagnosis was particularly prominent in those diagnosed with highly fatal cancers, cementing the power of the iatrogenic effect of disease labels.[14] That the divinations of the doctor have the power to predict a person's imminent demise shows us how the words and rituals of Western medicine create potentially harmful power dynamics between physician and patient.

At a cellular level, the terror that accompanies the cancer diagnosis can drive the pathogenesis of cancer, both precipitating and perpetuating the disease process. Within this view, it is possible that our culturally conditioned beliefs about our vulnerability to cancer sow the seeds of symptoms that are ultimately diagnosed as disease. The antidote requires reframing the lived experience of illness in a new light, bringing curiosity to the conditions the body is seeking and those that it is crying out for you to transform. In order to reverse any illness, we must figure out what the body is demanding through the symptoms it is expressing. Shedding the fear and psychic conflicts underpinning cancer will help to carve out space for its spontaneous resolution.

Overdiagnosis: The Problem with Early Screenings

When we consider the inexactitude of cancer diagnoses and prognoses, the effect of the psychology of fear is especially tragic. The truth is that the most common cancers, such as those of the breast, prostate, and thyroid, have been massively overdiagnosed and overtreated.

This trend of overdiagnosis is confirmed by data from the *Journal of the American Medical Association* (*JAMA*) showing significant increases in incidence of early-stage disease without proportional declines in incidence of later-stage disease,[15] alongside statistics showing a rapid rise in cancer diagnosis in the absence of an accompanying rise in death from cancer.[16] Patients may have "the disease," but it may never cause symptoms or death during their expected lifetimes. If cancer were truly being caught earlier, we would expect to see a decline in both later-stage cancer and cancer mortality. These findings suggest that widespread cancer screening has led to detection of "incidentalomas," false positives, and overdiagnosis, which, according to researchers in the *British Medical Journal*, may wholly offset any disease-specific advantages of screening.[17]

In cancer overdiagnosis, we find normal human variations and pathologize these variants as disease. Data published in the *Journal of the National Cancer Institute* indicates that computerized tomography (CT) colonography scans find abnormalities outside the colon in up to half of examinations.[18] It also reveals that when chest x-ray or mucus samples are used to screen for lung cancer, overdiagnosis occurs 51 percent of the time. In addition, an analysis of 12 randomized trials of cancer screening concluded that overall mortality was unchanged or increased in comparison to unscreened populations in the majority of studies.[19] Another systematic review found that only one-third of screening trials produced reductions in disease-specific mortality, and yet none of the studies exhibited reductions in overall mortality.[20] While cancer screening measures have been touted as lifesaving interventions, a sober cost-benefit analysis raises serious concerns.

Despite public confidence in x-ray mammography, a Cochrane Review of mammography following over 600,000 women concluded that there is no definitive mortality benefit with mammographic screening procedures.[21] This is significant because the Cochrane Collaboration is a relatively independent and unbiased panel of experts with minimal industry affiliations that reviews the strongest evidence available from the medical literature about health care interventions. The *International Journal of Epidemiology* reports that a high proportion of women have been shown to overestimate the benefits from screening mammography.[22] Even when true cancers are detected, any disease-specific mortality reductions may be wholly negated by deaths due to the downstream harms of screening and the effects of overdiagnosis.[23] That such a cavernous divide exists between the efficacy of mammography and public perception is a testament to the lack of informed consent around the procedure.

Cancer screening can beget identification of nonprogressing cancers or occult tumors that may never have threatened the life of the person who harbors them. For example, the cancer might be inherently nonaggressive, or the cellular abnormalities might either fail to progress or naturally regress. Or perhaps the immune system might contain the cancer, or the cancer may outgrow its own blood supply and succumb to starvation.[24] In one study, 14 percent of diagnosed solid renal tumors regressed on their own,[25] and adenomatous polyps and cervical dysplasia, the precursor lesions of colorectal cancer and cervical cancer, respectively, oftentimes reversed with no treatment at all.[26] Even neuroblastoma, a rare childhood cancer, was shown to regress in all 11 subjects who took a watchful waiting strategy in a small trial.[27] Prostate cancer overdiagnosis is also common, constituting 60 percent to 67 percent of prostate cancer diagnoses. Further, the tripling of melanoma rates in the context of a generally stable death rate illustrates that most of the increase in melanoma diagnosis is emblematic of overdiagnosis.[28]

In 2013, a National Cancer Institute–commissioned expert panel published a report in *JAMA* that concluded that millions of individuals who were diagnosed with cancer and treated aggressively with chemotherapy, radiation, and surgery as a result actually did not have cancer after all. These patients underwent preventive cancer screening programs to "find cancer early." The results revealed tissue abnormalities or lesions that, while mis-identified as "cancer" or "precancer" in the past, are now known to have been benign, representing little to no threat to health. This report confirmed what many leading-edge researchers have been saying for years: that millions of people have been wrongly diagnosed with early cancer of the breast, prostate, thyroid, and lung through screening programs—underscoring that campaigns for universal screening recommendations may do more harm than good. The working group of the National Cancer Institute announced that what had been—and still often is—labeled as "cancer" should really be termed "indolent or benign growths of epithelial origin,"[29] meaning that these "cancers" often represent harmless morphological variations that often regress on their own without intervention.

As a team of scientists has pointed out in the *American Journal of Epidemiology*, statistics about the success of screening can be warped by lead time and length bias, concepts that are still familiar mostly to medical experts.[30] Lead time is the differ-ence between when a variation is detected "early" by a screening and the moment when it would present with symptoms and be detected through other methods, such as a breast exam. This lead time generates the statistical illusion that the screening program extends survival time, but the reality is that screening merely moves up the date of diagnosis. Length bias, in contrast, refers to the fact that screening-detected cancers tend to be the ones that grow the most slowly. These indolent cancers create few if any symptoms, and they may never progress to harm if left undiagnosed and untreated. In the realm of clinically sig-nificant findings, fast-growing tumors (i.e., life-threatening cancers) are of the greatest concern, yet these are precisely the ones that are the most difficult to detect early. It's a recipe for misplaced trust: screening tools can find the growths that don't become aggressive cancer, but they are less likely to find the ones that will. The result is overdiagnosis and overtreatment on an astounding scale.

The phenomenon of overdiagnosis is compounded by the propensity of the medical specialties, compartmentalized into their respective silos, to view the patient through the myopic lenses and constructs of their reductionistic training. Just as everything looks like a nail if all you have is a hammer, everything looks like cancer to a radiologist whose explicit expertise is to search for anomalies. This profound shift in priorities from understanding and treating a patient's subjective, first-hand, experiential complaints to screening and, through diagnostic parameters, finding diseases that often present with no symptoms at all is at the heart of the problem today. Cancer treatment, which was once focused on alleviating the patient's suffering, has become a juggernaut-like force creating arbitrarily circumscribed disease entities and increasingly invasive treatments, often in symptomless patients, which may result in more harm than good in those it claims to serve. The following represent some of the cancers that are most often overdiagnosed.

BREAST CANCER

The holy grail of the breast cancer industry, mammography has been the primary instrument in the conventional toolbox for more than three decades. Sixty-eight percent of women believe that mammography will slash breast cancer risk, and 62 percent believe that mammography will cut the risk of breast cancer in half.[31] Research, however, points to more complex answers. The Swiss medical board, for instance, has based their decision to no longer recommend mammography on research that showed that only one breast cancer death is averted for every 1,000 women screened.[32] Another set of statistics, as published in the *New England Journal of Medicine* (*NEJM*), show that without breast cancer screening, 5 out of 1,000 women die from breast cancer, whereas 4 out of 1,000 women died from breast cancer for every 1,000 screened. That is, for every 1,000 women who undergo screening, one breast cancer death is averted, but non-breast-cancer deaths may either remain at 39 or increase to 40. In other words, all 1,000 women are at increased risk of exposure to mammography radiation and overdiagnosis, and even if one woman's life is saved from breast cancer, it is possible that one in addition will die from a non-breast-cancer-related death from the screening, canceling any net positive effect. Women may essentially, then, "simply be trading one type of death for another, at the cost of serious morbidity, anxiety, and expense."[33]

According to *NEJM*, over the last 30 years, an estimated 1.3 million people were wrongly diagnosed with breast cancer. In 2008 alone, researchers Archie Bleyer and H. Gilbert Welch approximate that 31 percent of all diagnosed breast cancers represented overdiagnosis.[34]

Bleyer and Welch argue that mammography has failed as a screening tool, having not met the first prerequisite for a screening modality to reduce cancer-specific mortality: a decline in the number of individuals presenting with late-stage cancer. In their study, they underscore that in order to avoid one breast cancer death, "between two and 10 women will be overdiagnosed and treated needlessly for breast cancer," that "between five and 15 women will be told that they have breast cancer earlier than they would otherwise yet have no effect on their prognosis," and "between 200 and 500 women will have at least one 'false alarm' (50–200 will be biopsied)."[35] Another study in the *Journal of the American Medical Association* indicates that 60 percent of women receive a false positive result when they have undergone screening for a decade or longer.[36]

Especially troubling is the existential and psychological toll in the wake of misdiagnosis, as explored in a study published in the *Annals of Family Medicine*. False-positive breast cancer diagnoses were consistently associated with negative psychosocial effects, even three years after patients were declared cancer-free, relative to women who never received a cancer diagnosis. The researchers concluded, therefore, that "false-positive findings on screening mammography causes long-term psychosocial harm."[37]

Ironically, the "low-dose" radiation incurred from mammography itself represents a potent mammary carcinogen, capable of planting the seeds of cancer deep within irradiated tissue. Radiobiological studies demonstrate that risks of radiation-induced breast cancers from mammography x-rays have been significantly underestimated.[38] Evidence from *BJR*, the British journal of radiology, shows that the low-energy x-rays employed in mammographical screenings are four to six times more effective in damaging DNA than high-energy x-rays,[39] which underscores that mammography may play a causative role in precipitating the very outcome it is designed to detect.

In their efforts to avert cancer by complying with medical recommendations and undergoing regular mammography, women are being exposed to cancer-generating radiation. Ironically, *BRCA1* and *BRCA2* gene mutations—the "breast cancer susceptibility genes"—greatly increase the risk of cancer from exposure to radiation because they inhibit the breasts from repairing DNA damage. According to the international GENE-RAD-RISK study, any diagnostic use of radiation before age 30 increases breast cancer risk by 55 percent for carriers of *BRCA1* or *BRCA2* mutations,[40] yet those undergoing breast screening are rarely, if ever, told about these risks.

Debunking the Power
of the Breast Cancer Gene

The story that *BRCA1* and *BRCA2* mutation is a death sentence, which is harrowing enough for some to lead to prophylactic organ and tissue removal, is patently false. A *BRCA1* "mutation" should be more accurately termed a "variation" that does not slate someone for breast cancer. The spotlight on cancer risk has been affixed to *BRCA*, as its gene product helps cells repair damaged DNA and ensures preservation of the genetic material. Therefore, *BRCA* gene "mutations," technically known as single nucleotide polymorphisms, or SNPs, can result in dysfunctional or inactive *BRCA* protein production, which can prevent our bodies from fixing damaged DNA.

The same inherited *BRCA* variants, however, confer certain advantages, as reinforced by the recent review "The Case Against *BRCA1* and *2* Testing," which concludes that some of the over 500 identified polymorphisms in these genes may elicit protective effects.[41] A recent systematic review and meta-analysis concluded, "In contrast to currently held beliefs of some oncologists, current evidence does not support worse breast cancer survival of *BRCA1/2* mutation carriers in the adjuvant setting; differences if any are likely to be small."[42] Furthermore, *BRCA2* mutation carriers and noncarriers have similar rates of breast cancer–specific death.[43] Other studies conclude that although *BRCA-positive* patients have more frequently negative prognostic factors, their prognosis appears to be equal to or better than that of patients with normal, also known as wild-type, *BRCA* alleles.[44]

BRCA is not necessarily a hereditary defect, as epigenetic mechanisms, including exposure to the environmental pollutant known as 2,3,7,8-Tetrachlorodibenzo-p-dioxin

(TCDD), are implicated in *BRCA* gene silencing. This carcinogen, which participates in initiating lymphomas, soft-tissue sarcomas, lung cancer, and stomach carcinomas, is a by-product of incomplete combustion formed during the chlorine bleaching process used by pulp and paper mills, the incineration of municipal and industrial wastes, and the combustion of wood and fossil fuels. It is so persistent that this dioxin has been found in the global food supply and in breast milk.

This calls into question the value of using *BRCA1* and *BRCA2* gene status to determine breast cancer survival prognosis. For instance, it has been found that the rate of mutation carriers within Ashkenazi Jewish women by age 50 born before 1940 was only 24 percent, whereas the rate of those born after 1940 was 67 percent.[45] This indicates that environmental factors and not genetic ones are driving the breast cancer epidemic. Another review challenging the presumptive link between *BRCA* status and mathematically calculable disease risk certainty stated, "In contrast to currently held beliefs of some oncologists, current evidence does not support worse breast cancer survival of *BRCA1/2* mutation carriers in the adjuvant setting."[46]

The linear and deterministic path from gene to trait to disease risk or prognosis is an archaic way of thinking, whereas epigenetics reflects the complexity and nuance behind the etiological origins of breast cancer more than our genes alone can reveal. "Early detection" does not necessarily equate to prevention, and it is important to consider other environmental and dietary factors.

Prostate Cancer

Similar to breast cancer, prostate cancer is subject to the trends of overdetection, overdiagnosis, and overtreatment, even more so than cancers of the breast, cervix, or colorectum.[47] Screening for prostate-specific antigen (PSA) is the culprit, as it has doubled the likelihood that a man will be diagnosed with prostate cancer in his lifetime.[48] The incidence of prostate cancer overdiagnosis due to PSA screening has been estimated to be as high as 50 percent in some studies[49] and up to 67 percent in others, depending on the screening protocol, population characteristics, and study methodology.[50]

Discovered in 1986, the serine protease PSA protein was initially used to monitor prostate cancer progression and was only later adopted as a surrogate marker for prostate cancer, despite evidence that PSA is not independently prognostic or diagnostic of cancers of the prostate. An enzyme secreted by prostatic epithelial cells that contributes to the liquefaction of seminal fluids, PSA can increase with prostate enlargement and metastatic disease, but it is not cancer-specific, as it can also be elevated with benign prostatic hyperplasia, the latter being a noncancerous condition that commonly afflicts older men.[51] There are also reports of PSA-negative aggressive prostate tumors.[52] Though higher levels can predict the pathological stage, there is no direct correlation between PSA levels and increasing grade or stage of prostate cancer.[53] In effect, the clinical utility of PSA lies mainly in its use as an indicator of prostatic volume and as a tool to monitor cancer progression, regression, or recurrence.[54]

Despite these findings, the American Cancer Society and American Urological Association both still recommend offering annual PSA testing to men aged 50 or older and to those younger who are deemed at risk.[55] This recommendation directly opposes the results of the Prostate, Lung, Colorectal, and Ovarian (PLCO) Cancer Screening Trial, which showed that PSA screening conferred no reduction in prostate cancer mortality at seven years of follow-up.[56] The European Randomized Study of Screening for

Prostate Cancer (ERSPC) trial, on the other hand, demonstrated that screening reduced risk of death from prostate cancer by 20 percent, but at the cost of significant overdiagnosis.[57] In order to prevent a single prostate cancer death, 48 men would have to be treated unnecessarily,[58] exemplifying the broader trend of prostate cancer overdiagnosis. Researchers in the *Journal of the National Cancer Institute* estimate that over 1 million men have been needlessly treated for prostate cancer since 1986.[59]

Prostatic growths often categorized as prostate cancer may occur as an artifact of aging, as revealed by the Arnold Rich autopsy study. Rich found that a substantial proportion of male cadavers aged 50 or older that were autopsied contained clinically insignificant occult carcinomas of the prostate.[60] These growths, however, also occur in young men. In one 1996 study, 8 percent of healthy men in their 20s who had died from trauma were found to harbor these prostate cancers.[61] This begs the rhetorical questions of Willet Whitmore, M.D.: "Is cure possible? Is cure necessary? Is cure possible only when it is not necessary?"[62]

Abnormal PSA results are often followed by invasive biopsies, which pose the risk of hemorrhage and infection, as well as needless radical prostatectomies—partial or complete surgical removal of the prostate—which carry a high risk of impotence, alongside the risks of thrombosis, hemorrhage, bowel injury, infection, and incontinence.[63] The ERSPC trial also brings into question the validity of the biopsy itself. Of the men who underwent a biopsy due to elevated PSA, 75.9 percent had a false positive result.[64] Thirty percent of tumors removed via radical prostatectomy, surgical removal of the prostate gland and surrounding tissues, are found to be clinically insignificant.[65] In almost one-third of cases, then, when radical prostatectomy is undertaken, research has shown there could be a survival benefit from watchful waiting instead.[66]

Indolent prostate cancers may also be treated with androgen blockade therapy, which increases the likelihood of impotence by 267 percent after one year of treatment alongside 500 percent increases in hot flashes and gynecomastia (enlargement of the male breast gland).[67] Androgen deprivation therapy likewise increases risk of fracture, coronary artery disease, heart attack, diabetes, and sudden cardiac death.[68] Since endogenous testosterone is an indicator of health in men and inversely related to all-cause mortality, cancer-related deaths, and cardiovascular mortality,[69] the testosterone suppression therapy that is often prescribed could be adverse to promoting one's longevity.

The widespread screening efforts for prostate cancer have not translated into significant declines in prostate cancer mortality, as illustrated by comparison with figures from the United Kingdom, where widespread PSA screening has not been implemented.[70] This is further affirmed by the results of the Cochrane Collaboration (2013), which found that "prostate cancer screening did not significantly decrease prostate cancer–specific mortality in a combined meta-analysis of five RCTs."[71] In addition, men diagnosed with prostate cancer have a significantly elevated risk of suicide and myocardial infarction in the year following diagnosis.[72]

Collectively, this research points to PSA screening as a flawed endeavor. Even Thomas Stamey, M.D., a professor of urology at Stanford who first advocated PSA screening in 1987, stopped recommending PSA screening for prostate cancer as of 2004.[73] Because prostate cancer is slow-growing, with only .003 percent of men over the age of 65 dying of the disease,[74] it can be significantly suppressed or slowed using dietary and nutritional strategies. For example, before undergoing surgical resection of the prostate gland, we can consider removing dietary risk factors for prostate cancer, such as dairy consumption, first.[75]

Other food-as-medicine interventions can also be impactful. Flaxseed supplementation, for instance, reduces prostate cancer proliferation rates after just one month.[76] Other bioactive phytonutrients obtained from a whole-foods diet rich in fruits and vegetables can also be protective. Soy proteins, as well as zinc, selenium, vitamin E, and various other antioxidants, may serve as natural inhibitors of prostate carcinogenesis and growth.[77] When a small study of men with biopsy-proven, organ-localized prostate cancer who had refused conventional treatments were treated with prostate-nutritional supplements from plant-based sources alongside a modified Mediterranean diet, 87 percent experienced clinically significant improvements in PSA levels in an average of approximately three years.

Prostate Cancer–Defying Nutritional Supplements

In the previously described Mediterranean diet–involved study, subjects were administered a supplement containing the following ingredients: vitamins C, B$_6$, and E; zinc and selenium; the amino acids L-glycine, L-alanine, and L-glutamic acid; and herbs, including pumpkin seed, stinging nettle, ginkgo biloba, garlic, saw palmetto, *Echinacea purpurea*, and *Pygeum africanum*.

LUNG CANCER

Another category of highly overdiagnosed cancer is that of the lung, the leading cause of cancer death worldwide. Low-dose helical computed tomography (CT) has been deployed in the realm of lung cancer to catch tumors at early stages, with potentially disastrous consequences for overdiagnosis. Researchers from the National Lung Screening Trial (NLST) randomly assigned 53,454 people at high risk for lung cancer from 33 United States medical centers to undergo three annual screenings with either low-dose CT or single-view posteroanterior chest radiography to explore how low-dose CT reduced lung cancer mortality. As reported in the *New England Journal of Medicine,* they found "a total of 96.4% of the positive screening results in the low-dose CT group and 94.5% in the radiography group were false positive results."[78]

Further analysis showed that the likelihood that any lung cancer, non-small cell lung cancer, or bronchoalveolar lung cancer detected by low-dose CT represented overdiagnosis was 18.5 percent, 22.5 percent, and 78.9 percent, respectively.[79] This means, overall, approximately one in five people were told they had treatment-necessary cancer when their lesions may never have caused harm or death if left undiagnosed. Given that lung nodules are often found incidentally during x-rays for unrelated issues such as respiratory complaints and that they present asymptomatically (meaning that the patient does not experience symptoms), they fall into the category of an illusory "disease" that exists only via the lens of modern diagnostic technology. Again, an embedded irony is that CT scans rely on highly carcinogenic radiation, administering 200 times more than a chest x-ray per reading, and it has been estimated that about 0.4 percent of all cancers in the United States may be attributable to the radiation from CT scans.[80]

THYROID CANCER

Thyroid cancer is the fastest-growing cancer, with its rates quadrupling in the past four decades,[81] and it is projected to be the most common cancer by 2030.[82] Between 1998 and 2012, a doubling in the age-standardized annual incidence of thyroid cancer among women was observed.[83] That being said, several studies have highlighted that the increased rates of thyroid cancer diagnoses were limited to the most indolent form of thyroid cancer, the papillary carcinoma subtype, which are clusters of thyroid cells that form into a mass. Furthermore, the epidemic of thyroid cancer diagnosis occurs without a corresponding increase in thyroid cancer deaths, according to researchers in *PLOS ONE*.[84]

Papillary lesions of indolent course (PLIC), which are often characterized as "thyroid cancers," have been found to potentially be benign morphological variations that "do not evolve to cause metastatic disease or death."[85] The vast majority of these thyroid cancer diagnoses are small papillary cancers, the most indolent type of thyroid cancer, with a mortality of less than one percent after 20 years of post-surgical follow-up.[86] Autopsy studies indicate that many of us harbor these thyroid cancers in our thyroid glands.[87] When discovered as a postmortem finding, scientists have found that these occult papillary carcinomas (OPCs), which arise from normal follicular cells, should be "regarded as a normal finding which should not be treated when incidentally found."[88]

Radiographic investigations for nonthyroid issues, for example, can detect as incidental findings thyroid abnormalities that would have otherwise gone unnoticed.[89] Other mechanisms of overdiagnosis include opportunistic screening, where the thyroid is examined in asymptomatic patients, and diagnostic cascades, where multiple tests are conducted in the evaluation of nonspecific health complaints.[90] Aggressive use of thyroid ultrasounds is particularly implicated. For example, although it is not universally recommended, some centers in South Korea conduct routine ultrasonography screening for thyroid cancer in patients undergoing follow-up after breast cancer surgery. As a result, within a 14-year time period, incidence of thyroid cancer diagnosis increased tenfold in South Korea, a rise that is unparalleled worldwide.[91] The most likely explanation for these skyrocketing rates is not from genetic or environmental causes but from overdiagnosis secondary to unprecedented increases in advanced thyroid imaging and systematic exploration of small thyroid nodules.[92]

Increasingly tragic is the three- to fourfold parallel rise in unnecessary thyroidectomy that has accompanied thyroid cancer overdiagnosis and the lifelong synthetic thyroid hormone replacement that often ensues.[93] In Switzerland, researchers estimate that at least one-third of thyroidectomies, surgical procedures that remove all or part of the thyroid gland, may be unnecessarily performed each year as a consequence of thyroid cancer overdiagnosis.[94] Thyroidectomy is accompanied by risk of the electrolyte imbalance postoperative hypocalcemia, as well as vocal cord injury and the thyroid replacement therapy upon which the thyroidless patient becomes dependent, and it has its own burden of monitoring and treatment.[95] Moreover, the overdiagnosis of thyroid lesions often leads to unwarranted treatment with radioactive iodine, which puts patients at risk of secondary malignancies.[96]

In 2016, an international panel of doctors did an about-face in reclassifying the encapsulated follicular variant of papillary thyroid carcinoma as "noninvasive follicular thyroid neoplasm with papillary-like nuclear features" (NIFTP), removing the word "carcinoma" and effectively acknowledging that these tumors were never cancer after all. The name is a mouthful, but at the heart of the matter is that this revised diagnosis no longer includes the recommendation for aggressive treatment, and it comes with the implication that papillary lesions of the thyroid should not be characterized as lethal cancers. According to *JAMA Oncology*, this reclassification is estimated to affect over 45,000 patients per year. The change therefore significantly reduced "the psychological burden, medical overtreatment and expense, and other clinical consequences associated with a cancer diagnosis."[97] Sadly, medical treatment may be slow to reflect these new guidelines, since it takes on average 17 years for research to be translated into clinical practice.[98]

The Problems with Conventional Cancer Treatment

The National Cancer Institute report that sounded the alarm on overdiagnosis was published in 2013, though since then conventional practice of cancer diagnosis, prevention, and treatment has not undergone radical change. The conventional cancer industry continues to promote chemotherapy and radiation, even though they compromise genetic material. Their genotoxicity fits into the prevailing gene mutational theory of the origin of cancer, as we are targeting cancer cells with cancer-causing therapies.

First deployed in 1946, the original chemotherapeutic agents were derived from nitrogen mustard gas, which was originally used in chemical warfare.[99] By the early 1990s, anticancer drug development had been transformed from a low-budget, government-supported research effort into a high-stakes, multi-billion-dollar industry.[100] Today, the anticancer drug industry accounts for 10.8 percent of the total market share of the pharmaceutical industry, valued at $100 billion.[101]

Chemotherapy and radiotherapy are a deadly game of roulette, wherein we rely upon these intrinsically carcinogenic treatments to kill tissue lesions, growths, and abnormalities labeled "cancer" faster than they kill us. As in modern warfare, these modalities are indiscriminate in their propensity to inflict harm, and the decision to strike is based upon how much collateral damage is deemed permissible to the "civilian populations" of noncombatant healthy cells. This approach stands in stark juxtaposition to natural, plant-based anticancer compounds and whole plant extracts that are favorable in their selective cytotoxicity, or the ability to target cancer cells while leaving healthy cells intact. For example, graviola, from the seeds of the soursop fruit, is up to 10,000 times more cytotoxic to colon adenocarcinoma cells than the chemo agent Adriamycin, the trade name for doxorubicin, which is also known as the "red devil" because of its color and cardiotoxic side effects. Even though cell culture studies demonstrate that graviola elicits selective anti–prostate cancer, anti–pancreatic cancer,[102] antihepatoma,[103] and anti–breast cancer activity,[104] there is still a lack of fiscal incentive for further studies. Because the medical-pharmaceutical-industrial complex revolves around control over synthetic, patentable medications, and because natural products cannot be patented, further research on graviola has stalled.

Another fundamentally faulty premise continues to guide the treatment industry: the belief that tumor regression equals survival. The approval of anticancer drugs is contingent upon demonstration of clinical benefit, which is measured by objective measurements of tumor regression, quality of life improvements, and elongation of the time duration until recurrence.[105] These parameters for measuring success, however, have not translated into a significant benefit to life-span and cannot be taken as sur-rogate markers, or indicators, of survival.[106] The contribution of cytotoxic chemotherapy to survival is minimal, improving five-year survival by only 2.1 percent and 2.3 percent in the United States and Australia, respectively.[107] The simple fact that response to therapy does not necessarily prolong survival has been established by scientific literature and research,[108] leading a study published in the journal *Blood* to conclude, "Objective clinical responses to treatment often do not even translate into substantial improvements in overall survival."[109]

The study notes numerous examples where response and survival do not track together:

> Indolent lymphoma patients who achieved complete remissions (i.e., elimination of all detectable disease) with conventional-dose therapies in the prerituximab era did not experience a survival advantage over similar patients treated with a "watch and wait" approach. In multiple myeloma, neither the magnitude nor the kinetics of clinical response has an impact on survival. Similarly, significant clinical responses in pancreatic and prostate cancer have not translated into survival benefits.[110]

And then there is tamoxifen, the frontline treatment deployed to treat estrogen receptor alpha (ERα)–positive breast tumors in premenopausal women. By blocking estrogen receptors, tamoxifen prevents estrogen signaling and the expression of genes involved in cell proliferation and survival.[111] However, the success of this antiestrogen is often short-lived, as described by Viedma-Rodriguez and colleagues in *Oncology Reports*: "Patients with estrogen receptor-positive breast cancer initially respond to treatment with anti-hormonal agents such as tamoxifen, but remissions are often followed by the acquisition of resistance and, ultimately, disease relapse."[112]

Metabolites of tamoxifen elicit cancer-causing genotoxic effects, damaging genetic material[113] due to overproduction of reactive oxygen species (ROS) during metabolic activation of the antiestrogen agent.[114] Tamoxifen has been demonstrated to increase incidence of secondary primary malignancies including endometrial cancer,[115] as well as stomach cancer[116] and colorectal cancer,[117] and there are even reports of development of acute myeloid leukemia (AML) following tamoxifen therapy for breast cancer.[118] Tamoxifen use, then, may lead breast cancer patients to simply trade one form of cancer for another. So strong is the link between tamoxifen and endometrial cancer that researchers in the *International Journal of Cancer* call for an immediate long-term evaluation of the risk-benefit ratio of tamoxifen use.[119]

Not only that, but tamoxifen is associated with a host of adverse side effects, including subjective complaints of memory[120] and cognitive deficits,[121] nonalcoholic fatty liver disease,[122] cataracts,[123] stroke, and pulmonary embolism.[124] Tamoxifen was touted as lifesaving after the release of the ATLAS study in *The Lancet*, but close examination reveals a major conflict of interest from the study's funding by major pharmaceutical industry sources, including AstraZeneca, and a relatively low magnitude of impact, with a 3.9 percent reduction in breast cancer recurrence and a 2.8 percent reduction in breast cancer mortality.[125] Thus, the purported differences in breast cancer morbidity and survivability in the five-year versus extended tamoxifen treatment group may reflect the differing degrees to which women were subjected to overdiagnosis and overtreatment.

Rather than representing intrinsic therapeutic value in targeting breast cancer cells, tamoxifen may reduce the likelihood of detection and subsequent risk of overdiagnosis. Given the antiestrogen effects of tamoxifen, longer tamoxifen treatment suppresses growth of estrogen-sensitive tissues within the breast, whether benign or malignant, reducing the likelihood of mammography-detectable lesions, benign tumors, or "abnormal findings." Lower mortality, then, could result from avoiding the psychological and physical trauma that would ensue from a treatment that was inappropriate and misapplied in the first place.

The Old Cancer Paradigm

At the heart of the Old Cancer Paradigm are these three words: burn, cut, poison. Framing cancer as an irrational and irrepressible force of destruction presents what seems like the only option: to attack it with highly toxic weaponry and potentially deadly procedures. However, this scorched-earth policy fundamentally decimates the very immune defenses designed to protect against cancer.

The old thinking behind the origin of abnormal tissue growth, including cancer, is dominated by the somatic mutational theory, which is described by an article in the journal *BioEssays* as a three-legged stool. The first leg is the assumption that cancer happens when a somatic, or body, cell acquires too many genetic mutations of the wrong kind. The second leg posits that healthy cells are normally inactive, abstaining from the ceaseless proliferation observed in all cancers. Finally, the third leg is the belief that cancer is caused by defects in particular genes that control the cell cycle (the process of DNA duplication and cellular division that results in two identical daughter cells), which prevents cells from dying at appointed times. In this paradigm, mutations happen at random through a combination of inherited defects and environmental exposures, though the former cause is far more emphasized than the latter. This emphasis on genetic causes is not an accident; in the mid-20th century, much of the early research focused on a genetic cause to distract from the increasingly indicting signal of harm around commercial cigarettes.

There are several problems with the genetic cancer theory. One glaring deficiency is that many of the proto-oncogenes that are found to contribute to cancer, at least 40 of which have been discovered in our genome thus far, have evolutionary origins that can be traced back eons to earlier rudimentary life forms and were not produced by sheer chance through the chaos of strictly mutational forces. In fact, when functioning correctly, these proto-oncogenes carry out crucial functions, especially in embryogenesis, cellular growth and proliferation, and regenerative processes.

The idea inherent in genetic theory that cancer represents a collection of cells gone rogue—"a mosaic of mutant cells [that] compete for space and resources"[126]—flies in the face of modern cancer biology, failing to account for the extent of cooperation among cancer cells.[127] For example, cancer cells collaborate in the processes of angiogenesis and lymphangiogenesis, or the growth of a new vascular network and lymphatic vessels to supply the tumor with nutrients, oxygen, and immune cells and to remove waste products.[128] Cancer cells likewise exchange chemical mediators with each other and with exogenous tissue, and there is even evidence that less malignant cells can temper the expansion of populations of more malignant cells, restraining and governing their activity.[129] This phenomenon is best illustrated by the sudden proliferation of metastatic tumors after a primary tumor is surgically resected or by the flourishing of a malignant subpopulation of cells after chemotherapy targets the dominant population of cancer cells.[130]

The "cell gone rogue" theory fails to account for the ability of cancer cells to "deploy a formidable array of survival tricks, sometimes all at once," such as immune system evasion, penetration of the circulatory systems, invasion of organ membranes, colonization of distant body sites, silencing of tumor suppressor genes, and inhibition of cell senescence and apoptosis, the processes by which cells commit suicide or cease to divide, respectively.[131] It also fails to explain how cancer cells generate an arsenal of mitogenic signals and growth factors that prompt cell division, adapt to oxygen-poor and acidic conditions, remove surface-receptor proteins to escape detection by white blood cells, and alter the viscoelastic characteristics of cells to promote tissue infiltration and metastasis (the spreading of cancer cells to other tissues).[132]

These advantageous traits of cancer cells can be explained by the biomedical paradigm in terms of internal Darwinism, described as a series of fortuitous accidents of evolution where random genetic mutations occur secondary to normal blind Darwinian trial-and-error that, by happenstance, confer a selective advantage to cancer cells, allowing cancer cells to accrue a veritable multifaceted armory that renders them virtually immortal in the face of conventional treatments.[133] Researchers Paul Davies, Ph.D., ASU Regents' Professor and Director of the Beyond Center for Fundamental Concepts in Science, and physicist Charles Lineweaver, Ph.D. of the Australian National University poke holes in the internal Darwinism argument by underscoring that random mutations in healthy cells are often detrimental, leading to maladaptation and cell death. It is paradoxical that cancer cells can still thrive with deformed nuclei, gross structural alterations, dramatic chromatin reorganizations, and chaotic karyotypic configurations, including full-blown aneuploidy (the presence of an abnormal number of chromosomes in a cell). There is far more to the story than genetic scrambling producing reprobate cells that forget how to behave.

CANCER STEM CELLS

For decades it has been observed that tumors treated with chemotherapy and radiation initially shrink and sometimes appear to go into remission, only to come back with a vengeance. When they do, it is virtually impossible to treat these tumors again. Solid tumors are organized hierarchically with the self-renewing cancer stem cells (sometimes called "mother cells") at the apex, each individually capable of forming entirely new tumors, and less harmful populations known as the "daughter cells" arising from the mother cells. The progeny of cancer stem cells, however, are not themselves capable of the type of malignant growth and metastasis we fear most about cancer. In the 1990s, Dr. John Dick at the Ontario Institute for Cancer Research discovered that many malignancies arise from self-renewing cancer stem cells (CSCs), which sustain the tumor and give rise to all the daughter cell types found within the tumor colony.[134] And as articulated by Wang and colleagues in the journal *Oncotarget*, "Cancer stem cells are solely capable of self-renewal and unlimited replication and responsible for maintaining the whole tumour."[135]

This reconciles the discrepancy between response to therapy and survival. Treatments that eradicate nonstem cancer cells may be woefully ineffectual against cancer stem cell subsets,[136] because it is the cancer stem cells which drive cancer recurrence and metastasis.[137] Carol Ann Huff and colleagues liken this to "the dandelion phenomenon," wherein a dandelion cut off at ground level will continue to regrow unless the root itself is eliminated.[138]

Because of their slow replication rate, cancer stem cells are exceptionally resistant to conventional treatments that target rapidly dividing cells.[139] Researchers consider cancer stem cells virtually unreachable by chemotherapy, as they have shown resistance to platinum drugs, 5-fluorouracil, paclitaxel, and doxorubicin.[140] Moreover, because less than 1 in 10,000 cells within a particular cancer represents a cancer stem cell, they are exceptionally difficult to stamp out without destroying the vast majority of other tumor cells.[141] Finally, conventional chemotherapies target cells that are differentiated or differentiating, meaning that they are already specialized cells or are in the process of becoming specialized. But cancer stem cells, by definition, are still undifferentiated. The conventional therapies, then, simply aren't designed to reach the very cells that are at the root of cancer.[142]

The existence of cancer stem cells accounts for why conventional cancer treatments are misguided, as these treatments selectively extinguish the less harmful populations of daughter cells while having very little effect on the powerfully malignant cancer stem cells that give rise to them. Chemo and radiation may look successful at first, but most of the cells that are killed are the benign ones, which are weaker and more vulnerable. Meanwhile, the tiny, invisible population of cancer stem cells survive, and the heart of the cancer beats on. This invasive population comes back— sometimes even stronger than before. All it takes is a few remaining cancer stem cells for the tumor to grow back, given time and the right conditions. Since conventional treatment neither addresses nor alters the root causes of cancer, the cellular environment that remains after treatment continues to be conducive to regrowth and recurrence of cancer. Analogous to the use of antibiotics, which can annihilate commensal gut flora, chemotherapy decimates the patients' immune systems, leaving them more vulnerable to the infection, making disease recurrence a likelihood. Surgery, on the other hand, may provoke cancers toward increased invasiveness by disrupting mechanisms of cancer stem cell sequestration.

Even worse, radiation treatment has been shown to convert breast cancer cells into treatment-resistant breast cancer stem cells and may actually transform nonmalignant tumor cells into highly malignant ones. It has been found that the very radiation wavelengths used to treat cancer activate cellular pathways that convert normal cells into what are known as induced pluripotent stem cells. These radiation-induced, reprogrammed breast cancer cells have been found to have over a 30-fold increased ability to form tumors relative to nonirradiated breast cancer cells.[143]

Breast cancer is just one example where this phenomenon occurs. According to an article in the journal *Cancer Letters*, radiation therapy has been shown to increase cancer stem cells in the prostate, which may contribute to cancer recurrence and worsened prognosis.[144]

Therefore, traditional response criteria, which assesses tumor bulk, is flawed in that it fails to discern whether treatments elicit any effect on the cancer stem cell populations that are the progenitors, or forebearers, of cancer cells. This research illuminates that tumor-spawning properties of cancer stem cells should be the primary target of cancer treatments. As stated by Jim Moselhy in the journal *Anticancer Research*, "The failure to eradicate CSCs during the course of therapy is postulated to be the driving force for tumor recurrence and metastasis."[145] Collectively, conventional therapies make the tumor even more malignant, with radiotherapy wavelengths transforming non-cancer stem cells into those that have the property of "stemness," making them potentially much more aggressive and deadly. Our very anticancer treatments, then, make the cells at the heart of cancer harder to kill.

Since Dr. Dick's initial discovery of leukemia CSCs, other medical researchers around the world have confirmed that CSCs are at the root of cancer malignancy in the blood, breast, lung, prostate, colon, liver, pancreas, and brain. While the vital role of CSCs in cancer malignancy is no longer questioned by most authorities, the origin of CSCs is still debatable. Because cancer stem cells are relatively undifferentiated, meaning that they don't look like liver, breast, or brain cells but look more like other stem cells, it is difficult to determine what tissue they derive from. Nonetheless, there are two prevailing theories about their origins: the trophoblast theory and the oncogerminative theory.

THE TROPHOBLAST THEORY

The trophoblast theory derives from the work of the early-20th-century Nobel Prize–winning histology embryologist John Beard. It was elucidated almost a century later by Drs. William Kelley, Linda Isaacs, and Nicholas Gonzalez.[146] Over his 27-year career, Dr. Gonzalez, a journalist turned physician who trained at Memorial Sloan Kettering in New York City before striking out on his own, put hundreds of cases of terminal cancer into long-term remission through lifestyle medicine. He is best known for cases of multidecade recoveries from the notoriously fatal metastatic pancreatic cancer. To this day, conventional medical treatments have not succeeded in producing a single clinical outcome matched by one of his published cancer remission cases.[147]

The centerfold of this theory are trophoblasts, the cells that compose the outermost layer of a blastocyst, a structure in mammalian embryonic development that eventually forms the embryo. The trophoblast theory originated from Beard's observation that the conversion from trophoblast to stable placenta occurs at the same time as the appearance of the pancreas and its subsequent secretion of enzymes around day 56 of fetal gestation, which led to his speculation that these enzymes govern this transformation.[148] This theory has led to the discovery that in the absence of this regulatory signal, a gestational trophoblastic disease known as a choriocarcinoma, an aggressive cancer of the womb, develops.[149]

Beard drew the parallel between the trophoblast, or the placenta in its early stages, and cancer.[150] The former exhibits cancer-promoting properties in the following ways: the trophoblast initially displays proliferation without restraint, infiltrating and disseminating throughout the epithelial lining of the uterus into underlying stream tissue, which creates a dense network of blood vessels connecting to uterine vasculature in order to maintain embryonic life.[151] At the molecular level, cancer cells and trophoblasts share similar cellular markers and secretory products, such as human chorionic gonadotrophin (hCG), which is a hormone secreted by the fetus in pregnancy and by cancer cells.[152] Cancer employs many of the same molecular mechanisms as trophoblasts, including using the same matrix metalloproteinases to chew through the connective tissue, the same transcription factors to modify gene expression, and the same ability to travel through the dense underlying stroma and invade the basement membrane of cell linings.[153]

Beard's second observation concerned "wayward trophoblasts," which migrate throughout the fetal body during embryogenesis, deposit in distant tissues and organs, and remain in undifferentiated nests for the lifetime of the organism.[154] Although they are maintained in dormant or quiescent forms, they may be stimulated into replicative activity via environmental signals conducive to cancer.[155] These "ectopic trophoblasts"—ectopic meaning "in an abnormal place"—are now recognized as adult stem cells and can become cancer cells when they evade regulatory mechanisms and adopt characteristics of the local tissue as a by-product of local signals.[156]

Like the cancer stem cell theory, the trophoblast theory suggests the potential of a single primitive cell to form a tumor when stimulated into replicative activity by maladaptive cellular conditions. Thus, cancer can be recognized as evolving from stem cells that lose their overarching regulatory restraints rather than healthy cells gone molecularly berserk. The trophoblast hypothesis is compatible with the stem cell hypothesis, suggesting that a subset of adult stem cells are ectopic trophoblasts. In the journal *Alternative Therapies*, Nicholas J. Gonzalez, M.D., explains that when these misplaced trophoblast cells are "stimulated into reproductive activity through inflammation or infection, in the wrong place and at the wrong time, they become the invasive, exponentially growing tissue we identify as cancer."[157]

What makes Beard's theory so interesting is his observation that at about 12 weeks of pregnancy, the fetal pancreas begins to secrete pancreatic enzymes, a regulatory signal that causes the trophoblast to stop growing and the placenta to take over the function of nourishing the fetus. It was this discovery that led others to use pancreatic enzymes, such as trypsin, to inhibit the growth of cancer. Beard predicted that trypsin could be harnessed as a cancer treatment since it would elicit the same effects it does on the embryonic trophoblast, impeding the out-of-control cell division, angiogenesis, invasion, and metastasis while restoring normal cell adhesion and differentiation.[158] He initially tested his hypothesis in mice with a sarcoma-like malignancy, in experiments that showed total regression of tumors with injection of trypsin.[159] Later, medical literature referred to pancreatic enzyme therapy in reports of stabilization or regression of inoperable cancers, including uterine, colorectal, metastatic breast, tongue, and head and neck cancers. Dr. Gonzalez would later refine this enzyme approach to cancer in his practice, ushering a wide range of so-called incurable cancer patients into remission, further reinforcing the efficacy of this approach. For instance, in a pilot study, Gonzalez and Isaacs demonstrated that high-dose proteolytic enzymes, detoxification procedures, nutraceuticals, and an organic diet significantly prolonged survival in patients with inoperable, biopsy-proven pancreatic adenocarcinoma.

The trophoblast theory explanation is compelling, as it indicates an effective cancer framework. But there is also a growing body of research that suggests that somatic cells can begin to behave like more primitive cancer stem cells even if they do not originate embryologically. This means that cancer stem cells can emerge from normal, terminally differentiated cells having been "hit" multiple times by genotoxic agents or having had to adjust to inhospitable conditions (such as low oxygen or chronically acidic or low pH), reverting back to a germline or undifferentiated stem cell type. The theoretical framework that melds the three viewpoints—trophoblast, mutational, and cancer stem cell theories—is known as the oncogerminative hypothesis.

THE ONCOGERMINATIVE HYPOTHESIS

The oncogerminative hypothesis, which proposes that cancer is a dynamic, self-organizing process that mimics the reproducible, orderly succession of events in early embryonic development, was first advanced by Ukrainian oncologist Vladimir Vinnitsky in 1993.

In this model, cancer passes through five discrete stages resembling those of early embryonic development, with the end product being a tumor rather than a fetus. This theory differs from the trophoblast theory in that somatic cells can be malignantly transformed to activate the "germinative cell genome," enabling them to become deathless yet—ironically—deadly to the body as a whole.[160] In this way, the oncogerminative hypothesis merges and reinforces both the cancer stem cell and trophoblast theories in a way that maintains their validity while extending upon both theories with added nuance.

CANCER TAPS THE GENES OF ANCIENT ANCESTORS

Even with the trophoblast and oncogerminative hypotheses, lingering questions remain. Namely, how did such a highly complex program, latent within every cell of the body, endure the evolutionary test of time? How is it that by reverting to a more primitive, less differentiated cell type, body cells can unleash the incredible resilience and hypercomplexity of cancer? Since nothing in the body happens by accident, it makes sense to dig deeper and understand what adaptive benefit cancer has afforded us over the course of evolution.

The adaptive value of unleashing the system of uncontrolled cell growth typifying cancer remained a mystery until the pioneering work of Paul Davies and Charles Lineweaver, who painted a portrait of cancer as a living fossil—a subterranean layer of primordial genes that becomes reawakened with exposure to postindustrial environmental threats.[161] In their seminal work, "Cancer Tumors as Metazoa 1.0: Tapping Genes of Ancient Ancestors," published in *Physical Biology*, they propose that cancer is actually an ancient survival response buried deep within our genome that is recruited when genetic and epigenetic malfunctions reach a critical mass. Within this evolutionarily consistent context, we can understand cancer as symptomatic of disturbance in the internal physiological milieu and the logical defense against a carcinogen-saturated world that our bodies perceive as inherently dangerous.

Given the failed war on cancer and the vast body count it has left in its wake since its inception 50 years ago, it is abundantly clear that we need to examine the very essence of cancer, which has thus far eluded us. It must first be acknowledged that the mutational explanation of cancer has its place. Genotoxic, or DNA-damaging, substances such as formaldehyde, diesel engine exhaust, coal tar, asbestos, and tobacco smoke can play a role in cancer initiation and progression. But mutational processes alone do not explain everything, and cancer is not solely driven by random environmental exposure.

The quasi ubiquity of cancer, which occurs in nearly all metazoan life forms, implies that the mechanisms from which oncogenesis is born are deeply woven into the fabric of our evolutionary history. There is evidence that oncogenes, or genes theorized to be responsible for cancer, are ancient and highly conserved, dating back in some cases 600 million years.[162] That oncogenes have endured since time immemorial, with oncogene precursors dating back to the primitive metazoans, suggests that they serve fundamental roles in cellular and organismic physiology and confer some sort of survival advantage.[163]

In their pivotal paper, Davies and Lineweaver flesh out a connection between cancer and the evolution of multicellularity, proposing that cancer is an atavistic state of multicellular life.[164] Atavisms, or reversions to ancient or ancestral traits, often possess morphological features of the developing zygote of the species in question.[165] Atavism occurs when traits believed to be lost in evolutionary history, such as tails, gills, webbed feet, or supernumerary nipples in humans, reappear.[166] These ancient or ancestral traits are often preserved in an inoperative state in the genome or relegated to what was formerly called the "junk" or "noncoding" segment of DNA, suppressed in a quiescent state by regulatory elements that inhibit their expression. The dormancy of these atavisms, however, is reversed when more recently evolved genes designed to inactivate the traits malfunction.

Within their model, Davies and Lineweaver discuss how evolutionarily complex modern metazoan organisms—multicellular animals characterized by cellular specialization and organ differentiation—"were preceded by colonies of eukaryotic cells in which cellular cooperation was fairly rudimentary, consisting of networks of adhering cells exchanging information chemically, and forming self-organized assemblages with only a moderate division of labor."[167] Thus, these loose-knit colonies, which the authors call Metazoa 1.0, operated in the same fashion as neoplastic tumor cells. During Metazoa 1.0, the beginnings of which stretch back several billion years, cell life, for all intents and purposes, was immortal. The conditions on Earth at that point were so harsh that cells needed to focus on mere survival, which is why proliferative immortality was their default state. They didn't have the luxury of the programmed cell suicide of apoptosis, which is a prerequisite for the cell turnover required in biological regeneration and for the selective pruning that makes it possible for highly differentiated body tissues to evolve and exist. These cells are believed to have formed primitive "clumped-together" communities, which would look in today's terminology much like a tumor.

Metazoa 1.0 and its proto-metazoans fell by the wayside 600 million years ago with the emergence of Metazoa 2.0. The latter represented complex multicellular organisms with the highly specialized cell types, sophisticated communication and command networks, highly refined regulatory pathways, well-defined tissue architecture, and more advanced biological compartments and repertoires typical of modern humans.[168] With the evolution of modern complex organisms, the needs of the individual cell became subordinate to the whole, and cellular differentiation and organization developed. In the interest of expediency and specialization, functions were delegated to specific tissues, and the cells of different organs came to look and behave in dramatically different ways due to cellular differentiation.

The key to this theory lies in the genetic apparatus of the second incarnation of metazoa being overlaid atop the existing genetic framework of the Metazoa 1.0 system, meaning that evolutionarily, over the past billion years, our species has solidified a fatal pact with its individual members: your bodies will die, but the germline cells within you will remain immortal and can be passed down intergenerationally forever. This means that "death"—in the form of apoptosis and the finite life-span of individuals—is built into life through our progeny and future descendants. This hallmark feature of multicellular, complex animal life has made it essential that "immortality" does not erupt in our somatic cells in the form of cancer.

We carry our ancient genetic programs around with us, in nearly every cell in our body. And when we treat our bodies poorly from chemical and radiation exposures, mechanical damage in the form of wounds and inflammation, chronically low pH from excessively acid-forming foods, high-sugar diets, or low oxygen from inactivity and pollution, our cells sense a massive environmental threat. And then our old Metazoa 1.0 kicks in, making an opportunity out of what would otherwise be a deadly combination of changes. The implication, then, is that the subterranean genetic layer of Metazoa 1.0 activates within us in response to an increasingly inhospitable, unforgiving, and nutrient-depleted cellular climate mirroring that of over 600 million years ago, one that would favor the expression of genes designed for the singular imperative of replication and survival. Thus, it can be surmised that cancer represents our reversion to a primitive defense mechanism that serves the sole purpose of circumventing death and that evolved before protective adaptations meant to contend with environmental threats emerged. This is at the root of the irony that cancer's very lethality is tied to its remarkably regenerative, resilient, and quasi-immortal properties.

Cancer Reimagined

Examining the atavistic nature of cancer may give us hope, as it allows us to understand cancer as a natural adaptation to a lifetime of nutrient deprivation, environmental poisoning, and psychospiritual distress. This model allows a fresh perspective on the origin of cancer as not a curse but a protective mechanism, a vehicle to regain homeostasis within suboptimal conditions, when no other viable option remains. It is an infinitely resilient and life-promoting property buried deep within our biological infrastructure, one that has been stirred awake in modern times in response to the intense postindustrial challenges our bodies face.

As a corollary, by removing the bioenergetic and biochemical adversities that compel a cell to revert to a more primitive, despeciated phenotype characteristic of the ancestral proto-cell, we may remove the impetus for the survival mode that this prepackaged atavism provides. We can provide these cues of safety via an ancestral lifestyle regimen and a nutrient- and information-rich, evolutionarily appropriate diet, which may allow reinstatement of regulatory mechanisms that restore appropriate cell cycle controls and stop cancer in its tracks.

Going Forward: A More Humane Approach to Cancer Treatment and a Wiser Approach to Prevention

The New Biology tells us that enlightened practitioners should learn to address the root causes of the cancer atavism instead of violently suppressing the symptoms. We should focus on creating the conditions that support our genetic and epigenetic blueprints of health and wellness. We should take control and make daily choices that provide a healthy environment for our cells and boost our bodies' natural ability to target cancer stem cells before they even have a chance to become malignant cancerous tumors.

The Regenerate Rx details dietary practices you can follow to provide your cells with the support they need to thrive. You'll boost your cells' ability to engage in healthy apoptosis and engender homeostasis (bodily equilibrium) by provisioning nutrient density, sending a signal of safety to every cell in your body and preventing reversion to the ancestral Metazoa 1.0 phenotype. As it has done for hundreds of thousands of years and is encoded to do going forward, your body will use these traditional foods to facilitate healthy cell turnover and the clearance of aberrant cells before cancer develops.

Cancer through a New Lens

When we explore the natural pharmacopoeia of anticancer compounds available to us, we can transcend the image of cancer as an unconquerable, unassailable adversary.

Instead, we can carve a path forward by adopting a clear-headed, evidence-based approach and remaining focused on prevention by embracing the healing power of nature in full consonance with the Hippocratic principle of doing no harm.

The mainstay of a truly preventive strategy for all cancers is an evolutionarily compatible diet and avoidance of exposures to chemicals and radiation. These are accessible approaches we can implement in our daily lives to reclaim agency in our medical decisions and to regain responsibility for our health. We do not need to relinquish our power or surrender ourselves to the whims of our "genetic destiny." When we recognize our limiting beliefs, outdated narratives, maladaptive coping mechanisms, and unproductive patterns, we clear the cobwebs of fear and confront cancer with a newfound clarity.

FIRST, LET GO OF FEAR: HOW STRESS AND PSYCHIC WOUNDS BEGET CANCER

Whether you are fleeing from a predator on the African savannah or facing what is presumed to be a fatal cancer diagnosis, your physiology is primed to react in the same way. Your body does not know the difference between a perceived threat and actual physical danger. When we are gripped by a relentless foreboding feeling that catapults us into fight-or-flight response, the stranglehold of fear causes our bodies to react in a predictable manner. Glucose is released from the liver as a quick energy source, and blood flow is diverted from the digestive system to the extremities in anticipation of an energy-demanding escape. Increased respiratory depth and bronchiolar dilatation occur in tandem with enhanced cardiac output and blood pressure to improve oxygenation and energy delivery to the musculature. Stress hormones such as catecholamines, glucocorticoids, growth hormone, and prolactin flood our systems in order to mobilize energy reserves.[169] It's a precarious compromise; reproduction and immunity are put on hold in favor of more primordial impulses to elude predators and to evade immediate danger.

Cognitive processes inherent to the frontal lobe, the brain region governing the executive functions of learning, memory, problem-solving, and decision-making, are forestalled in favor of instinctual reflexes activated in pursuit of survival. The mass activation of the sympathetic nervous system results in stimulation of the reticular activation system, the brain area responsible for heightened alertness and sensory amplification,[170] to put us in touch with the potential hazards in our surroundings. The paraventricular nucleus of the hypothalamus, the ancient core of the brain that has its roots in the last common ancestors of vertebrates, flies, and worms, coordinates and orchestrates the response to stress,[171] meaning that we revert to autopilot when confronted with a stressor.

Stress-induced disorders were once branded as psychosomatic, a relic of the Freudian concept called hysteria, now rebranded as "conversion disorder." The underlying assumption of these disease labels is that your concerns are all in your head, leaving you questioning the legitimacy of your symptomatology, the compass of your innate intuition, and the veracity of the diagnosis your trusted practitioner provides. But there still is a two-way dialogue between mind and body. Stress is a profoundly impactful vector of physiological dysfunction, prompting maladaptive neuroendocrine responses that can either initiate or progress bodily illness,[172] and cancer is no exception.

At a physical level, the neuropeptides released during exposure to stressors affect both the cell-mediated and humoral (antibody-mediated) poles of our immune responses. According to researchers, data from animal and human studies indicate an adverse immune system response to the release of adrenaline during episodic stress.[173] Primary lymphoid organs such as the thymus and bone marrow, where our immune cells mature, as well as secondary lymphoid organs such as the spleen and appendix, are innervated (supplied) by noradrenergic nerve fibers, meaning that immune tissue is directly responsive to messaging from our stress-governing sympathetic nervous system.[174] Other signaling molecules released from peripheral sensory nerve fibers triggered by stress regulate different aspects of immune cell function such as differentiation, activation, recruitment, chemotaxis (migration), and vascular (blood vessel) responses.[175] And perceived stress has been shown to mobilize inflammatory immune cells from the bone marrow into action.[176]

Our fight-or-flight response can suppress the type of cell-mediated immunity needed to neutralize cancer and can cause other deleterious effects. Adrenaline, one of the hormones released during the stress response, makes colon cancer cells more resistant to several types of chemotherapy. One of the first biomedical studies revealing a direct mechanistic link between cancer and stress showed that adrenergic activation (adrenaline production) produced dose-dependent increases in the oncogene *ABCB1* gene and its gene product, P-glycoprotein, which protects cancer cells from anticancer compounds.[177] Since our immune systems serve as both sentinels that surveil the body for cancer and a loyal clean-up crew that degrades and disposes of cancerous cells, the ability of stress to derail our immune system is key to the pathogenesis of cancer. Conversely, remediating stress can help promote optimal immune function and clearance of cancerous cells.

The implications of this body of literature are important, as they lend support to the proponents of the mind-body connection. One such pioneer is Hungarian-born Canadian physician Gabor Maté, who collates research on how emotions like anger profoundly affect cancer risk and prognosis in his book *When the Body Says No*. Another expert is Dr. Candace Pert, the mother of the vanguard discipline of psychoneuroimmunology. Her book *Molecules of Emotion* elucidates how our feelings—our past disappointments, failures, heartaches, and traumas—are concentrated in "nodal points" that are lodged and encoded within our body tissues and systems. Pert was one of the first neuroscientists to show that our endocrinological and immunological systems are united in a bidirectional network of communication via mediating information carriers called neuropeptides. These systems engage in a multilingual crosstalk of chemicals and energy, thereby overturning the antiquated notions that the mind and the immune system are independent and confirming that our body is a storage depot for unresolved emotions that can translate into disease. Stated plainly, your body hears everything your mind says.

Dr. Mario Martinez's work on biocognition has been pivotal in providing a semantic grounding for the way in which psychospiritual stress can lead to illness. He described how three archetypal human wounds—shame, abandonment, and fear—are stitched into different illness challenges, producing corresponding bodily patterns and energetic fields. Each of these wounds is inflicted and co-created by different cultural settings. For example, shame can be the product of teasing, bullying, judgment, criticism, ridicule, or guilt trips, and it manifests as a hot, humiliated, pro-inflammatory phenotype that is characteristic of autoimmune disease. Betrayal is associated with broken promises, infidelity, abuse, or lack of integrity and causes an angry fight-or-flight reaction involving adrenaline and cortisol, leading to the phenotype of heart disease. Abandonment can result from neglect, lack of support, and invisibility. It is represented by a cold and fearful, adrenaline-based fight-or-flight reaction, and it is oftentimes associated with cancer.

By cultivating our complementary healing fields, however, with honor in the place of shame, commitment in the place of abandonment, and loyalty in the place of betrayal, we can change our neural maps, alter the way our emotions are archived, and heal our biology. For cancer, specifically, commitment in the form of making yourself a priority, keeping your word, and honoring your promises can make room for expansive emotions that heal the wound.

DELETE CANCER-PROMOTING TOXICANTS

The best way to avoid cancer is by creating a microenvironment that does not activate our more primitive Metazoa 1.0 layer, where the "cancer program" resides. The Regenerate Rx will give you an extensive list of foods in which to bathe your cells' informational signals to promote optimal immune function. But part of adopting a more evolutionarily compatible ancestral microenvironment is becoming more aware of products that contain cancer-promoting toxicants, whether you ingest them or come into external contact with them.

Consider glyphosate, the world's most widely used herbicide, with about 2 billion pounds being applied to the surface of the planet annually. Also known commercially as Roundup, it's used to kill weeds in our front lawns, our parks, and a good number of crops that provide the world's food supply. The problem is that when we apply glyphosate indiscriminately, we don't just kill the weeds but also the microbes, earthworms, insects, plants, and rodents that are part of the bioaccumulative food chain that leads to human beings. Further, the use of glyphosate has given rise to genetically engineered plants that are not limited to the botanical variety. If you eat a food that's been genetically modified, you're likely eating food that's contaminated with glyphosate. And even foods that aren't genetically modified, such as wheat, potatoes, and oats, are often sprayed with glyphosate as a preharvest desiccant. For example, Cheerios are labeled as non-GMO, but in 2015, it was revealed that their oats supplier, Richardson Milling, used glyphosate as a desiccant, virtually guaranteeing contamination of this product with glyphosate.[178] Thus non-GMO project certification labels can't be the only guide to avoiding this toxic chemical.

Glyphosate has a wide range of modes of toxicity, for which I have indexed over two dozen on the GreenMedInfo.com glyphosate database alone.[179] But its carcinogenicity as an estrogen-mimicking endocrine disruptor is one vector of toxicity that is still widely overlooked. Two-thirds of all breast cancers are found to be estrogen-dependent or estrogen receptor positive. When certain estrogens or estrogen-like chemicals attach to a cancer cell's receptor, they can stimulate proliferation, which, in extreme cases, can lead to the type of unregulated growth found in cancer.[180] The article "Glyphosate Induces Human Breast Cancer Cells Growth via Estrogen Receptors" in *Food and Chemical Toxicology* revealed that glyphosate drives the growth of hormone-dependent breast cancer cells.[181] And it doesn't take a whopping dose for glyphosate to induce cancer cell proliferation. These effects occur in the parts per *trillion*, which is an infinitesimal amount.

A larger dose of the same chemical can cause the cell to die via programmed cell death as a defense mechanism to protect the body as a multicellular whole, whereas a lower dose can keep it alive but transform the cell's phenotype toward a more cancerous set of traits. This finding invalidates the age-old toxicological risk model "the dose makes the poison" for toxicants like glyphosate, where sometimes *the lower the concentration, the more likely* it is to induce hormone-disruptive and carcinogenic effects.

How to Limit Exposure to Glyphosate

Glyphosate is so pervasive that none of us can completely escape its reach. It's in the air. It's in the rain.[182] It's in the groundwater.[183] It's in our hair. Unless we radically transform our agricultural practices, we're all subject to its subtle yet powerful effects. That doesn't mean that we're helpless, though. We can significantly reduce our exposure to this toxicant by choosing the following:

- Eating food that is organically grown

- Avoiding GMO foods

- Becoming more educated about foods that are at risk for contamination (one place to start is The Detox Project at detoxproject.org, an organization that tests for and certifies glyphosate-free products)

BE AN INFORMED CONSUMER

In addition to becoming more aware of the toxicants entering our bodies surreptitiously, consider the personal care chemical products that we apply consciously. Clever marketing and poor regulatory oversight have obscured grave dangers associated with the use of the vast majority of deodorants, cosmetics, shampoos, and skin creams that contain known carcinogens and endocrine disruptors such as heavy metals and/or petrochemicals. When we slather these products onto our skin, they enter directly into our lymphatic and circulatory systems, depositing in internal organs and body fat. Unlike products you ingest orally, substances that are applied to your body topically bypass the exquisite filter that is your liver. This is why *you should never put on your body anything you cannot or would not eat.* (Hint: if you need a chemistry degree to identify an ingredient and/or it is not found in nature, avoid it.)

Mainstream antiperspirants are filled with toxicant compounds, the worst of which is aluminum, a heavy metal that acts as an estrogen mimic. One study shows that regular application to the underarm area may contribute to aluminum-associated disease processes, including breast cancer.[184] Another study revealed that aluminum found in breast tissue of cancerous breasts is more prevalent in the outer breast, which matches the most common location of breast cancer, the upper outer quadrant, where underarm antiperspirants are routinely used.

The problems get worse if you use an aerosol spray as an antiperspirant. Then you are breathing in the aluminum as well as coating your skin with it. In addition, antiperspirants inhibit sweat, which is the body's primary means of eliminating toxicity. Both the carcinogenic effects of aluminum and the secondary inhibition of sweat detoxification escalate the harmful impact.

Commercial lotions, even those from commonly trusted brands, are usually full of petrochemicals (crude oil derivatives). One such crude oil derivative, mineral oil, has so fully infiltrated our tissues that a 1985 study of 465 autopsies found that nearly half the subjects' livers and spleens exhibited signs of lipogranuloma, which is the body's way of establishing a barrier against the deposit of oily substances.[185]

Commercial detergents and cleaners are typically rife with toxic ingredients. One European study found that household cleaning products have a high level of impact on the overall respiratory function of women who used them. Researchers summarized that the extent of measured damage for women who performed cleaning tasks was equivalent to smoking a pack of cigarettes every day for 20 years.[186]

Even the part of your skin that touches your clothing may be absorbing residue from the detergent you use. The risk increases with clothing you exercise in, as sweat and open pores make you even more susceptible to pulling in chemicals.

As an alternative, consider products that are made from exclusively natural ingredients. For example, extra-virgin coconut oil has been found to be equally effective at moisturizing dry skin and hair as mainstream oils and creams.[187] Use the following resources for more information on the problem and suitable alternatives:

1. Environmental Working Group's Skin Deep
    (ewg.org/skindeep)

2. IReadLabelsForYou.com

3. WellnessMama.com

CHAPTER FIVE

LIFESTYLE MEDICINE FOR BRAIN HEALTH

Toxicants to Avoid and Practices to Keep Your Mind Vibrant for Life

In the comedy *As You Like It*, Shakespeare depicts the aging process as a circular path. We start as babies, grow through various points of adulthood, and then finally reach old age. It's all good until the very last stage when, as Shakespeare tells us, we end up in a second babyhood—toothless, disoriented, and unable to care for ourselves. A descent into the oblivion of dementia is a fate we all dread. Alzheimer's disease, which currently afflicts 5.6 million people, and other neurodegenerative brain disorders are terrifying because, unlike other maladies, they seem to rob us of our personhood and sever us from our agency. Who are we without our memories and our ability to reason, care for ourselves, or interact with others?

Few, if any, conventional treatments have been proven to work for neurodegenerative disorders. Billions of dollars have been expended in 1,246 human clinical trials, and we still do not have a single FDA-approved drug that offers anything more than mild and temporary symptom reduction.

Increasingly, Alzheimer's disease diagnoses are being made for not just the very old but also those under the age of 65. There are now almost a quarter of a million cases of early-onset Alzheimer's diagnosed in the U.S.[1] And it carries with it a dismal prognosis: an incurable, progressively degenerative brain disease with a 100 percent fatality rate. The New Biology, however, offers us a different and far more promising vision of what is possible. Because the brain tissue *can* regenerate and heal itself, no one is without hope.

THE OLD PARADIGM OF NEURODEGENERATION

According to the old paradigm, Alzheimer's-associated neurodegeneration is caused by the accumulation in the brain of beta-amyloid plaque, a "sticky" protein that is toxic to nerve cells. It is believed to interfere with cognition and memory by inhibiting the proper functioning of the neurotransmitter acetylcholine. A class of chemical drugs known as acetylcholinesterase inhibitors are used to treat the symptoms of the disease. These drugs, such as Aricept, have received FDA approval as palliative treatment, even though they have not been demonstrated to slow the progression of the disease. As with so many pharmaceutical approaches to symptom suppression or management, the root cause of the pathological process is neither identified nor corrected.

But the New Biology may end up revolutionizing the way we understand and treat the disease. In only the past few years, it has been discovered that the brain has both a lymphatic system and a microbiome, which means that the immune system, the brain, and the gut are directly connected. These discoveries require the reexamination of thousands of once authoritative textbooks that long held the brain was an immunologically privileged and sterile organ.

Add to these paradigm-shifting discoveries the accumulating evidence that nerve cells *are* capable of regeneration and regrowth, and you will begin to appreciate just how questionable these long-held assumptions may have been and how urgent it is for us to update them. Perhaps one of the most exciting examples of this is the new research that indicates that beta-amyloid plaque, once presumed to be the villain in the fight against neurodegeneration, may protect the brain from toxic exposures and/or pathogens that operate at the root-cause level of the disease.

THE NEW PARADIGM OF NEURODEGENERATION

We know that in addition to the structural and functional degradation of brain cells, Alzheimer's and other age-related neurodegenerative diseases appear to be marked by the calcification of the brain. With this knowledge, the pineal gland emerges as one of the primary keys to the Alzheimer's mystery.

The pineal gland is found deep inside the human brain, with evidence of its calcification now found in two-thirds of the adult population.[2] While they are related to neurological injury and innate repair processes, the exact causes of these calcifications are mostly unknown. One of the gland's primary functions is to secrete melatonin, a powerful regulatory hormone best known for its role in sleep that also functions as an antioxidant and affects every cell in the human body. A recent study found that the degree of pineal gland calcification (and pineal cyst volume) in study participants correlated inversely with sleep rhythm disturbances. Also, the less calcified their pineal glands, the more melatonin was found in the participants' saliva.[3]

Alzheimer's disease patients are often deficient in melatonin levels, which is likely related to the higher levels of oxidative stress commonly associated with the condition.[4] We don't know which comes first, the low melatonin or the pineal gland damage and calcification, but it has been established that Alzheimer's patients have been found to have a higher degree of pineal gland calcification than patients with other types of dementia.[5]

A 2009 study published in *Medical Hypotheses* succinctly sums up the theory of the pineal gland dysfunction–Alzheimer's disease connection: Calcification of the gland leads to loss of function, which causes melatonin levels to drop. This likely contributes to the formation of deposits of beta-amyloid, the hallmark of Alzheimer's, within neuronal tissue.[6]

While the pineal gland/Alzheimer's link was being researched, another theory was gaining ground. In 2005, studies revealed a correlation between insulin levels and brain cell deterioration so convincing and provocative that health practitioners began to wonder whether Alzheimer's disease might simply be type 3 diabetes.[7] We already know that diabetics are at least twice as likely to experience dementia.[8] It turns out that the cells of your brain can become insulin-resistant just like other cells in the body. And since the brain is a massive energy sink, capable of only a few minutes of glucose deprivation before it becomes alarmed, it is especially sensitive to the problems associated with insulin resistance.

Several studies have shown that brain cells shrink and become tangled from high blood sugar levels over time.[9] This means that your carbohydrate intake (especially sugar and high glycemic processed grain products) could be dramatically affecting your long-term brain health, increasing your likelihood of developing those beta-amyloid lesions in the brain. Simply switching from insulin-dependent, glucose-driven metabolism to a more fat-based diet could dramatically improve neurological health and, subsequently, cognition and memory. My friend and colleague Dr. David Perlmutter dove deep into this topic in his best-selling book *Grain Brain*.

Beta-amyloid plaque, which has been vilified as the brain's enemy, may be an innocent bystander or even the hero of the story, forming as part of the body's self-healing mechanism. According to groundbreaking research published in 2009 in response to almost a quarter of a century of failed treatments based on viewing plaque as the cause of the disease, researchers at the

Department of Pathology, University of Maryland, Baltimore, led by R. J. Castellani, proposed a different explanation. Referencing the problem of a poor correlation between the presence of plaque and the level of dementia (plaque is often found within the cognitively intact), they proposed that the beta-amyloid protein precursor and beta-amyloid may in fact have a protective role against heavy metals and toxicants, as well as certain bacteria and fungi. In fact, they point out that amyloid protein fragments have antioxidant properties. The researchers suggested that until the focus of Alzheimer's research shifts to the upstream processes that lead to lesions, progress will be hampered.[10]

The New Biology asks us to shift from a perspective that the body is inherently faulty and turn our attention instead to how its innate intelligent and resilient responses can be properly understood and appreciated. Our industrialized society has spawned an ever-expanding array of toxic exposures, many of which accost our nervous systems daily. It would make sense to look to these factors first and learn how to avoid and mitigate them instead of blaming the victim (our bodies) as is commonly done.

BRAIN CELL DEGENERATORS

There are plenty of neuroprotective agents out there, as you'll see in this chapter and in Part III (The Program). But first, let's perform the vital task of identifying the neurotoxic agents that compromise our brain health.

STATINS

Let's start with statins, an excessively prescribed class of drugs used to suppress cholesterol production in patients believed to be at risk of cardiovascular disease. You may know them by brand names like Lipitor and Crestor.

Statins have been shown to be myotoxic, which means that they damage muscle tissues, causing pain, weakness, and, in some cases, muscle tissue death. Statins have also been shown to interfere with the proper functioning of nerve tissues throughout the body, but most alarmingly in the central nervous system. This is no surprise when you consider that one-quarter of the cholesterol found in the human body is in the brain. And about one-third of that cholesterol is used as a component in myelin, the insulating sheath that surrounds the nerve tissues in the brain and speeds conduction of electrical impulses. Interference with myelin plays a starring role in neurodegenerative diseases like Alzheimer's, Parkinson's, and multiple sclerosis. These two primary side effects—muscle and nerve tissue toxicity and damage—taken together are a huge red flag for heart health, given that the heart is the most nerve-dense muscle in the body. Indeed, a 2009 study published in the *Journal of Clinical Cardiology* shows that statin drugs actually weaken the heart muscle.[11] Additional research shows that statin drugs increase the prevalence and extent of coronary artery plaques possessing calcium[12] and increase microalbuminuria, considered a predictor of cardiovascular events.[13]

An accumulating body of biomedical literature on the adverse effects of statin drugs now links them to over 300 different signals of harm,[14] not the least of which is that their use is linked with higher risk of cancer, especially breast, thyroid, and prostate.[15] But most important to point out for the purposes of this chapter is their well-known neurotoxicity, which is why the FDA now warns memory loss has been reported with their use based on postmarketing surveillance of the drug's many side effects.[16]

None of this should be surprising when you consider that the "bad" low-density lipoprotein (LDL) delivers fat-soluble nutrients, antioxidants, and energy production co-factors like coenzyme Q10 throughout the body, particularly the brain. Without adequate LDL in our bodies, we would die.

Rather than quantity, the quality of your LDL is the key factor in determining if it is "good" or "bad," and LDL quality depends almost entirely on your diet, lifestyle, and chemical exposures.

Reducing LDL cholesterol unnaturally with pharmaceuticals can therefore directly interfere with nourishing and protecting the brain. This may be why low cholesterol has been associated with neuropsychiatric conditions such as morbid depression, suicide, homicide, accidental deaths, and Alzheimer's disease.

The efficacy of statins has been framed in a grossly overstated manner by drug companies looking to maximize sales. Take the ASCOT-LLA trial on atorvastatin (trade name Lipitor). The trial found that in the placebo group, 3 percent suffered a heart attack versus 1.9 percent in the atorvastatin group. Yet in a semantic sleight-of-hand, Pfizer marketed the drug to the public with its 36 percent *relative risk* reduction rather than its *absolute risk* reduction of 1.1 percent. In other words, only an insignificant number of people appeared to benefit, even though we can assume everyone in the trial was adversely affected by statin side effects in some way.

Given the many adverse effects of this drug class, is the one percent reduction of absolute risk of cardiovascular disease worth the heightened risk of cancer and Alzheimer's disease?

An Apple a Day
Keeps Statins Away

As reported in the *British Medical Journal*, researchers at Oxford found that the vascular benefits of eating one apple a day were equivalent to the benefits of taking modern statin drugs,[17] making apples a simple and inexpensive alternative treatment.

PROTON PUMP INHIBITORS

Proton Pump Inhibitors (PPIs), one of the highest-selling classes of drugs in the U.S., may be particularly bad for brain health. PPIs such as Nexium, Prilosec, or Prevacid reduce the amount of gastric acid secreted in the stomach wall by chemically blocking fundamental cellular processes in the parietal cells (acid-producing stomach cells) and are marketed to the public as a palliative remedy for indigestion, heartburn, and acid reflux. Available with or without a prescription, acid blockers are a $10 billion business in the U.S. Their use is so ubiquitous that they were prescribed at nearly 270 million hospital trips made by adults via ambulance from 2006 to 2010,[18] and millions more prescriptions were filled for regular outpatient visits. Our Western-style diet of sugar-laden and highly acid-forming processed foods and accompanying stress-filled lifestyle ensure that PPIs are among the most highly prescribed drugs in Western medicine.

PPIs are fundamentally xenobiotic chemicals, so taking them could adversely impact *any* cell in your body, not just those in your stomach. A growing body of research shows that PPIs increase the risk of kidney disease, heart disease, and digestive disorders, including inflammatory bowel disease and liver disease. They have also been shown to compromise immunity and have been linked to diminished brain function. PPIs increase the brain burden of amyloid-beta, an amino acid that is the main component of beta-amyloid plaque and are known to contribute to vitamin B_{12} deficiency, another important factor in Alzheimer's disease.[19]

A large study conducted in 2016 analyzed more than 73,000 dementia-free participants, aged 75 years or older. The patients receiving regular PPI medication had a significantly increased risk of incident dementia compared with the patients not receiving PPI medication. Researchers made the forthright conclusion that "the avoidance of PPI medication may prevent the development of dementia."[20]

The good news for sufferers of gastric distress who want to avoid PPIs is that clinical research shows that something as simple as drinking water reduces stomach acid more effectively than these drugs and does so safely, without negative side effects.[21]

CALCIUM SUPPLEMENTS

Calcium supplements are used by many people, especially women, because they believe it will strengthen aging bones. However, osteoporosis is not caused by a deficiency of limestone, oyster shell, or bone meal, substances from which most of the mass-market calcium supplements are produced. The reality is that most people do not need extra calcium from sources other than food and that the risks of most inorganic calcium supplementation far outweigh the benefits. The ingestion of excess calcium does not always address the main concern, and it can contribute to a host of other problems, most notably heart disease and accelerated Alzheimer's disease–linked neurodegeneration.[22]

A provocative study published in the *British Journal of Nutrition* found that calcium supplementation may be associated with brain lesions (known on MRI scans as hyperintensities) in older adults.[23] These brain lesions, visible as brighter spots in MRI scans, are known to be caused by lack of blood flow (ischemia) and subsequent neurological damage.

PAINKILLERS

Over-the-counter painkillers may seem like convenient and harmless ways to take the edge off aches, pains, and injuries, but they have been shown to profoundly affect heart health and emotional well-being and contribute to the etiology of neurodegenerative disease.

A 2013 review of 754 clinical trials published in the prestigious British medical journal *Lancet* found that nonsteroidal anti-inflammatory drugs (NSAIDs) were associated with roughly double the risk of heart failure.[24] In particular, ibuprofen (e.g.,

Advil and Motrin) has been estimated to cause thousands of heart disease–related deaths each year. Another highly concerning discovery made in 2015 was that acetaminophen (Tylenol) dulls the emotional responses of its users, particularly empathy, at the same time as it dulls pain.[25]

Furthermore, acetaminophen poses risks to developing brains. Studies in rodent models demonstrated that acetaminophen used during a sensitive period of brain development caused long-term alterations in the brain that manifested as problems with social function. At least eight published studies have evaluated the long-term effects on children of acetaminophen use during pregnancy or during childhood.[26] Two studies were published in *JAMA Pediatrics*, one of the most highly respected pediatric journals, and all the studies pointed toward acetaminophen use being associated with long-term problems with neurological function on developing brains, including autism spectrum disorder.[27]

FLUORIDE

Since the 1940s, much of the municipal water in the United States has had fluoride added to it in an effort to eradicate tooth decay. Tooth decay rates have indeed declined since then, but this decline has happened in communities both with and without fluoridated water, which means the improvement in dental health may have been misattributed to water fluoridation. It has also come at a high cost to our brain health.[28] While it is considered normal in the U.S. to medicate our entire population through its drinking water, consider that Great Britain, Ireland, Spain, and Serbia are the only member nations of the European Union that fluoridate their water. That is only 12 million people of a population of three-quarters of a billion, or 3 percent.[29]

Fluoride is a potent neurotoxin without any known natural biological role in the human body, and it has been linked to a wide range of adverse effects. Of particular concern to neuroscientists is its well-established association with lower IQs in children[30] and suspected contribution to the calcification of the pineal gland.[31] While pineal gland calcification is linked to neurodegenerative disorders, it's also thought to be a culprit in circadian dysregulation, hormone imbalances, low back pain, insomnia, bipolar disease, and increased risk for hypothyroidism.

Fluoride-Free Options for Water

Distilled water is low in dissolved solids (one part per million or less), which means it is least likely to have fluoride and other contaminants compared to tap water, which on average has between 140 and 400 ppm of what can amount to hundreds of contaminants and naturally occurring but potentially toxic, minerals. For whole-house application, a reverse osmosis system is ideal, as it will remove the majority of these contaminants, sometimes including fluoride. Another choice is to buy bottled spring water, such as Mountain Valley, which comes in glass containers, though it will contain naturally occurring fluoride. The saving grace is that it is far less toxic than the fluorosilicic acid used in municipal fluoride treatments, which contains radionuclides, or highly toxic radioactive elements, as well as heavy metals such as lead. If you do distill your water, add back a natural source of minerals such as a pinch of Himalayan sea salt or trace mineral concentrate from the Great Salt Lake of Utah.

Be aware that your water supply may not be your only source of fluoride exposure. Fluoride is present in antibiotics such as Cipro, in Teflon-coated dental floss, and in nonstick cooking pans. It's in your swimming pool and your hot tub (unless you install a whole house reverse osmosis system, which I highly recommend). It may be in your infant formula and conventional produce like lettuce and commercially baked goods. It's used in textiles like Gore-Tex, and, of course, it's proudly advertised as an ingredient in toothpaste.

One of the best ways to counteract overfluoridation may be to make sure your diet has sufficient iodine, for which one of the best dietary sources is seaweed. Seaweed is a nutritional powerhouse loaded with minerals and is an ideal addition to the diet of anyone concerned about fluoride consumption. It also provides iodine in a form that enables your body to take what it needs versus accosting it with excessive doses of the isolated form.

WHEAT

We've already discussed the evolutionary incompatibility of wheat with the human diet given the intestinal damage and disruptive immune system changes that 23,000-plus different proteins colloquially known as "gluten" can cause. But gluten also has deleterious effects on the brain in at least three ways: (1) by acting as an excitotoxin due to its high aspartic and glutamic acid levels, (2) by acting as an opioid due to the presence of gluten exorphins and gliadorphin, and (3) by disrupting the gut-brain connection, a bidirectional superhighway that is a conduit for mutual information exchange conducted by the microbiomes. Gluten grain consumption has been implicated in a wide range of brain-related neuropsychiatric conditions, including cerebellar ataxia (a disorder relating to involuntary movements), epilepsy, autism spectrum disorder, psychosis, multiple sclerosis, headaches, and schizophrenia.[32]

COW'S MILK

Got health problems? In addition to cow's milk intolerance, of which I have firsthand experience, the biomedical literature has identified cow's milk consumption as a contributing factor to a wide range of disorders ranging from acne and autism to diabetes and multiple sclerosis.[33]

A study in 2000 found that one key mechanism behind the pathogenesis of multiple sclerosis is the production of antibodies to a protein in cow's milk known as butyrophilin.[34] This protein can cross-react with myelin oligodendrocyte glycoprotein, a major component of the central nervous system. A 2004 study found that people with MS exhibited statistically significant elevations in IgA antibodies to the milk protein casein versus controls.[35] Cross-reactivity linked to cow's milk protein has also been identified in people with autism.[36] Another study found that a milk-free diet downregulates folate receptor autoimmunity in cerebral folate deficiency syndrome, a condition that involves decreased folate transport to the central nervous system.[37]

Given the evidence of the potential for cow's milk to incite neurological autoimmunity and damage, anyone concerned about brain or immune conditions should consider eliminating this food as a precautionary step. Calcium deficiency concerns can be addressed by such dietary means as eating green, leafy foods, like kale, which have more calcium per milligram serving than milk. Also, consider the obvious but often overlooked fact that cow's milk is intended for calves to consume, not humans. Because it contains a wide range of informational molecules specific to that species (such as bovine microRNAs), it isn't just a problem of incompatible proteins and lipids. It is an example of evolutionary mismatch where we are consuming something that is not designed for us, and we experience adverse effects as a consequence.

MONOSODIUM GLUTAMATE FLAVORINGS

Monosodium glutamate (MSG), despite its near ubiquitous use and acceptance in mainstream products, is far closer to a toxic chemical and drug than a benign food additive. It contributes to illness in two ways: First, it makes food that is bad for us taste good by tricking our taste buds and intuition into consuming unhealthy products beyond satiation. Second, it *directly damages* neurological tissue via its neuronal excitotoxicity. It also induces the body-wide generalized endocrine disruption known as metabolic syndrome, the symptoms of which include hypertension, insulin resistance, elevated blood lipids, visceral adiposity (belly fat), and/or elevated blood sugar.[38] (Metabolic syndrome is often a harbinger of diabetes, and diabetes has a lot in common with Alzheimer's disease.)

ARTIFICIAL SWEETENERS

Despite its well-established neurotoxicity and carcinogenicity,[39] aspartame is a sweetener that has been used in the U.S. since 1981 and has been approved in over 90 countries. More than 40 adverse health effects of aspartame have been documented in hundreds of studies,[40] one of which found that chronic (90-day) administration of aspartame to rats at ranges close to what the FDA considers safe for human consumption resulted in neurological changes consistent with brain damage.[41]

While it's wise to cut back on consumption of refined sugar, it doesn't make sense to replace refined sugar with a toxic chemical. Splenda, also known as sucralose, isn't necessarily any better than aspartame. When heated, sucralose degrades and releases both dioxins and dioxin-like compounds,[42] persistent organic pollutants that are so toxic that the International Agency for Research on Cancer (IARC) classified them as a Group 1 carcinogen in 1997. It's also linked to other systemic consequences, from GI issues to hormone disruption and, ironically, weight gain and obesity.[43]

LOW-FAT DIETS

People often adopt low-fat diets in pursuit of good health. But your body needs fat to thrive. By weight, 60 percent of your brain is made from fat.[44] By definition, we must obtain *essential* fatty acids from food since our bodies can't produce them on their own. Thus, a low-fat diet can basically starve the body of the essential substrate that it must obtain from food in order to maintain optimal health, which also explains why there are hundreds of studies that indicate essential fatty acids, such as omega-3s, prevent and mitigate over 300 different conditions.[45]

PESTICIDES

While most people would not intentionally consume chemicals designed to kill living things, we still often eat foods sprayed with highly toxic chemicals intended to do so. Pesticides are almost universally carcinogenic, and most are also neurotoxic,[46] making conventional food a kind of self-abuse in which we unknowingly participate. Organic, pesticide-free food is essential for promoting the conditions of true health, and one can understand why by examining just how profoundly different the conventional blueberry is from its organic or wild-harvested version. Although the berries may look identical on the surface, a 2008 report from the U.S. Department of Agriculture discovered that over 50 pesticide residues were present in conventional blueberries alone.

Economics plays an important part of this picture, as organically grown food can be cost-prohibitive and is not universally available. But in the relative scheme of things, the premium paid for nontoxic food is orders of magnitude lower than the price we pay to treat the diseases caused by eating conventionally.

AIRPLANES

Air travel exposes us to all manner of health assaults, including radiation, oxygen deprivation, bad food, and prolonged close contact with strangers who may be sick. But the most toxic exposure on board is in the air that we breathe. Aircraft manufacturers decided decades ago to pull air for the cockpit and cabin of planes from the jet engine exhaust as "bleed air." This air travels to a compressor for cooling but is not filtered properly and brings with it a toxic mix of engine oil, lubricants, and various hydrocarbons. What has us feeling woozy after a long flight may not be jet lag but instead chemical poisoning.

Perhaps of greatest concern is the engine turbine lubricant tricresyl phosphate (TCP). TCP is an organophosphate with known neurotoxic effects in the same category as the weapon of chemical warfare sarin gas. TCP and other noxious agents can be toxic at small doses and often cannot be detected through smell. High TCP exposure can cause neuropathy, paralysis, and damage to myelin sheaths, similar to what happens in multiple sclerosis. This constellation of symptoms has been termed "aerotoxic syndrome,"[47] and it is gaining increasing recognition within the medical community. We may receive a high dose of exposure if our flight happens to have a "fume event," in which high levels of engine contaminants leak into the cabin air, but even low-level exposure can be damaging in the long run from frequent flying.

Limiting Exposure to
Airborne Cabin Contaminants

What can a frequent flyer do to try to stay healthy? Your best bet is to wear a mask while flying, though I have yet to identify one that has been validated by a third-party organization to filter out the petrochemicals of concern. I encourage you to do your own research and share what you learn, as ultimately it will be bottom-up consumer pressure that will drive industry reform.

When I fly, I always turn the vent above my seat off, and I stay well hydrated with water. Whenever possible, book your travel on a Boeing 787. Boeing's Dreamliner uses "bleedless" technology and incorporates fresh air drawn through inlets at the wing roots. However, 787s represent less than 2 percent of commercial aircraft in operation, and they are mostly used for intercontinental flights. Until this technology is widely implemented, as famously stated by Alisa Brodkowitz, a prominent lawyer representing claims by sick pilots against the airline industry, "the only thing filtering this toxic soup out of the cabin are the lungs of the passengers and crew."[48]

CELL PHONES

Even though it is common knowledge that cell phone radiation is powerful enough to disrupt sensitive equipment within an airplane or hospital, there is still resistance to acknowledging it may adversely affect the human brain, a highly electrochemically and electromagnetically active organ that is sensitive to electrical impulses.

A recent study of 3G phones reveals that they disrupt brain wave activity when pressed against the ear for as short a time as 15 minutes. Significant radiation effects were found for the alpha, slow beta, fast beta, and gamma bands,[49] meaning 3G mobile phone exposure resulted in electrophysiological changes in nearly the entire brain's structure and function. Scientists believe that 4G phones are even more problematic, as they are more powerful. And we can only imagine what 5G phones will do once this technology is implemented.

How to Control Cell Phone Damage to Your Brain

Distancing your cell phone from your brain (and while we're at it, your reproductive organs) can help to reduce cell phone damage to your body. You can also use headphones, avoid pressing the device to your skull, and opt for downloading content like audio books or music so that you can keep your phone in airplane mode. Avoid bringing your cell phone into the bedroom, and sleep far away from any source of radiation—cell phones, tablets, and Internet-connected TVs. Using the built-in Night Shift function on iPhones, Night Mode on Androids, or other similar functions will minimize blue wavelengths during phone use in the evening. These actions will go a long way toward preventing, or at least mitigating, nervous system overstimulation and circadian rhythm dysregulation and dysfunction.

BRAIN CELL REGENERATORS

The good news is that the food we choose to eat every day—packed with flavor, variety, and color—can help our brains to function optimally. Some foods are uniquely poised to nourish our brains and to facilitate brain cell regeneration. Here are just a few examples of these must-have staples.

HERBS AND SPICES

Seasoning food with fresh herbs and spices loaded with natural medicinal properties enhances flavor and carries extraordinary health benefits—not just for the central nervous system but also for decelerating the aging process, reducing inflammation, protecting against aches and pains, and improving digestion. If you want to harness these health effects, use 1 teaspoon dried or 2–3 tablespoons fresh herbs and spices daily in your salads, soups, sides, and/or main dishes.

Unless the herbs and spices are labeled as certified organic/nonirradiated or wild-crafted, they have likely undergone gamma irradiation, or "cold pasteurization." This process uses hundreds of times more than the human lethal dose of nuclear reactor–culled radiation to ionize spices and herbs, which destroys nutrients and beneficial biomolecules and eradicates their innate beneficial energetic and informational properties. With this in mind, below are the essential regeneration-promoting spices to include in your diet.

TURMERIC

This rhizome plant plays an essential role in cancer protection and staving off Alzheimer's disease. Curcumin, turmeric's most powerful biomolecule, imparts the signature golden color. A robust body of literature documents the therapeutic potential of curcumin for Alzheimer's patients.

Two studies reveal curcumin's capability to enhance the clearance of the pathological beta-amyloid plaque in Alzheimer's disease patients.[50] When combined with vitamin D_3, the neurorestorative process is further enhanced.[51] Additional preclinical research indicates curcumin and its analogs elicit inhibitory and protective effects against Alzheimer's disease as measured by a reduction in the formation of beta-amyloid proteins.[52]

GINGER

Research shows that ginger boasts more than 80 distinct pharmacological actions.[53] It has cancer-preventative properties, mitigates the toxicity of chemical exposures, and alleviates nausea, migraines, and menstrual pain. It also stimulates digestion, eases gastric distress, and lowers inflammation. Neurodegenerative diseases may also be aided by ginger's ability to inhibit production of nitrous oxide and pro-inflammatory cytokines.

A study published in the *Indian Journal of Experimental Biology* suggests that ginger may be an excellent natural anti–Alzheimer's disease treatment. Researchers at the Department of Neurochemistry at the National Institute of Mental Health and Neurosciences in Bangalore report that ginger "influences multiple therapeutic molecular targets of Alzheimer's disease and can be considered as an effective nontoxic nutraceutical supplement for Alzheimer's disease."[54] The study follows from an already established body of research[55] demonstrating ginger's antioxidant and anti-inflammatory properties, both of which have value in addressing the underlying causes of neurodegeneration associated with Alzheimer's disease. Exosomes from ginger have the ability to positively modulate inflammatory processes.[56] Because exosomes can cross the blood-brain barrier, ginger may have therapeutic effects on the brain through downregulation of inflammatory pathways.

You can add ginger to tea, soups, stir fries, salad dressings, and smoothies for better brain and immune system health.

ROSEMARY

This small perennial shrub in the mint family has been revered since ancient times for its brain-boosting powers. Greek scholars wore rosemary in their hair to aid in memory and mental performance. An accumulating body of research has shown the herb can enhance cognition, memory, and sensory awareness.[57] A revealing study published in the *Journal of Medicinal Food* confirmed the traditional lore about rosemary's powers. The elderly people enrolled in the study who took small doses of dried rosemary leaf powder were found to have significantly improved memory speed relative to the placebo group. Another group of participants who took high doses of the herb showed impaired cognition, revealing that culinary doses may be far more therapeutic than heroic ones.[58] Rosemary leaves, fresh or dried, enhance the flavor of sauces and cooked meats and vegetables.

COFFEE

The debate on whether coffee is good for you continues to rage on, but there are a large number of studies that show coffee has potential health benefits for the brain. An article in *Clinical Nutrition* showed that drinking between one and two cups of coffee (versus less than one cup a day) was inversely linked to the incidence of cognitive disorders such as Alzheimer's disease, dementia, cognitive decline, and cognitive impairment.[59] In Japan, a study of over 23,000 adults over age 65 showed a 20–30 percent reduction in advanced dementia in those who consumed two to four cups of coffee daily. Even decaffeinated coffee can improve cognitive function.[60] Another study showed that coffee consumption is associated with a longer life.[61] Ultimately, moderation and timing are key, as noted by the Hungarian proverb "coffee before noon is medicine; after noon is poison."

GREEN TEA

Tea, especially green tea, is even more beneficial than coffee because it reduces oxidative stress, feeds the microbiome, and slows the aging process. Daily consumption of green tea catechins (the polyphenols in tea) delays memory regression and brain dysfunction in aged mice.[62] An excellent example of one of the many studies on green tea comes out of Japan, where a group of scientists confirmed that higher consumption of green tea is associated with better results in cognitive testing in elderly subjects.[63] Tea provides flavonoids, caffeine, and L-theanine, an amino acid that features a range of health benefits, including stress reduction and cognitive improvement.

One of the more compelling experiments relevant to brain health showed that very low doses of epigallocatechin-3-gallate, the primary polyphenol found in green tea, increase the activity of brain-derived neurotrophic factor, or BDNF, which is an important player in the growth of nerve cells. These doses are equivalent to single servings of green tea.[64] The potential for green tea–induced neurogenesis is an intriguing possibility, and because green tea has proven to be safe for millennia, there's no reason to wait for further research to enjoy its regenerative benefits.

Many teas are good for you, but perhaps the best tea for your brain is a specific form of green tea called matcha, as it has the highest quantity and absorption of L-theanine and has been demonstrated to reduce stress in both experimental and clinical trials.[65] It can also be used in cooking or added to smoothies, making it a versatile ingredient and not just consumable as a beverage.

LION'S MANE MUSHROOM

Hericium erinaceus is a shaggy mushroom common around the world and particularly beloved in Asia, where it has been eaten traditionally for centuries to boost memory, creativity, and attention. Buddhist monks have consumed lion's mane tea for centuries before meditation in order to enhance their powers of concentration. Paul Stamets, who is my go-to mycologist, believes it is a powerful regenerative agent, as it is capable of encouraging neuroplasticity and the release of endogenously produced nerve growth factor, a neuropeptide that plays a role in the regeneration, differentiation, and survival of neurons.

Lion's mane possesses two potent nerve growth factors, so it is the best mushroom to add to your diet to support your nervous system. You can find it in supplement form as a powder or tincture in many health food stores. I prefer Paul Stamets' brand Fungi Perfecti for personal use, not just because I want to support his work but because he certifies the mushrooms have genetic integrity from their wild-harvested state. If you'd rather enjoy the mushroom's meaty texture in a meal, sauté it in clarified butter (also known as ghee) to intensify the flavor or use it to replace meat in soups and stews.

WALNUT

Consider the exquisite design of the walnut. Its skull-like shell encompasses its bi-hemispheric "brain," which is chock-full of the omega-3 fatty acids that are essential to the human brain. Its design points to its symmetry with the anatomical brain, beautiful and reassuring in its implicit promise to nourish and heal the body. The Greek physicians Galen (A.D. 129–216) and Dioscorides (A.D. 40–90) noted in their "doctrine of signatures" that herbs that resemble organs in appearance are particularly beneficial.

This doctrine has been rejected as a form of magical thinking, but the New Biology explains a possible scientific mechanism by which these two seemingly unrelated entities—the walnut and the human brain—mirror one another so literally and poetically. Because plants and animals have co-evolved intimately over countless millennia and have become dependent on one another for various functions, the visual homologies may speak to the existence of an informational bridge through which genetic/ epigenetic information has flowed. Thanks to the New Biology, we now know that exosomes allow plants and animals to share RNA-coded genetic information of significant impact with one another. As the entire biosphere participates in this exosome-based information-sharing network, it is plausible the resemblance of walnuts to the mammalian brain reflects their intimate genetic connection and interdependency.

Not surprisingly, abundant research has established that walnuts boost cognition, including inferential verbal reasoning abilities,[66] especially supporting the brain health of the elderly when consumed daily. Researchers from Harvard University and Brigham and Women's Hospital estimated that women who are 70 years or older saw a reduction in cognitive decline equivalent to two years.[67] Clearly, greater intake of high-antioxidant foods such as walnuts may increase health span and enhance cognitive and motor function in aging.

GINKGO BILOBA

Ginkgo biloba is a plant that can live for 1,000 years or longer, and its traditional medicinal uses reflect how it has helped humans optimize their own longevity in the face of many adversities, including predators, infections, radiation, and fluctuations in nutrient availability and climate. Consuming ginkgo biloba allows us to absorb some of its age-defying phytochemical power, with multiple studies now underscoring its power to improve memory and cognition.[68]

Ginkgo biloba protects neurons from oxidation through its function as a free-radical scavenger, improves microcirculation in the brain, and reduces platelet aggregation (which may prevent stroke).[69] It also stimulates brain-derived neurotrophic factor, which improves brain and cognitive function and encourages regeneration.[70] The best way to take it is through dietary supplement form, as directed on the label, such as in standardized products containing 24 percent of flavone glycosides and 6 percent terpenes (ginkgolides and bilobalides), and, when possible, certified to be free of a naturally occurring neurotoxin known as ginkgotoxin. This antivitamin is structurally related to vitamin B_6 and can cause neurological problems in vulnerable people deficient in B_6, or who consume high amounts. The leaves are generally considered harmless, but it never hurts to be careful, especially if you have a history of seizures.

CANNABIDIOL

Cannabidiol (CBD), the most extensively researched active ingredient in marijuana, also found in hemp, can help turn the tide against the accelerating Alzheimer's epidemic. There are over 100 studies on CBD demonstrating its neuroprotective properties. And even the compound found in marijuana known as delta-9-tetrahydrocannabinol (THC), to which the plant's characteristic "high" is attributed, has been found to provide therapeutic value in two ways: (1) by competitively inhibiting the enzyme acetylcholinesterase (AChE), similar to the drugs currently used to treat Alzheimer's symptoms, and 2) by preventing AChE-induced beta-amyloid peptide aggregation, which is considered the key pathological marker of Alzheimer's disease.[71] This is an ironic finding, considering that the prevailing stereotype is that using marijuana "fries" the brain, leading to debilitating memory issues.

COCONUT OIL

Coconut oil is a widely consumed traditional food and a leading preventative tool in cognitive health. Coconut oil positively affects the brain after just *one* 40-mL dose (about two and one-half tablespoons). Medium chain triglycerides (MCTs), the primary class of easily digestible fat found in coconut oil, help to boost brain metabolism with near-immediate improvements in cognitive functioning. Recent research has shown that patients experienced significant neurological healing after four to six weeks of using the oil.[72] The MCTs in coconut oil increase energy production in the brain by providing neurons with ketone bodies as an alternative to glucose. The oil also contains potent antioxidant polyphenols that may reduce oxidative stress, improving blood circulation in the brain and reducing neuroinflammation. Coconut oil can easily be incorporated in moderate amounts into your daily diet as an alternative to olive oil and butter in stir-fries, sautés, and braised dishes.

COCONUT WATER

Coconut water contains a range of essential biomolecules needed for health, including vitamins, minerals, antioxidants, amino acids, enzymes, growth factors, and other nutrients that have yet to be fully characterized. It also contains cytokines, classes of phytocompounds that modulate cell division and are believed to have anti-aging properties. One cytokinin known as trans-Zeatin has been investigated as a possible new treatment for Alzheimer's disease.[73]

Coconut water is one of nature's best forms of hydration due to its isotonic properties: it is able to pass through cell membranes easily and may thereby help to restore hydration to the brain, potentially translating to increased energy production in the tissues that sustain cognition. Drink it plain or diluted with water after a workout or add it to a fruit smoothie as a flavor enhancer.

Helpful Neuroregenerative Habits

SLEEPING WELL

A good night's sleep is crucial to good health. Sleep consolidates memories, balances hormones, regulates emotions, and flushes out metabolic waste products that make it harder for your brain to self-regulate. With restorative sleep, this functional waste disposal pathway enhances the convective exchange of cerebrospinal fluid with interstitial fluid, which in turn may increase removal of beta-amyloid plaques and other nerve cell–poisoning waste products that accumulate in the central nervous system.[74]

One mechanism that may help you get enough sleep is alignment with the sun's cycles and the body's regulation of melatonin. Cycles of light and darkness influence our metabolism and our hormones. Sleep disturbances have been identified as a primary driver of Alzheimer's disease pathogenesis, because wakefulness increases the brain protein beta-amyloid, while sleep reduces it.[75] Melatonin has been identified as a factor inhibiting the progression of beta-amyloid brain pathology as well as the formation of the protein itself.[76] Furthermore, infrared light therapy has been shown to have brain-regenerative effects for Parkinson's and Alzheimer's diseases in animal models, marking the beginning of a new way to address neurodegenerative prevention and care.[77]

The bottom line is this: get as much sleep as your body needs—at the very least six hours a night and perhaps as much as eight to nine, as I do. Sleep in a cool, dark room—I recommend blackout curtains—away from electronics and noise. Expose yourself to tolerable levels of sunlight as much as you can during the day, emphasizing early-morning outdoor light, which will regulate your circadian rhythm via effects on the suprachiasmatic nucleus of the brain. As little as 10 minutes a day will have significant health impacts. If you live in a climate where that is not possible, consider investing in a light therapy box.

AEROBIC EXERCISE

As we age, it can be tempting to take it easy on ourselves physically and let our fitness slide. But a growing body of research highlights the importance of staying as fit as possible, for as long as possible, to ensure a healthy body, and especially a healthy mind.[78]

Research indicates that improvements we make to our fitness throughout midlife can create long-term benefits for our brains. A 2016 study on the benefits of midlife exercise and how it relates to brain volume later in life determined that poor cardiovascular fitness and high diastolic blood pressure and heart rate during exercise were associated with a smaller total cerebral brain volume almost two decades later.[79] A 2017 study exploring the benefits of good cardiovascular health during young adulthood found that it affects midlife brain structure. Researchers concluded that "maintaining ideal levels of cardiovascular health in young adulthood is associated with greater whole brain volume in middle age."[80]

A recent editorial published in *Neurology* stated that "cardiovascular dysfunction and vascular aging are systemic conditions that affect all major target organs, including the brain. It follows that cardiovascular disease . . . and cardiovascular risk factors are associated with an elevated risk for developing dementia."[81] Vigorous exercise has been explored for its neuroprotective properties against Parkinson's disease and may significantly inhibit its progression.[82] Researchers recommend integration of physical fitness programs as adjunct therapy and advise structured, graduated fitness instruction for deconditioned patients with Parkinson's disease.

If you are looking for an aerobic fitness regimen beyond the conventional offerings of a gym, try dancing. A recent study published in *Frontiers in Human Neuroscience* demonstrated that while most forms of exercise slow down age-related decline, dancing has even more profound benefits. Considered a psychosocial intervention, dancing combines the mood-elevating effects of increased social interaction with improvements in brain function, cardiac fitness, and overall quality of life. Mastering new rhythms, steps, and formations, in combination with increased social engagement, provides a boost to brain activity that creates additional cognitive benefits.[83]

MEDITATION

In animal models, stress has been shown to contribute to calcifying the pineal gland.[84] Yoga and meditation are two of the best-studied modalities for stress relief and offer significant benefits with few risks. Yoga, which combines meditation, controlled breathing, and some movement, promotes a healthy mood. Meditation promotes healthy blood flow to the brain, which means oxygen and nutrients are reaching this precious tissue. A Harvard researcher found that meditation increases the gray matter of the hippocampus, the part of the brain associated with learning and memory, and decreases the gray matter in the amygdala, the part of the brain associated with stressful events.[85] And a study of people with subjective cognitive decline found that after six months of practicing Kirtan Kriya meditation, the volunteers reported improved memory and tested better on measures of cognitive performance.[86] Most researchers have found that even short 5- to 10-minute sessions of meditation confer benefits. Furthermore, the deeper self-insight and present-moment awareness that will emerge once you do it more regularly can have a profound impact on your overall quality of life and relationships. Daily meditation should be a goal for anyone seeking to develop a more resilient body and mind.

MUSIC

Music, which may be the most ancient form of human expression and ecstatic experience, has the potential to restore hormonal and immunological balance and improve neurodegenerative disorders by stimulating the formation of new brain cells and neural connectivity.[87]

Music is primal. It is an enveloping sanctuary that consoles us in our desperation and liberates us from the dark abyss of alienation and despair. It is a reprieve from the burdens we carry and a force of solidarity, one that narrows the chasm between cultures and engenders sacred union and spiritual experience.

Music has been demonstrated to affect the cerebral nerves in humans from our fetal stage to adulthood. Research has found that music facilitates cerebral plasticity, the expansion of neural networks and connectivity,[88] likely mediated by steroid hormones, which are generated by nerve cells and elicit neuroactive and neuroprotective roles.

The processing of emotionally laden experiences in the brain, which can be impaired in those diagnosed with psychiatric disorders, dementia, Alzheimer's, and other neurodegenerative diseases, may be engaged when music is incorporated into neurologic remediation therapies. Studies of Alzheimer's patients have proven that listening to music from one's past can act as a catalyst for the recall of other long-term memories via reconfiguration of existing neuronal networks. Other studies show that listening to music can enhance the recovery of cognitive function post-stroke, mitigate symptoms of mood disorders, improve emotional intelligence, and enhance executive brain functions.[89]

CHAPTER SIX

UNDERSTANDING YOUR HEART

Myths and Facts about Medications, Cholesterol, Fat, and the Inflammation Connection

Within the long-standing paradigm of cardiology, cardiac regeneration has been deemed the stuff of science fiction. The mammalian heart has been regarded as a terminally differentiated or "postmitotic" organ, and replenishment of heart cells has been thought to be an impossibility. New research, however, has cast doubt on this antiquated view, showing that cardiac muscle cells retain some capacity for division.[1] Scientists have also discovered endogenous cardiac progenitor cells residing in the heart and bone marrow that can be transformed into various tissue types within the heart, comprising as they do endothelial cells, smooth muscle cells, and cardiac myocytes.[2] This makes for the good news that, despite all the abuses that come with contemporary lifestyles, the human heart can renew itself.

The not-so-good news is that heart disease remains the leading cause of death in the developed world. The Global Burden of

Disease Study approximated that in 2001, 12.45 million deaths worldwide were caused by cardiovascular disease and cerebrovascular disease. For those who survive a heart attack, the treatment options may seem severely limited since it has long been assumed that the heart does not have the capacity to heal itself.

The fear of heart disease is a real physiological factor in heart disease, as it is with cancer. One meta-analysis concluded that anxiety is an independent risk factor for incident coronary heart disease and cardiac mortality,[3] and another systematic review and meta-analysis found a significant association between panic disorder and incident heart disease.[4] Epidemiological data also illustrates that chronic stress is predictive of heart disease and that chronic exposure to career-related stressors increases risk of a first heart-related event.[5] High levels of psychological stress lead to excess production of reactive oxygen species (ROS), which causes dysfunction of cardiac endothelial cells, hypertension, atherogenesis (the deposition of plaque), and remodeling of blood vessels.[6] Even short-term stress can trigger an acute myocardial infarction, or heart attack, due to stress-induced disturbances in inflammatory, hemostatic, and autonomic nervous system processes.[7]

UNDERSTANDING ATHEROSCLEROSIS

Heart disease is an umbrella term often used to describe a range of cardiovascular system disorders, including coronary artery disease, which encompasses myocardial infarctions and angina pectoris, as well as stroke, congestive heart failure, high blood pressure, peripheral artery disease, and other vascular disorders. Despite the nomenclature, all these diseases point a finger at the same pathophysiological mechanism known as atherosclerosis.

First coined by German pathologist Felix Jacob Marchand to describe the buildup of plaque within the arteries into a "porridge-like hardening," atherosclerosis is found most notably in the walls of the arteries that feed the heart in a condition known as coronary artery disease. Before we had the tools to examine the precise histological changes in atherosclerotic lesions, the view that prevailed for most of the 20th century was the lipid theory of atherosclerosis. Positing atherosclerosis as a simple fat storage disease, it implicated dietary cholesterol and saturated fat as primary causes. More recent discoveries, however, reveal that atherosclerosis is a chronic immuno-inflammatory condition rather than simply a localized narrowing of the arteries. Both the innate and adaptive immune systems play a role in the early formation of fatty streaks, in the infiltration of immune cells into the subendothelial layers, and in the onset of adverse clinical vascular events.[8] One of the main links tying the immune system to heart disease is soluble factors called cytokines, which are both secreted by and act upon cells in the atherosclerotic process.[9]

Atherosclerosis starts when the endothelial cell lining of blood vessels becomes damaged or is otherwise rendered dysfunctional as a result of injury or infection, initiating the formation of atherosclerotic lesions within the arterial walls called fatty streaks. Specialized immune cells called macrophages, or "big eaters," engulf lipids, becoming activated foam cells that produce growth factors, perpetuating an inflammatory response and recruiting more lymphocytes to the lesion. This initial fatty streak is not problematic from a clinical perspective, as the arterial wall can enlarge to accommodate the growth of the plaque without compromising the artery diameter.[10] When this happens within the coronary arteries, however, deep trouble may follow. The repetition of this cycle leads the lumen of the arteries to narrow and harden as the plaque grows and develops a fatty core covered by a fibrous matrix, which can erode or rupture in processes responsible for 70 percent of all fatal acute myocardial infarctions and sudden coronary deaths.[11]

Conventional thinking blames cholesterol levels—more specifically, low-density lipoprotein (LDL), which delivers cholesterol to cells—as the drivers of vessel damage and blockage. The "cholesterol myth" or "cholesterol hypothesis" revolves around the premise that LDL cholesterol is the villain. But while it is true that the presence of LDL and VLDL cholesterol in the bloodstream is required for the creation of the early nonfatal atherosclerotic lesion, this conclusion is a case of mistaking correlation for causation. Cholesterol may be present at the scene of the crime, but it is not necessarily the perpetrator. LDL modified by certain inflammatory processes, though, can be deleterious to both endothelial and vascular smooth muscle cells.[12] Oxidized LDL signals for the support of the immune system, and white blood cells rush to the scene. The oxidized LDL causes all the players to secrete inflammatory chemicals that attract more white blood cells, with the endothelial cells lining the blood vessels expressing "cell adhesion molecules"—ICAM-1 and VCAM-1—which allow circulating white blood cells to stick to their surface and facilitate their entry into the intima (the middle section of the blood vessel).

Scientists have discovered, however, that the most important factor in determining risk is the LDL particle number of lipoproteins that ferry cholesterol and fats around the body rather than the concentration of LDL within the particle. The more LDL particles in the blood superhighway, the greater is their opportunity to collide with the fragile lining of the artery, penetrate the endothelium, and set off the process of plaque formation within the artery wall. Particle size is also important, as small and sticky LDL is more likely than big and fluffy LDL to trigger the process of plaque formation and increase cardiovascular risk.[13]

Chances are that your doctor is measuring your cholesterol concentration rather than the particle number. Fixation on LDL concentration is like a traffic report broadcasting the number of passengers per vehicle on the road rather than the number of cars on the road, which determines the likelihood you will encounter a traffic jam. Measuring LDL concentration alone while neglecting LDL particle number will miss cases in which there is discordance between the concentration and particle number, a pattern that oftentimes occurs in those with metabolic syndrome, who are already at higher risk for cardiovascular events.[14]

Pharmaceutical companies selling cholesterol-lowering drugs have promoted a polarized dichotomy, with LDL cholesterol as the enemy and high-density lipoprotein (HDL), a scavenger that removes cholesterol from the bloodstream, as the hero. People who are diagnosed with high cholesterol are routinely prescribed statin drugs, a class of medications that reduces the levels of LDL cholesterol by interfering with the enzymatic pathway known as the mevalonate pathway and disturbing the intricate cellular machinery of your body. Doctors prescribe statins to roughly one in four American adults over the age of 45, and some U.S. health authorities have gone so far as to push for the addition of statins to the water supply.[15] This is despite studies showing that approximately half of people hospitalized with coronary artery disease have levels of LDL classified by current guidelines as optimal.[16]

There is a growing awareness that the unintended, adverse health effects of statin drugs, with 28 distinct modes of toxicity, may far outweigh their purported benefits. Statins can cause nerve damage,[17] muscle damage,[18] liver damage,[19] and birth defects.[20] They are associated with endocrine disruption[21] and cognitive impairment[22] and are diabetogenic[23] and carcinogenic.[24] In fact, statins represent a perfect storm of cardiotoxicity despite their purported lifesaving cardioprotective qualities.[25] A network meta-analysis of 170,255 patients from 76 randomized trials showed an increased incidence of diabetes with statin treatment.[26] Not only that, but statins disturb the metabolism of essential fatty acids that are so important for prevention of cardiovascular disease[27] and foster major deficiencies in micronutrients, including zinc and copper,[28] selenium,[29] and vitamin E,[30] among over 30 other documented troubling pharmacological actions.[31] Statins have shown such small reductions in absolute risk in middle-aged men who have already had a heart attack that their use as a cardioprotective, in practical terms, is highly questionable.[32]

THE BIG FAT LIE:
CHOLESTEROL, SATURATED FAT,
AND HEART DISEASE

Cholesterol is not the all-out bad guy it has been made out to be. In fact, low cholesterol poses its own risks, since cholesterol plays so many indispensable roles in the body. It is an important precursor to our steroid hormones and bile acids, the latter of which we need to digest fats. It also helps maintain structural integrity and fluidity and is an essential component for transmembrane transport, cell signaling, and nerve conduction. So important is cholesterol that women with a total cholesterol below 195 mg/dL have a higher risk of mortality compared to women with cholesterol above this cut-off.[33]

The cholesterol myth was busted as far back as 1973, in the Minnesota Coronary Experiment, where the saturated fat in the diets of approximately 9,000 institutionalized psychiatric patients was replaced with polyunsaturated fats in the form of corn oil. A 2010 re-evaluation of the data from this experiment published in the *British Medical Journal* found that these patients experienced a 22 percent higher risk of death for each 30 mg/dL reduction in serum cholesterol.[34] While substituting omega-6 fats in place of saturated fat may have led to reductions in blood cholesterol levels, these patients actually suffered worse health outcomes.

Saturated fat is another scapegoat. A recent meta-analysis in the *American Journal of Clinical Nutrition* that compiled data from 21 studies, including 347,747 people who were followed for an average of 14 years, concluded that there is no appreciable relationship between saturated fat consumption and incidence of cardiovascular disease or stroke.[35] Another meta-analysis published in the *British Journal of Medicine* determined no association between saturated fat and risk of cardiovascular disease, coronary heart disease, ischemic stroke, Type 2 diabetes, or all-cause mortality (the risk of death from any cause).[36] Moreover, a recent trial showed that eating a diet high in fat and deriving a large proportion of calories from saturated fat improved biomarkers of cardiometabolic risk and insulin resistance, such as insulin, HDL, triglycerides, C-peptide, and glycated hemoglobin. Another systematic review and meta-analysis on low-carb diets, which tend to be high in saturated fat, found that low-carb approaches have beneficial effects on multiple parameters of cardiovascular health, including body weight, body mass index, blood pressure, abdominal circumference, fasting glucose, plasma insulin, triglycerides, HDL cholesterol, and a biomarker of inflammation called C-reactive protein.[37]

Even international health agencies like the World Health Organization (WHO) have changed their tune on saturated fat. In a recent article in the *Annals of Nutrition and Metabolism*, an expert panel held jointly between the Food and Agriculture Organization (FAO) and WHO reviewed the relationship between saturated fat and coronary heart disease and found that saturated fatty acid intake was not significantly correlated with cardiovascular events or mortality. Similarly, from their investigation of intervention studies, they found that the incidence of fatal coronary heart disease was not reduced by low-fat diets.[38]

Dispatches from the Blue Zones

What works for one person may not for another, so this data should not be collectively taken to mean that everyone does well with copious amounts of fat. People with specific genetic variants, like the *APOE4* genotype linked to insulin resistance and metabolic syndrome, may be more sensitive to changes in dietary cholesterol, total fat, and fatty acid composition.[39] In some cases, dietary saturated fat can increase the permeation of endotoxins (the outer cell membrane of gram-negative bacteria) into systemic circulation, creating the inflammatory condition endotoxemia.[40] Endotoxemia, in turn, is a predisposing factor for atherosclerosis, sepsis, fatty liver, obesity, and diabetes.

Whether this is problematic is likely dependent upon the bacterial composition of your gut ecosystem and the endotoxin content of foods you consume; pre-packaged, pre-chopped produce is higher in endotoxin and far more prone to microbial spoilage. Other variables at play in determining how much fat we should eat include the sufficiency of our bile acids, which break down fats into fatty acids.

Our ability to tolerate dietary fat and our degree of bile acid production may be influenced by our ancestral heritage. Populations descended from the Inuit, who have historically consumed a high percentage of dietary fat from seal blubber, or the Maasai tribe, who have derived 60 to 70 percent of their calories from meat, milk, and blood of animals, may tolerate higher levels of fat. People of other ancestral lineages, such as the Kitavans, who consume almost 70 percent of their calories as unrefined carbohydrates such as yam, sweet potato, taro, and cassava and derive only 20 percent of their calories from fat, may find high-fat diets more problematic. Similarly, the elder Okinawans of Japan, who inhabit a "blue zone" with a disproportionately high number of centenarians, consume an estimated 10:1 carbohydrate-to-protein ratio, with two-thirds of their daily caloric intake coming from starchy carbs.

When we vilify any macronutrient or isolated constituent of real food out of context, we lose. Health and longevity are less about the macronutrient ratio of carbs, fats, and proteins in the diet and more about the micronutrient density and quality of the food. Regardless of the macronutrient ratios they consumed, the shared commonalities of "blue zone" populations are their emphasis on real foods from the earth and their virtual freedom from obesity, diabetes, stroke, and heart attacks.

How Belly Fat Sets You Up for Heart Disease

To better understand the constellation of factors that give rise to heart disease, we must explore metabolic syndrome, the condition from which heart disease is often born and that is present in one of every four adults.[41] Metabolic syndrome is an aggregate of risk factors that predict the development of atherosclerotic cardiovascular disease, hypertension, central adiposity (excess upper body fat that can accumulate around internal organs or subcutaneously), "visceral adiposity" (belly fat), and elevated plasma glucose.[42] Another defining feature of metabolic syndrome is the various lipoprotein abnormalities that characterize dyslipidemia, including reductions in HDL cholesterol and increases in markers such as serum triglycerides, small, dense LDL particles, and apolipoprotein B.[43] At their core, these seemingly disparate criteria are united by biochemical mechanisms such as insulin resistance as well as dysfunction in endothelial cells, cardiac cells, and the smooth muscle cells of the vasculature (blood vessels).[44] In addition, oxidative stress (an excess of free radicals), inflammation, and autoimmune mechanisms, in which the immune system has become misdirected against your own tissue, mediate and propagate these adverse changes.[45]

According to researchers, the crux of metabolic syndrome may be deviations in fat metabolism and in the arrangement of fat in the body, with excess abdominal fat implicated in the etiology of the disorder.[46] Central adiposity is one of the cardinal indicators of the metabolic syndrome presentation that is strongly associated with insulin resistance.[47] Insulin resistance occurs when your cells become desensitized to the effects of insulin, leading to a condition of excess glucose in the blood known as hyperglycemia. Too much sugar in the blood is damaging, causing microvascular complications that augment risk for cardiovascular disease.[48]

The deposition of belly fat that occurs with central adiposity also leads to production of adipokines, or signaling molecules secreted by the fat tissue itself. Increased genesis of inflammatory adipokines and decreased production of a protective adipokine and adiponectin, a protein that increases insulin sensitivity, exacerbate insulin resistance and dyslipidemia, leading to a vicious cycle.[49] Upper-body obesity also leads to ectopic accumulation of nonesterified fatty acids in the muscle and liver,[50] setting the stage for fatty liver disease. Accumulated fatty acids in the liver of a person with fatty liver disease are packaged as triacylglycerides (TG) and distributed into the bloodstream as a component of very-low-density lipoproteins (VLDL) and apolipoprotein B, both transporters of fat in the bloodstream that are predictive of coronary artery disease.[51] These increased VLDL concentrations, in turn, reduce the number of HDL cholesterol particles and generate more small, dense, atherogenic LDL particles, which are more prone to lodging in arterial walls.[52]

The excess lipids that become disseminated in the bloodstream as high concentrations of VLDL in nonalcoholic fatty liver disease cannot be burned as fuel due to a condition known as metabolic inflexibility, or the inability to switch between fat and glucose as the primary fuel source depending on nutrient availability—a hallmark of metabolic syndrome.[53] When glucose is plentiful in the diet, the body should burn it via glycolysis, and when fat is readily accessible, the body should be able to readily increase beta oxidation to metabolize fat for fuel. This nutrient sensing and substrate switching is blunted by the metabolic inflexibility[54] that precedes full-blown heart disease.[55] As if coronary artery disease and fatty liver disease were not enough, metabolic syndrome also increases the rise of polycystic ovary syndrome (PCOS), gallstones, sleep apnea, and diabetes and may even contribute to the etiology and progression of certain cancers.

Getting to the Heart of Cardiovascular Disease: Endothelial Dysfunction

The primary cause of heart disease is not cholesterol abnormalities but inflammation associated with the repeated injury and repair of the endothelium, the single vessel layer that represents the ultimate barrier between the blood and the other tissues in the body. Endothelial dysfunction keeps your blood vessels from dilating properly. When blood vessels don't fully dilate, your blood can't flow where it needs to go. Once thought of as the "'cellophane wrapper' of the vascular tree,"[56] the endothelium is one of the largest organs in the body—and is in fact the largest endocrine organ in the body—weighing about one kilogram and covering a surface between 4,000–7,000 square meters in an adult human. Rather than merely the passive border of the vasculature, standing guard between the circulating blood and organ systems, the endothelium is an active organ lining the entire circulatory system that regulates the delicate balance between pro- and anti-inflammatory processes. The endothelium interacts with almost every organ system in the body and responds to various stimuli, including temperature, transmural pressure, shear stress, mental stress, and neurohumoral responses.[57]

This ability of your blood vessels to relax and contract as physiology and life situations demand is what determines your blood pressure and how hard your heart must work to pump blood to the rest of your body. The endothelium also acts as a semiselective barrier, determining the transit of fluids and electrolytes and the trafficking of leukocytes and other cells between the vessel lumen and surrounding tissue. In a healthy state, the blood flowing through the heart, arteries, veins, and capillaries remains fluid as it interfaces with the healthy endothelial cells lining the vessels. But various factors, including tobacco use, obesity, a sedentary lifestyle, hypertension, dehydration, hyperlipidemia, and poor dietary habits can lead to injury or dysfunction of the endothelium, activating the blood clotting system so that the macromolecules of the basal lamina, a layer of the extracellular matrix synthesized by the endothelial cells, become strongly thrombogenic, or favorable to the formation of a clot.[58]

In this setting, platelets and white blood cells adhere to the vessel and can promote the creation of a thrombus, a blood clot that sits in the blood vessel and impedes blood flow, depriving tissues of normal circulation and oxygen. Depending on its location, the thrombus can cause deep vein thrombosis, a type of chest pain called unstable angina, peripheral arterial limb ischemia, heart attack, ischemic stroke, or a pulmonary embolism if a piece of the clot breaks free and lodges itself in the bloodstream to the lungs.

Damage to the endothelium and its subsequent dysfunction is an initiating step in the development of atherosclerosis, setting off a chain of events that lead to what we call heart disease. The dysfunctional endothelium leads to an imbalance between nitric oxide (NO) production and consumption, favoring the latter at the expense of the former, enhancing the structural damage to the arteries and increasing plaque formation.[59]

Common Threats to Your Endothelium

Repeated injury, inflammation, and recruitment of the body's healing mechanisms can spiral out of control, causing endothelial lesion formation. The following are some of the main causes of repetitive injury to the endothelium:

- Opportunistic infection by bacteria or viruses

- Environmental irritants, such as tobacco

- Oxidative stress due to excess production of reactive oxygen species (ROS)

- Hypoxia

- Hyperlipidemia

- Poor oral health

- Emotional stress, which can induce constriction of blood vessels

- Chronic increased heart rate and blood pressure

- Pharmaceuticals such as ibuprofen

- Elevated blood sugar and associated sticky "blood caramelization" (glycation), which damages the blood vessels

- Frequent consumption of wheat, fried foods, oxidized fats, refined sugars, flours, and other items in the Western Pattern Diet

- Vegetable and fruit deficiency[60]

Because your body's primary interest is self-protection, epithelial injuries mobilize an immune-mediated response to repair damage. There is an entire category of regenerative stem cells released from the bone marrow called endothelial progenitor cells, which ceaselessly heal the damage to the lining of your blood vessels. But because the root causes of damage and dysfunction often continue, the body can only do so much before a fatal failure occurs. We ask our bodies to patch up damaged blood vessels at a frantic pace, and they do, but after decades of consistent, persistent self-injury followed by self-healing attempts, lesions on the vessels become bulging areas of plaque, narrowing the vessel lumen, mucking up the flow of blood, and causing the body to increase blood pressure in an attempt to overcome the increased resistance. As time goes on, plaque deposits accumulate and develop a "cap" of calcium in a potentially fatal transition in the disease process.

The plaque can become so brittle that a sudden increase in blood pressure can cause a piece of plaque to break off, block the artery, and result in a stroke or heart attack. But you don't have to have an arterial obstruction to be mortally affected by cardiovascular disease. In the case of cardiac arrest, which can be caused by electrical disturbances in the heart, too much calcium can cause a "cramping" of the heart muscle.

These complex variables—which are not merely due to eating meat and eggs—are the ultimate antecedents that tip the scales in favor of cardiovascular disease. The key to reducing the risk of heart disease is to prevent the development of the true underlying cause of cardiovascular disease, namely, the inability of the inner lining of blood vessels to dilate fully as a consequence of mostly symptomless damage that can start early in life. When the underlying disease continues forward unabated with the additional risks associated with the use of synthetic drugs, the side effects are often deadlier than the condition they treat. For example, antithrombotic agents such as warfarin are associated with cerebral microbleeds,[61] intracerebral hemorrhage,[62] reduced bone density,[63] and major bleeding. Even a single dose of aspirin can increase permeability of the gastrointestinal tract through "leaky gut syndrome," opening the floodgates for microbes, toxins, and undigested food proteins to permeate into systemic circulation and incite inflammation. A baby aspirin a day, which conventional allopathic wisdom goes so far as to recommend for healthy individuals over a certain age, is not necessarily better.[64]

The New Biology implies that in many instances the true causes of heart disease can be prevented through adequate hydration, the regular consumption of foods that stimulate myocardial regeneration, and avoidance of foods and habits that promote endothelial dysfunction. By consuming the right fruits and vegetables, you are providing your body with the highest quality structured water, essential micronutrients, and microRNA-messengered information that can modify your gene expression in an anti-inflammatory direction. The opposite happens when you consume products that compromise your endothelium.

Good Fats
for the Heart

- Avocado oil (raw, organic)

- Chia seed oil (raw, organic)

- Clarified butter, also known as ghee (organic)

- Coconut oil (extra-virgin, raw, organic)

- Flaxseed oil (raw, organic)

- Macadamia oil (raw, organic)

- Olive oil (extra-virgin, organic)

- Red palm oil* (wild-harvested, raw)

* Look for the RSPO "Certified" label for palm oil products that do not contribute to deforestation, destruction of peatlands, and habitat loss.

THE PROBLEM WITH CALCIUM

The idea that calcium supplementation can be toxic to cardiovascular health is not new, as many advocates of whole food sources of nutrition have long warned against the use of supplements made from limestone, oyster shell, eggshell, or bone meal (hydroxyapatite). There have been at least three studies,[65] including two meta-analyses, performed over the past few years showing a statistically significant increase in heart attack risk among users of calcium supplements.[66]

Food—whole, fresh, and from plants and animals—is an intelligent delivery system that your body is ingeniously designed to receive. But elemental calcium, decoupled from real food, doesn't contain any of the amino acids, lipids, microRNAs, or other factors that enable your body to use it in a biologically appropriate manner. When calcium is separated from nature's delivery system, it doesn't go toward strengthening your bones. Instead, it can end up accumulating within your body's soft tissues, a process known as ectopic calcification. It can also end up in your bowels contributing to constipation or in your kidneys as stones. It can find its way into your blood, potentially contributing to the dangerously brittle calcium "cap" that forms on arterial plaque at the most lethal stage of atherosclerosis. Excess calcium may cause the heart muscle to become overly contractive (hypertonic), which is why conventional medicine uses calcium channel blockers to reduce blood pressure. In very large amounts, calcium can even stimulate unnaturally accelerated cell divisions of your bone cells known as osteoclasts, which can exhaust the cells' regenerative potential over time.

It is best to avoid all mass-market calcium supplements. But if you do decide to take calcium via dairy, supplements, or fortified products, consider balancing it with additional magnesium. Magnesium stimulates the production of calcitonin, a hormone that removes calcium from the soft tissues and blood, thereby reducing the risk of heart attack and several other diseases,[67] and sends it to your bones, where it's most needed.

Plant-Derived Sources of Bone Minerals

I believe that it is better to bypass supplementation altogether and get your calcium packaged inside the real food that your body knows how to process. Consider these sources instead:

- Bone-in sardines

- Kale and other greens

- Miso soup

- Plums

- Pomegranates

RED WINE: IT'S NOT THE ALCOHOL THAT MAKES IT HEALTHY

You might have already heard that red wine can be good for your heart due to its natural antioxidant, resveratrol. But the New Biology shows that it's a more potent cardiovascular tonic than we had originally thought—and why.

Resveratrol does, in fact, help lessen the oxidation (which is, essentially, biological rust) that can be harmful to your heart. In addition, now we know that resveratrol does more than reduce damage. It appears to help heart cells regenerate. A study in *Molecular Medicine Reports* showed that when rats were injected with resveratrol, the markers that indicate stem cell proliferation in their hearts increased. Better yet, these stem cells differentiated into brand-new heart cells.[68] Preliminary research shows that resveratrol modulates a wide range of RNA profiles in the heart consistent with cardio protection and increased resilience against injuries such as oxygen deprivation.[69]

Before you pour a glass of hearty red wine with dinner, though, ask yourself a few questions. First, be honest with yourself about your alcohol habits. If you find yourself giving that glass of wine too much power, or if you have trouble stopping with just one glass, it may be better to avoid wine and find an alternative. Chocolate and red grapes and blueberries, especially organic ones, contain physiologically significant quantities of resveratrol.

The second issue with red wine is that some varieties contain worrisome levels of arsenic, pesticides, and added sulfites that can have serious toxic effects. Arsenic is a natural metal that leaches out of rocks and into the water from which wine is made. Because of differences in geology, American wines tend to have more arsenic than European wines, and because more arsenic is pulled into the skin of red grapes, red wine tends to have more arsenic than white. A study at the University of Washington found that several American wines exceeded the levels of arsenic that the Environmental Protection Agency allows in drinking water.[70] But the problem isn't restricted to the United States; wines from around the world can contain heavy metals at up to 200 times the concentration considered safe for human consumption.[71]

GARLIC, NATURE'S ROTO-ROOTER

Research suggests that garlic can slash your risk of heart attack and stroke by half and cut your risk of general heart problems by 38 percent.[72] Garlic accomplishes this miracle via its direct effect on calcification. A study at UCLA focused on 65 people who were considered to be at intermediate risk for heart disease and were taking statin drugs. These volunteers were given either a placebo or aged garlic extract to take for one year. At the end of the trial, researchers measured the level of calcification in their coronary arteries. The group who had been taking the placebo experienced a progression of coronary artery calcification of 26.5 percent, but the group taking aged garlic extract had just a sliver of that progression at 6.8 percent.[73] If you'd like to take the same supplement as the volunteers in this study, you can. The researchers used Kyolic Formula 108 by the Wakunaga company, which is packaged with the additional vitamins B_{12}, B_6, folic acid, and L-arginine. The combination of aged garlic plus these vitamins appears to have deeply beneficial effects on the arteries, even for those who kept taking statins. Garlic's cardiovascular benefits are wide ranging, including anti-inflammatory, antioxidant, anti-hypertensive, anti-infective and even arterial calcium dissolving.

Don't forget to enjoy garlic as a whole food. Nothing beats the aroma of garlic and onions gently cooking in a bath of olive oil. And if you can handle the strong taste, try eating a little raw garlic every day. Chop it into small pieces and incorporate it into a dish like salsa. If you're worried about the garlic scent on your breath, eat some parsley or drink some fresh lemon water for a neutralizing effect.

CHOCOLATE: CANDY OR MEDICINE?

Dark chocolate's heart-opening and healing powers have been recognized for thousands of years by indigenous South Americans who used it ceremonially and considered it a "drink of the gods." Chocolate's components include theobromine, or "god food" in Latin from *theo* and *bromine*.

Chocolate consumption has a strong inverse association with cardiac mortality. A 2009 study found that those who ate chocolate twice or more per week had a 66 percent lowered relative risk of cardiac mortality compared with those who ate no chocolate at all. In the last decade, chocolate and cocoa (chocolate's primary ingredient) have been shown to lower blood pressure, dilate arteries, improve insulin resistance, reduce endothelial dysfunction, reduce stroke risk, and prevent cholesterol oxidation (which turns normal lipoproteins like LDL into oxidized-LDL, which can damage arteries).[74]

Chocolate is so pharmacologically active and powerful that it can be easy to fall into the habit of using it to self-medicate. It may be easier to moderate your intake if you choose a brand that is lower in sugar and higher in cocoa. And while raw chocolate often does not taste as good as more processed forms, I highly recommend it at a concentration of 65 percent cocoa or more due to its enhanced therapeutic profile. All of this being said, keep in mind that the chocolate industry has often been linked to child labor, human trafficking, and enslavement, particularly on the Ivory Coast.[75] If you want to make sure that the chocolate you are buying is made without exploitative labor practices, look for the Rainforest Alliance certification and avoid West African–sourced cocoa. Also, opt for USDA-certified organic products, as nonorganic chocolate can contain residues of glyphosate.[76]

HEALING YOUR ARTERIES WITH POMEGRANATE

Sometimes nature hands us obvious clues to a food's healing properties. Pomegranates, one of my favorite fruits for flavor and wellness, are full of such clues. This fruit is sweet but also pleasingly astringent. Drink a glass of pomegranate juice, and your mouth and gums will pucker up and feel cleansed. And even though you are drinking liquid, your mouth will feel a bit dry. That's because pomegranate shrinks and disinfects your mucous membranes, which are technically the same type of tissue that lines your blood vessels. Pomegranate offers visual clues as well: its juice looks like blood. The whole fruit even bears a resemblance to a multichambered heart.

One way that epithelial cells of the arteries benefit from pomegranate juice has to do with intima media thickness—a measurement of the thickness of tunica intima and tunica media, the innermost two layers of the wall of an artery. When the intima and media are inflamed and clogged with plaque, they grow thicker, leaving less room for blood to flow through the artery. One Israeli study showed that the intima media thickness of volunteers who drank pomegranate juice shrank in a single year by more than 30 percent compared to the placebo group, whose intima-media thickness increased by 9 percent over the same time period. This study also revealed that pomegranate juice reduced oxidized LDL by 90 percent, decreased antibodies against oxidized LDL by 19 percent, improved total antioxidant status by 130 percent, and reduced systolic blood pressure by 21 percent.[77] In addition, pomegranate soothes chronic inflammation and can help heal the viral and bacterial infections that can appear alongside heart disease.[78]

THE BEET/BLOOD CONNECTION

If you've ever prepared beets at home, you know that this vegetable turns your counter into a bloodbath—but one that's beautiful and dense with nutrients. Like the pomegranate, the appearance of a beet's juices poetically mirrors its counterpoint inside our bodies. A beet, as its juice loudly proclaims, is one of nature's finest tonics for your blood.

Beets are one of the original "superfoods." Eating beets helps you exercise at a higher intensity and reduces muscle fatigue.[79] Beets can ward off the flu and staph infections,[80] appear to protect against liver damage,[81] and may even have anticancer properties.[82] But they are especially good to your heart. A study published in the journal *Hypertension* found that beets contain pharmacologically significant quantities of nitrate, a natural inorganic compound that causes blood vessels to dilate. Three hours after volunteers drank 500 milliliters of beet juice (about two cups), their blood pressure dropped—a direct result of having more nitrate in their blood plasma.[83] You can buy drinks made with beet juice, but watch out for added sugar. To have more control over what goes into your body, consider investing in a juicer to make your own cardiovascular pick-me-ups at home. You can drink beet juice on its own or mix it with the juice of carrots, apples, kale, or ginger. Your blood vessels will thank you.

TURMERIC AND BLOOD VESSEL DILATION

Turmeric is unique among spices, with documented health benefits that number in the triple digits. But I was especially excited when I learned that this ancient Indian spice can protect the human heart. According to the *Journal of Nutrition and Metabolism*, healthy adults who took curcumin (turmeric extract) for two months experienced significant improvement in their blood vessels' ability to dilate,[84] suggesting that it is instrumental in the process that relieves endothelial dysfunction. Turmeric also produces many of the same cardiovascular benefits as exercise (though, to be clear, it does not replace it). In an eight-week study that compared groups of exercising women, the group that included curcumin in their diet had more elastic blood vessels[85] and therefore better endothelial function.

WATERMELON

One of nature's best medicines for the heart is watermelon, a delicious summer fruit. It contains a highly bioavailable source of the carotenoid lycopene[86] and high doses of the amino acid L-citrulline,[87] both of which are extremely beneficial for cardiovascular health. A study in the *American Journal of Hypertension* found that when middle-aged obese people with hypertension were given watermelon extract for six weeks, their arterial function improved and the blood pressure in their ankles reduced.[88] It has also been studied for alleviating many other heart disease–related comorbidities, such as dyslipidemia,[89] metabolic syndrome,[90] oxidative stress,[91] and arterial stiffness.[92]

OMEGA-3 FATTY ACIDS

Though I generally prefer food-based healing, there is one supplement I wholeheartedly recommend. Fish oil is a potent source of bioavailable omega-3 fatty acids, which are known to downregulate inflammatory processes throughout the body and have been shown to reduce the risk of sudden cardiac death.

Other excellent dietary sources of omega-3's include small, fatty fish such as sardines and anchovies, though be aware that fish likes tuna and mackerel, which are often recommended as sources of omega-3s, are often high in heavy metals such as mercury, so I cannot recommend them. I prefer wild-caught salmon because they still have relatively low levels of mercury when compared to other fish. You can use the FDA's handy table to identify the relative levels of mercury in fish sold on the global market today: https://tinyurl.com/mercuryfishfda.

But while there is a robust body of research supporting the connection between fish oil and cardiac health, more recent research calls it into question. At the possible root of this growing disparity in the biomedical literature is the role of statins; these widely prescribed medications may reduce the effectiveness of omega-3s and thus skew recent study results.[93]

Neutralizing Burgers
with Avocados

Is a beef burger healthy for your heart? If it's the usual kind, the answer is probably going to be no—but not for the reason you might think. The biggest problem is that most ground beef comes from cows that have been grain-fed. Grains are disproportionately high in omega-6 fats, versus grass, which is high in omega-3 fats. Since a cow's natural diet consists of grass, cows end up converting grain to a type of fat known as arachidonic acid, which, in excess, is pro-inflammatory. Additionally, when beef rich in polyunsaturated fats is heated, some of the fats are oxidized, producing deleterious effects including damaging fatty acid radical production. These factors can make something as simple as a hamburger adverse to the health of the cardiovascular system.

The avocado offers a solution. Researchers at the UCLA Center for Human Nutrition asked healthy volunteers to eat a hamburger patty. Half the volunteers ate plain burgers, and the other half ate burgers with avocado. Two hours after eating, the blood vessels of the plain burger group had narrowed. But the blood vessels of the avocado group were unchanged. Three hours later, both groups had blood samples taken. The volunteers who had eaten the plain burger had enhanced markers of inflammation; those who had eaten the burger plus avocado showed higher levels of a marker known as IκBα, indicating that its inflammatory pathway had not been activated. Finally, the plain burger group saw their triglyceride levels rise after the meal, while the avocado burger group's triglycerides remained stable. The researchers concluded that ingesting a burger with Hass avocado had some beneficial anti-inflammatory and vascular health effects.[94]

The Perfect Burger

Avocados are a rich source of the monounsaturated fatty acid commonly found in olive oil known as oleic acid, along with chlorophyll and potent antioxidants. These substances likely provide balance to the harmful omega-6 fats and lipid peroxidation found in burger patties. Recipes for foods and meals were the original medical prescriptions for healing, and the traditional culinary practices of adding side dishes, condiments, dressing, and spices to our dishes have reasons that go beyond adding flavor. These "extras" can protect and amplify the nutrition present in the main dish while negating or balancing out some of its less healthy effects. If you are going to eat a burger, choose one sourced from cattle that were humanely raised and allowed to graze. And put an avocado and other natural, traditional accompaniments on top of it.

MIND, BODY, AND HEART

The state of your mind and your heart are intimately connected. When we are relaxed, happy, or in a state of gratitude, we can feel it and see it in our bodies. Research shows there is a hardwired neurobiological basis for this intimate connection. Over the last 40 years, the HeartMath Institute has gathered research showing that the heart has neurons that form a two-way channel to the brain.[95] The two organs are in continual dialogue, with the heart sending more signals to the brain than vice versa! This is a profound departure from the Old Paradigm that has looked at the heart as simply a tireless blood pump, when, in fact, it turns out that your heart communicates to the brain in four major ways:

1. Neurological communication (nervous system)

2. Biochemical communication (hormones)

3. Biophysical communication (pulse wave)

4. Energetic communication (electromagnetic fields)

This has significant implications for the mind-body connection, or, more precisely, the "heart-mind" connection. Conditions that were once considered compartmentalized and exclusive to the head or heart must now be considered holistically in the context of cardiovascular health.

Consider our experience of "heartbreak." A bad health-related prognosis (e.g., cancer) confers up to 26.9 times higher risk of heart-related death in the week that follows diagnosis. Thus, it's not necessarily the diagnosed disease in and of itself that's lethal to your heart but your feelings about it instead. The mind-body and heart-body connection goes deep, and it is important for us to understand, accept, and learn how to express emotions in constructive ways in order to find health and balance in our bodies as a whole.

CHAPTER SEVEN

REVERSING METABOLIC DISEASE

Natural Remedies for Insulin Resistance, Belly Fat Accumulation, and Dietary Hormone Disruptors

One obvious sign of the metabolic syndrome epidemic is the fact that more than two-thirds of Americans are overweight and about half are obese.[1] Metabolic syndrome is a cluster of conditions that include high blood pressure, insulin resistance, elevated waist-to-hip ratio, and dyslipidemia (an unhealthy imbalance of blood lipid levels and triglycerides). If you have three or more of these symptoms, you already fall within this syndrome's category, alongside 23 percent of other American adults. Together, this constellation increases the risk of developing disabling, and even deadly, conditions such as diabetes, stroke, and heart disease, the rates of which have escalated worldwide.

Not all body fat is the same. Some body fat is brown and some white, and the former is healthier than the latter. But the question of *where* fat tissue gathers takes the discussion to the next level. Abdominal obesity, also known as belly fat, increases the risk of developing diabetes or cardiovascular disease, including stroke. Belly fat is the single most significant indicator of metabolic syndrome, itself an independent risk factor for all-cause mortality *that's stronger than smoking.*

The long-term consequences of a disordered metabolism include promoting the conditions that drive atherosclerosis. But there are simple changes you can make to your diet that can profoundly alter your metabolic trajectory and reduce your inflammatory load and propensity toward fat generation and storage. These changes will also help you regenerate cells that are constantly being damaged by exposure to toxins, chemicals, and stress-inducing behaviors.

In the Old Paradigm, metabolic disorders were treated with a combination of palliative, symptom-reducing drugs and often superficial lifestyle and dietary recommendations, the latter of which are based on outdated nutritional concepts, such as eating more complex carbs (whole grains) versus simple ones. Metabolic syndrome is an optimal example of a chronic disease category that can be mitigated and reversed through diet, lifestyle choices, and a healthier response to stress.

CONDITIONS LINKED TO METABOLIC SYNDROME

Type 1 diabetes is an autoimmune disorder that develops when the host's own immune system responds to injury in the beta cells in the pancreas. While there is a genetic component to Type 1 diabetes disease susceptibility, other factors, including chemical exposure, microbial imbalance, food intolerances and allergies, and stress, are influences that can induce a loss of immunlogical self-tolerance and overwhelm the body's innate regenerative repair mechanism. When the insulin-producing beta cells in the pancreas can't keep up with the higher cell turnover required, it can lead to organ damage. Without insulin, glucose will not get into your cells. Instead of fueling your metabolism, the glucose accumulates in the blood, binding to proteins and lipids and leading to the production of highly tissue-damaging glycation end products. Approximately 5 percent of diabetes cases are Type 1, where the damage to the pancreas is addressed medically with synthetic insulin replacement therapy. While metabolic syndrome is commonly considered to be linked to Type 2 diabetes, it also occurs in about one in three people with Type 1 diabetes.[2]

Type 2 diabetes is often identified as being caused by lifestyle factors—eating the wrong kinds of foods and at quantities beyond the body's capacity to process glucose in a healthy way. When these lifestyle conditions persist, the cells' insulin receptors develop lowered sensitivity, reducing how much glucose can enter while simultaneously leaving excess glucose and insulin to accumulate in the blood. This is insulin resistance. When glucose can't enter cells, it remains in the blood, creating a rise in blood sugar. Excessive blood sugar and its glycation end products cause damage to our tissue, particularly to the lining of the blood vessels. The pancreas thinks, "Ah, there's too much glucose in the blood. Better tell the beta cells to produce more insulin and whisk that glucose into the cells." The cells then become *even more* resistant to insulin, creating a vicious cycle, because *now* your insulin levels are so high that, if left unaddressed, they can disrupt the functioning of your heart, brain, and hormones. Insulin resistance can also interfere with satiety, often leading to increased appetite, which compounds the problem.

Of the 30.3 million Americans who have diabetes, about 95 percent are Type 2. That's not the worst news, though. When the cycle of rising blood sugar and insulin production continues over time, the beta cells can become exhausted and lose their ability to produce insulin completely. This condition, known as "double diabetes," is marked by beta cell damage, lower insulin production, high blood sugar, and insulin resistance. Throw in synthetic insulin and oral antidiabetic drugs,[3] both of which have been found, in some cases, to increase or accelerate metabolic disturbances linked to higher cardiac mortality,[4] and a downward cycle is created that can be hard to overcome.

Prediabetes occurs when blood glucose levels are higher than normal but not high enough for a diagnosis of diabetes. Technically, a diagnosis of prediabetes is based[5] on blood tests showing that a blood biomarker of glycation known as A1c is within the range of 5.7 percent to 6.4 percent. If you are at 6.5 percent or higher, you would be categorized as prediabetic. A jaw-dropping 84.1 million Americans fall within the prediabetic diagnostic category. The global statistics are far more alarming: close to half a billion people will be diagnosed with the condition by 2030, potentially representing health liabilities in the trillions of dollars.[6]

Of all the drugs that are prescribed for diabetes, metformin (Glucophage) is far and away the most popular. In the short term, metformin is effective at lowering blood sugar. But it's unclear whether metformin achieves the longer-term goal of reducing heart attack risk and all-cause mortality. Over time, doctors are prone to prescribing higher and higher doses to maintain blood sugar levels, often combining it with other drugs known as sulfonylureas. But that's not a sustainable solution either. A study by the University Group Diabetes Program (UDGP) showed that diabetics who took the sulfonylurea tolbutamide suffered two and a half times the death rate compared to people who were controlling their diabetes through diet alone.[7] A third class of drugs, known as thiazolidinediones, also appears to hasten mortality. A review of 42 different studies shows a 43 percent increase in heart attacks for people taking Avandia (a thiazolidinedione) and a 64 percent increase in death from heart disease when compared to people who were given a placebo.

Moreover, people who take metformin are sometimes tempted to believe that the drug is a safety net that allows them to eat whatever they want. This can lead doctors to note a failure of the diet and prescribe more drugs.

The New Metabolic Disorders Paradigm

Metabolic disease is our body's attempt to deal with the onslaught of a radically inappropriate diet, a vast array of toxicant exposures, inactivity, and persistent, health-degrading stress. Perhaps the most exciting finding of the New Biology is that lifestyle factors are the primary cause and therefore can be a cure for diseases like metabolic syndrome. By identifying and removing the causes, we activate the full potential of our default healing state of ceaseless regeneration.

Once you switch to an ancestral diet, introduce herbal remedies, and regularly practice intentional movement, insulin resistance can go completely put into remission. High blood pressure and high blood sugar will come down, lipid levels will normalize, and excess belly fat will melt away. Following this approach, insulin-dependent patients with Type 2 and, in some cases, Type 1 diabetes have been shown to gradually reduce their dependence on synthetic insulin. While much of this is anecdotal and yet to be proven in clinical trials, the plausibility of these cases is affirmed by a growing body of research showing that the insulin-producing beta cells in the pancreas can and do regenerate, especially when utilizing natural substances such as chard, bitter gourd, or curcumin.[8]

Toxicants and the Insulin Resistance Connection

Anyone at risk for metabolic disorders is immediately told to reduce their intake of fats and sugars. But that advice is far too general, and it's misleading. Some fats and simple carbohydrate sources can be exceptionally good for the metabolically disordered. If you want to improve your blood sugar, or if you simply want to shrink some belly fat, you could see concrete results simply by dramatically reducing the following.

WHEAT

The Old Paradigm encouraged the consumption of whole grains. The New Biology reminds us that the seeds of cereal grasses are incompatible with the ancestral diet designed to keep our metabolism in balance.

Wheat disrupts the metabolism by generating insulin resistance. Wheat starch is composed of approximately 75 percent amylopectin, which has been demonstrated to be particularly effective at inducing insulin resistance.[9] This is the reason that wheat bread, according to statistics produced by Harvard Health Publishing, is higher on the glycemic index than white sugar.[10] In addition, wheat disrupts the biological activity of the satiety hormone leptin. Leptin is produced by fat cells that travel through the bloodstream to the brain with the message for the body to stop eating. Wheat lectin, however, can bind to and antagonize the leptin receptors in your brain, reducing leptin's appetite-reducing effects and leading to leptin resistance. That's one reason wheat-based bread, pasta, cereal, crackers, and sweet-baked goods leave you hungrier after you've consumed them.

FRUCTOSE

All of us, especially people at risk for metabolic disorders, should avoid excess sugar. But not all sugars are the same. Fructose, which means "fruit sugar" in Latin, *is* pure and health-giving if it comes nestled within its raw, organic form of whole fruit.

But let's be candid. We are not suffering from an epidemic of people overeating fresh fruit. Quite to the contrary: we have a deficiency in the consumption of fresh, raw, organic fruit. Keep in mind that food is not just an energy source but also information and software for your body. Fruit contains wholesome molecules full of vitamins, fiber, plant stem cells, and antioxidants and delivers biologically indispensable information that is especially nourishing to the the mammalian cardiovascular and reproductive systems. This industrially processed fructose may be as addictive as alcohol,[11] and perhaps even morphine.[12]

According to USDA research into major trends in U.S. food consumption patterns during 1970–2005, we now consume fructose at the rate of at least 50 pounds a year. The biggest culprits are sugar and corn syrup (which is sometimes misleadingly labeled "corn sugar"), but pasteurized fruit juices are also a hidden threat, as they continue to be adulterated with additional sugar or HFCS.

Because high-fructose corn syrup contains free-form monosaccharides of fructose and glucose, it cannot be considered biologically equivalent to sucrose, which has a glycosidic bond that links the fructose and glucose together and slows its breakdown in the body.

Fructose can easily be converted into ethanol with a pinch of yeast in order to make alcoholic beverages. It bears great resemblance to alcohol (ethanol) in its capability of stimulating dopamine production in the brain. It also shares similar metabolic pathways and effects on the liver. So toxic is "purified" fructose that at GreenMedInfo.com, we have indexed research on over 70 adverse health effects associated with its excessive consumption.

The Sugar/Mood
Disorder Connection

While the parallels between fructose and alcohol consumption may not seem intuitive, the intimate connection between what we eat and our psychological health is beginning to gain wider recognition, especially considering new research that links aggression to trans-fatty acid consumption, episodes of acute wheat mania, and the widespread presence of opiate-like peptides in common foods. Fructose-opiate infatuation is deeply embedded within mammalian biology, and this has been the subject of scientific investigation since the late 1980s. A study published in the *European Journal of Pharmacology* found that both glucose and fructose were capable of antagonizing morphine-induced pain-killing effects,[13] likely due to the direct opioid effects of these sugars or their metabolic by-products on the central nervous system. In fact, the study found that fructose was more potent than glucose in accomplishing these effects.

To avoid fructose, it helps to become an educated label reader. HFCS is often hidden in products through the use of the following terms: glucose syrup, maize syrup, tapioca syrup, glucose/fructose syrup, fruit fructose, crystalline fructose, HFCS, and fructose. If you choose whole foods that don't come in packages, the only fructose you'll get is the kind that's naturally encapsulated in one of nature's most wholesome and delicious forms, such as fruit or honey.

MSG

The omnipresent ingredient of monosodium glutamate (MSG) in modern mass-market food takes advantage of our biologically hardwired taste receptors, particularly those that perceive savory flavors. The "Yummy!" sensation that occurs immediately after ingesting an MSG-laced morsel is the sensation the Japanese call umami (savoriness), which the Japanese consider to be one of the five basic flavors.

I consider MSG more of an addictive drug than a food additive, a concept that a growing body of research supports.[14] Our bodies, which have evolved complex sensorial and cognitive pathways to determine whether something is good or bad for us based on appearance, taste, and smell, are increasingly being chemically manipulated. MSG tricks our taste buds into finding a nutritionally vapid substance loaded with semi-synthetic ingredients designed to be ravishingly delicious. Inevitably, over time, real food appears less attractive and less satisfying of our cravings.

Technically, MSG is the sodium salt of glutamic acid, a naturally occurring nonessential amino acid. Glutamic acid-rich foods include wheat, dairy, corn, soy, and seafood. The problem is that when you isolate a single amino acid out of a complex food and increase the concentration to unnatural proportions, the resulting glutamic acid can have devastating health effects, not the least of which is an insatiable appetite for more of the very same chemical stimulating the craving.

Beyond MSG's addictive qualities, research from the U.S. National Library of Medicine highlights the connection between MSG and obesity. While excessive food cravings caused by MSG's taste-enhancing effects figure into this relationship, MSG may directly cause brain lesions, insulin resistance, and leptin resistance.[15] Therefore, MSG can no longer be considered simply a flavor enhancer. It's an intrinsically harmful chemical that can disrupt your hormones and actively contribute to metabolic syndrome, obesity, fatty liver, and dysregulated blood lipids, as well as a wide range of neurological problems.[16]

MSG's Many Disguises

Here are some of the many disguises of MSG on food labels:

- Autolyzed protein
- Autolyzed yeast extract
- Calcium caseinate
- Canned broth
- Gelatin
- Glutamate
- Glutamic acid
- Hydrolyzed plant protein
- Hydrolyzed protein
- Hydrolyzed vegetable protein
- Maltodextrin
- Modified corn starch
- Modified food starch
- Monopotassium glutamate
- Natural flavor
- Protein isolate
- Seasonings
- Sodium caseinate
- Soy sauce
- Textured protein
- Torula yeast
- Yeast extract
- Yeast food
- Yeast nutrient

BISPHENOL A (BPA)

If you're trying to lose weight, especially around the middle, first, look inside your pantry. Toxicant-laden processed and packaged food can lead to weight gain, as can their means of being stored. Food and drinks stored in thin, clear, shatter-resistant plastic containers or cans may provide exposure to BPA, an industrial chemical that's linked to obesity and metabolic syndrome. BPA is found almost everywhere, but it leaches into foods primarily through contact with containers made with the chemical. Other BPA sources include PVC piping, plastic dinnerware, compact disks, toys, dental sealants, and medical devices. It's found in virtually all currency throughout the world, as well as cash register receipts issued on thermal paper.

BPA is known to disrupt the human endocrine system, which regulates hormones like insulin and leptin. A Kaiser Permanente study has found that girls between 9 and 12 years of age with higher-than-average levels of BPA in their urine were twice as likely to be obese compared to girls with lower levels.[17] This study confirms findings from earlier animal studies that high BPA levels can increase the risk of weight gain and obesity.

Limiting Your Exposure to BPA

Here are some ways to minimize your exposure to BPA:

- Avoid canned foods. Even when the label says BPA-free, a can's liner can be made with the equally toxic bisphenol S (BPS) or bisphenol F (BPF), which are from the same chemical class.

- Opt for food sold in glass jars or the waxed cardboard cartons known as Tetra containers.

- Don't use baby bottles, cups, dishes, or food containers marked with "PC" (for polycarbonate) or recycling label #7.

- Don't microwave food in plastic containers.

- Don't touch cash register receipts from stores. Ask to have them dropped in your bag, take a photo of them for your records, or have the receipt emailed to you instead of being printed.

- Avoid eating and drinking from plastics whenever possible.

Natural Ways to Reduce Insulin Resistance

Several plant compounds, including many found within common foods, can stimulate your pancreas's regenerative process.

The medical community has invested heavily in researching and developing stem-cell therapies, transplants of islets (groups of pancreatic cells that produce hormones), and an assortment of synthetic drugs. Yet an effective treatment—and even a possible cure—for metabolic disorders might be sitting on your kitchen shelves or growing in your backyard garden as we speak.

One of the primary ways that natural alternatives to metformin and other diabetes drugs work is through restoring your cells' sensitivity to insulin, and in some cases they pull double duty as beta cell regenerators (helping to spark back up the body's insulin production). When taken in tandem with an ancestral diet and lifestyle and under the care of a licensed health professional, it's possible they can eventually replace diabetes drugs or, better still, help keep blood sugar so steady that they won't be needed in the first place.

1. Turmeric. In a groundbreaking study published in the American Diabetes Association's journal, *Diabetes Care*,[18] 240 pre-diabetic adult patients were given either 250 milligrams of curcumin or a placebo every day. After nine months, *none* of the participants taking curcumin had developed diabetes, but 16.4 percent of the placebo group had, suggesting that curcumin was 100 percent effective at preventing Type 2 diabetes.

2. Ginger. In a 2014 randomized, double-blind, placebo-controlled trial, 88 volunteers with diabetes were divided into two groups. Every day one group received a placebo while the other received three one-gram capsules of ginger powder. After eight weeks, the ginger group reduced their fasting blood sugar by 10.5 percent, but the placebo group *increased* their fasting blood sugar by 21 percent. In addition, insulin sensitivity increased significantly more in the ginger group.[19] In another study, researchers demonstrated that 1,600 milligrams per day of ginger improves eight markers of diabetes, including insulin sensitivity.[20] Since 1,600 milligrams amounts to about a quarter teaspoon, the results show you don't necessarily need a high dose to get impressive results.

3. Cinnamon. Cinnamon has been used for millennia as both a spice and a "warming" medicine to improve the blood. The *Journal of Medicinal Food* published a meta-analysis of eight studies that concluded that cinnamon (or cinnamon extract) lowers fasting blood sugar levels.[21] One way it works is by keeping your stomach from emptying too quickly after eating. Sprinkling just a half-teaspoon a day onto your meals or into your smoothies can reduce blood sugar levels, even if you have Type 2 diabetes.[22] Look for cinnamon labeled as Ceylon cinnamon, from the ancient name for Sri Lanka (Ceylon), where it was originally harvested. Anything else is likely not cinnamon at all but cassia, a mere cousin to real cinnamon.

4. Olive leaf extract. University of Auckland researchers proved that olive leaf extract increases insulin sensitivity. In a randomized, double-blind, placebo-controlled study, 46 overweight men were divided into two groups. One group received capsules containing olive leaf extract, and the other group received a placebo. After 12 weeks, olive leaf extract lowered insulin resistance by an average of 15 percent. It also increased the productivity of the insulin-generating cells in the pancreas by 28 percent. Supplementing with olive leaf extract yielded results "comparable to common diabetic therapeutics (particularly metformin)." [23]

5. Berries. If your meal includes berries, your body will need less insulin after eating. In a study of healthy women in Finland, volunteers were given white and rye bread to eat, either with or without a selection of pureed berries. The glucose level of the women who ate the plain bread spiked quickly after eating, but the women who ate the bread with berries had a much lower spike in their after-meal blood sugar.[24]

6. Black seed (*Nigella sativa*). Black seed is also known as Roman coriander, black sesame, black cumin, and black caraway. Just two grams of black seed each day can significantly reduce blood sugar and glycation end-product formation. The same dose can also improve insulin resistance.[25]

7. Spirulina and soy. Spirulina is a type of blue-green algae that's an excellent source of protein, calcium, iron, and magnesium. It can be eaten as a food, though in the United States, it's most often consumed in powder form and added to smoothies or shakes. In a study in Cameroon, spirulina and soy powder went head-to-head, as researchers tested which is better at controlling insulin sensitivity. In this randomized study consisting of volunteers suffering from insulin resistance related to treatment with antiretroviral drugs they were taking, one group received 19 grams of spirulina a day for eight weeks, while the other received 19 grams of soy. At the end of the trial, the soy group increased its insulin sensitivity by 60 percent, which is relatively good, but the spirulina group's insulin sensitivity leaped by an average of 224.7 percent. And although 69 percent of the soy volunteers experienced increased sensitivity to insulin—which, again, is relatively good—*all* the volunteers in the spirulina group saw an improvement.[26] This is a strong endorsement of spirulina's healing power, even when it's under an extreme challenge such as living with adverse effects related to taking HIV drugs.

8. Berberine. Perhaps the bitterness of berberine, a compound found in the roots of plants like goldenseal and barberry, is a clue to its effectiveness in stabilizing blood sugar. In a Chinese study of 36 patients, scientists found that three months of treatment with berberine was just as effective as metformin in bringing down blood sugar.[27] It should be noted that special caution should be taken with herbs like berberine, which, while generally far safer than pharmaceutical compounds, are not without side effects, and therefore should be used under the guidance of a medical herbalist or experienced integrative medical practitioner.

9. Resistant starches. Unlike other foods in their class, resistant starches are far lower on the glycemic index because they are broken down slowly in the large intestine. This "resistance" to digestion means that they are unlikely to cause spikes in blood sugar. And they have time to ferment, giving the beneficial gut bacteria of your microbiome an opportunity to flourish. As a source of fermentable fiber, resistant starches can help improve insulin sensitivity[28] and reduce body fat.[29]

Resistant Starches to Include in Your Diet

- Amaranth

- Cassava

- Chickpeas

- Millet

- Muesli

- Soaked beans (all varieties)

- Unprocessed oats

- Unripe bananas

A FINAL WORD ABOUT BELLY FAT

Nature has made us in a glorious variety of shapes and sizes, and those sizes can sometimes change with age. Particularly as you get older, you might develop more fat around the hips and thighs or find it harder to keep weight off. Within the bounds of moderation, these developments are healthy and normal, and you do not need to be small and slender to be healthy, but it is crucial to watch out for excess belly fat.

When you remove processed food, processed fructose and high-fructose corn syrup, wheat, and MSG from your diet, or when you prevent the accumulation of petrochemicals like BPA in your body from food or other sources, your reward may be a leaner belly, lower blood sugar, and a much better shot at staying free of disease into a healthy, lively old age.

To help make it a little easier to maintain a healthy level of belly fat and regulate your blood sugar, I offer the following tested strategies.

1. LEARN TO FAST

Many people find traditional fasting difficult and not sustainable. Research has shown, however, that you can receive the benefits of fasting without taking things to an extreme. University of Florida researchers have come up with what's known as the feast-or-famine diet. It involves alternating one day of eating about 175 percent of your normal caloric intake ("feasting") with one day of eating 25 percent of your usual calories ("fasting"). An average man would generally eat about 4,550 calories on feast days and 650 on fast days, and most women would eat a little bit less. Put the feasting and fasting days together, and your average number of calories is about what it would usually be. But it's the timing that makes all the difference.[30]

One study examining the effects of the feast-or-famine diet found that the participants' insulin levels significantly decreased after 10 weeks. If you're trying to reduce your blood sugar, feast-or-famine could be a good way to do it. On feast days, load up on wholesome, healthy, regenerative foods. On fast days, continue to choose foods from the Regenerate Rx, but keep your consumption down to just one meal and about a quarter of what you'd usually eat.

If feast-or-famine still feels too hard, you can take small steps toward fasting. It takes 8 to 12 hours for your body to burn through all the sugar stores from a meal, unless you ramp up your post-meal exercise, which can be a good idea if your time and schedule allow. If you don't let 8 to 12 hours elapse between meals, your body will only burn carbs, and it won't have the chance to burn fat, including belly fat.

Even short, simple fasts can allow optimal fat-burning to take place. The first step is to stop eating food after 8 P.M. Eat dinner and then call it a night in terms of food consumption. The second step is to stretch your breakfast time until 8 A.M., and voila, you're partaking in a 12-hour microfast every day. Since you'll spend most of those hours asleep, fasting should be easier and give your body an opportunity to do the deep regenerative work it cannot do when not burdened with excessive food from eating late. Once you're comfortable with your 12-hour fast, you can extend it. Walk away from the kitchen at 7:00 P.M., and don't return for breakfast until 11:00 A.M. the next day.

Fasting is *not* starving. If you feel yourself becoming sick or weak, stop. That being said, if spacing out your eating feels healthy to you, it may be able to help improve your metabolism, even if you don't change what you eat.

2. SUNBATHE TO SPEED UP YOUR METABOLISM

Sunlight can strengthen and build your bones and brighten your mood. When human skin is exposed to ultraviolet light, the body can speed up the metabolism of fat that's directly under the skin (subcutaneous fat).[31] Unlike belly fat, which is wrapped around your internal organs, subcutaneous fat is not considered a risk factor for metabolic disorders. But consider this: people who don't get enough vitamin D tend to have more belly fat.[32] And there's a solid body of research that links obesity with a deficiency of vitamin D.[33] Getting UVB radiation might be an essential and easy strategy to burn your belly fat away, because it helps your body manufacture vitamin D from cholesterol. Head out sunscreen-free for 15–20 minutes during the UVB-abundant two hours before and after solar noon. To protect yourself, use the internal sunscreens of increased chlorophyll, astaxanthin, and antioxidants.

Externally, you can apply titanium dioxide formulations, as long as they do not contain nanoparticles (make sure the label states "non-nano"), or sunscreens made with zinc oxide.

3. DEVELOP A HIGH-INTENSITY INTERVAL TRAINING ROUTINE

The definition of an ideal workout used to be 30–60 minutes of cardiovascular activity performed at a moderate pace. New research shows that very short blasts of high-intensity interval training (HIIT) can dramatically improve glucose metabolism and produce immediate effects. It's also the most effective exercise method for reducing belly fat for obese women with metabolic syndrome.[34]

Americans often hear from their doctors that when it comes to exercise, doing "something is better than nothing." That's true. It really is better to walk around the block than to sit on the couch, and it's better to take the stairs than to take the elevator. Exercise, or intentional movement, of any kind helps the body to use stored-up energy. It increases the number of insulin receptors in your muscle cells, which allows blood glucose to be delivered to the cell for energy, and can release hormones and neurotransmitters that help suppress your appetite. If you enjoy working out at a moderate pace for a half an hour or longer, don't let me stop you. But if you are at risk for a metabolic disorder or are serious about losing belly fat, doing HIIT can do the job twice as fast.

A Sample HIIT Workout

Consider building up a foundation of basic cardiovascular fitness through this HIIT workout, swimming or using a stationary bike or cardio machine:

DURATION	INTENSITY
10 minutes	Warm-up
30 seconds	All-out effort
4 minutes	Recovery pace (very slow)
30 seconds	All-out effort
4 minutes	Recovery pace (very slow)
30 seconds	All-out effort
4 minutes	Recovery pace (very slow)
30 seconds	All-out effort
4 minutes	Recovery pace (very slow)
5–10 minutes	Cooldown

When you rethink metabolic disorders through the lens of an evolutionarily appropriate lifestyle template, you will discover an array of preventive and curative options. By avoiding the toxic chemicals that ravage your metabolism and by consuming the foods and natural compounds that regenerate the beta cells of your pancreas, you might discover that over time, your symptoms will resolve themselves. Add in some fasting, high-intensity interval training, and targeted sun exposure, and you will feel your mood soar. And not only will your waistline contract, but your core will grow stronger. With lower blood sugar and an optimized cellular response to insulin, you can successfully beat back metabolic disorders, maintain a healthy weight, and extend your life.

CHAPTER EIGHT

THE NEW AGING PARADIGM

How to Rewind Your Biological Clock

Getting older is *not* a disease. Nor is it a guarantee that you will develop one. While our bodies *are* subject to an unprecedented level of toxic exposures, nutritional incompatibilities, and stress factors, all of which contribute to an accelerated rate of biological aging well beyond what is natural, the good news is that we have the power to decelerate, avoid, and even reverse our biological age and most chronic diseases by living, eating, and thinking differently.

The New Biology tells us that our habits determine our health future more than our genes do. Simple changes in diet and behavior can completely redefine your health, unleash your inner physician, and set up the conditions needed for deep self-regeneration. Don't think of this as an effort solely to extend your life-span; think of it as a way to extend your health span. Focus on the quality of those years—not just the number—so that you experience as many joyous moments of *being alive* as possible.

One of the first steps in taking back control of your biological destiny is understanding just how resilient and powerful your body is. It is a sacred vessel and miraculous technology, capable of performing trillions of intricate and precisely orchestrated biological operations each moment, somehow regenerating itself through the course of a lifetime. The New Biology's assertion that our bodies have the capacity to regenerate thanks to the seed of immortality planted deep within us eons ago is a fundamental shift in perspective.

You heard me correctly: immortality. Our bodies contain a population of cells that are deathless. While the human body is often considered the epitome of mortality, a biological thread of immortality lives in your testes if you are a man and your ovaries if you are a woman, in the form of the sperm and egg cells, respectively. These incredible cells, from which all the other cells in our bodies originated, came in the form of the original zygote (sperm-fertilized egg) donated by your father and mother, and theirs by their fathers and mothers, going back not just to the origin of our species but to the preceding mammalian and premammalian species from which we evolved.

Astoundingly, these germline cells reproduced over and over, in an immortal thread that runs back through billions of years, through a near-infinite number of replication cycles, to the first cell that spawned all living things. This mystery is at the heart of all biological systems today. And this original protocell, called LUCA, is believed to have appeared some 3.4 billion years ago. LUCA's legacy is found in every one of our cells, but especially the stem cells that inhabit our various tissues and work tirelessly to replace damaged and diseased tissue, creating it anew. These stem cells are responsible for our incredible regenerative potential and directly connect us to all other living things in the web of life.

We are immensely powerful and resilient biological entities, and it is this power that we recruit when we engage and capitalize upon regenerative dietary and lifestyle practices that help us to undo chronic disease and reverse premature aging.

This isn't a mystical belief but is instead an actionable longevity goal. Consider ginkgo biloba, the world's oldest living plant, whose very existence is an archetype of immortality and resilience. It can live well over 1,000 years, and like all plants, it contains stem cells known as meristematic cells, which give rise to the various tissues in the plant body. Gingko biloba is believed to have originated around a quarter of a billion years ago and is appropriately nicknamed a "living fossil."[1] Ginkgo biloba has survived the Earth's five mass extinction events and was the only plant species to survive the August 6, 1945, atomic bombing of Hiroshima. A month after the bombing, six ginkgo biloba trees were still standing at the epicenter of the blast. They budded shortly after and are still alive today.[2]

Amazingly, ginkgo biloba's incredible hardiness and cellular longevity transfer over to humans. At the cellular level, it works as an antioxidant, reducing the oxidative stress that can lead to diseases we associate with aging, including cancer, Alzheimer's disease, and heart disease. It also enhances mitochondrial respiration, one way in which the cells produce energy. And ginkgo biloba elicits this antiaging effect across several cell types: neurons, blood platelets, and fibroblasts (which produce the collagen needed to support the skin and make it smooth), as well as cells of the liver, heart, and endothelium.[3] And these are only a few glimpses into the mysterious power that ginkgo biloba wields and shares with those who consume it.

MAGNESIUM, CELL AGING, AND RESTFUL SLEEP

It has long been observed that astronauts experience accelerated aging while they're in space. They return to Earth with the same cardiovascular capacity you'd expect from someone who is aging at 10 times the normal rate. One of the likely culprits is the magnesium reduction that often occurs during space flights.[4]

Magnesium deficiency is common here on Earth as well because the Western Pattern Diet is low in magnesium-rich foods, the most archetypal of which are green, leafy vegetables saturated with magnesium-rich chlorophyll. Magnesium deficiency might underlie accelerated aging in the cardiovascular system, and it can prevent healthy cell regeneration in a way that leads to a host of other symptoms and disorders we associate with "normal" aging.

You need magnesium to keep the cells of your heart working. The heart's muscle cells know how to contract automatically, without a signal from the brain. These contractions help to keep your blood pumping. As an antioxidant, magnesium prevents free radicals from damaging your heart. And it can act as a natural alternative to calcium channel blockers, a class of blood pressure–lowering drugs that have significant side effects, including weakening the heart muscle by preventing it from fully contracting.

Magnesium's importance extends past the heart cells to the cellular regenerative process throughout your body. A deficiency of magnesium accelerates aging in several cell types, interfering with their ability to divide and renew themselves. These cell types include endothelial cells, which line the blood vessels and the heart. You also need magnesium to avoid premature aging in your fibroblasts, which are cells in your connective tissues such as bones, tendons, and cartilage. These cells aid in the production of collagen, which maintains the cell's structure and keeps your skin looking firm and elastic. When these cell types can't replicate as often as they should, their tissues can undergo changes similar to those seen in the aging process.[5] But with the right amount of magnesium, these tissues can thrive for a much longer time.

Magnesium is a true utility player with a staggering number of functions, binding to 3,700 different sites in the body.[6] It plays a role in mood and cognition, with studies showing that it improves mild to moderate clinical depression in as little as two weeks, and can act as a buffering agent during times of stress by helping to modulate the hypothalamic-pituitary-adrenal (HPA) axis.[7] When you're under stress, the body releases a cascade of hormones, sending dopamine, adrenaline, norepinephrine, and others streaming into your blood. This stress response, if sustained over extended periods, interferes with the body's regenerative, self-healing process.[8]

Another major benefit of magnesium is that it can improve sleep by partially reversing some of the changes that come with aging. According to a 2002 study published in *Pharmacopsychiatry*, magnesium supplementation restores sleep brain wave patterns and improves the neuroendocrine disruptions that happen in the night as we get older.[9]

Best Dietary Sources for Magnesium

We are designed to consume foods that contain magnesium, but modern monoculture crop practices and the use of magnesium-devoid fertilizers have led to soil erosion and compromised the magnesium content of our food. Many people will benefit from taking a supplement, but ideally you should strive to get magnesium mostly from food sources, such as chlorophyll-rich vegetables, which have a wide range of additional health benefits.

One of the richest sources of dietary magnesium might surprise you: it's coffee. An espresso, of the kind you'd get in a coffee shop, contains around 48 milligrams of magnesium.[10] Magnesium is a mineral that is finely regulated by the body, so take care to take it to bowel tolerance (too much and you'll get diarrhea). And if you are taking excess calcium via supplements, dairy products, or products fortified with calcium, you'll need more magnesium than you might otherwise. In addition to coffee, great sources of magnesium include leafy greens such as chard, spinach, and sea vegetables; tea; legumes; and whole pseudograins (dicots), such as quinoa.

Yoga and Your Stem Cells

Stress is inevitable and even health-promoting if allowed proper expression (positive stress is known as eustress). But much of what we stress about chronically is maladaptive. Sometimes the causes are unknown or are so deeply buried within our psyches that it is best to use meditation, yoga, exercise, or essential oils to soothe the jangled nervous system. The practice of yoga, which, according to a robust body of science, has more than 100 distinct health benefits,[11] is at least 5,000 years old and can help you live longer and happier.

Some of yoga's youth-promoting effects include increased physical flexibility, focused breathing, and deliberate, agile movement. But yoga goes much deeper—all the way to the marrow of your bones. Stem cells from your bone marrow periodically leave their "bone home" and enter the bloodstream. If you've torn a muscle, bone marrow stem cells can become healthy muscle cells, thereby fostering a regenerative process. If you have joint problems, they can convert into cartilage that pads your bones. A study published in the *Journal of Ayurveda and Integrative Medicine* found that people who practice yoga regularly have more of the markers in their urine that indicate the presence of stem cells.[12] The study suggested that all that bending, twisting, and deep breathing can release the stem cells from the bone marrow and send them into the bloodstream, where they search for tissue in need of repair. This process prevents premature cell senescence and death, and it reduces inflammation, possibly helping to explain why yoga is so astoundingly beneficial for aging bodies.

Age-Related Conditions that Yoga Can Improve

Here are just a few of the conditions related to aging that yoga can improve:

- Cardiovascular problems

- Cognitive decline

- Depression

- Eyestrain

- Hormone insufficiency

- Lower back pain

- Respiratory problems

- Sleep deficiency[13]

There's a yoga practice for everyone, from the sweaty and challenging power yoga to gentle classes that begin with students seated quietly in chairs, working on improving their basic mobility skills. Even those who don't feel they are flexible can reap these benefits with gentle versions of yoga.

Like ancestral foods that feed our DNA with information they need, yoga is a time-tested discipline that appears to have deeply regenerative effects. But to really understand all that it can do for you, you need to *experience its benefits directly.*

Younger Skin

Our outsides reflect our increasingly toxified inner physiology as early wrinkles, prematurely sagging skin, age spots, and general dullness. We can pay hundreds or even thousands of dollars for harsh beauty treatments but that will only make the underlying toxicity worse. Instead of Botox, which has recently been proven to numb the emotions and alter cognition,[14] we can choose natural and sustainable approaches to slow and even reverse the effects of premature aging.

ADD GOOD FATS AND PLANTS
TO YOUR DIET

A large Japanese study of more than 700 women showed that women who ate more total fat, including saturated and mono-unsaturated fat, had better skin elasticity.[15] Quality is the most important factor. When consuming plant-derived fats, go for raw, organic, or extra-virgin pressed, if available. Avoid vegetable oils, including soy, corn, canola, cottonseed, safflower, and sunflower, which have nothing to do with the kinds of vegetables we should be eating and are and disproportionately rich in easily oxidized and pro-inflammatory omega-6 fatty acids, which can accelerate skin aging. For the best fats, I recommend grass-fed meats, wild-caught salmon, pastured poultry and eggs, avocados, coconut oil, and olive oil.

The same study mentioned above revealed that women who ate more green and yellow vegetables had significantly fewer wrinkles. Green and yellow vegetables are wonderful sources of antioxidants and beta-carotene, which promote clear skin. Make sure to enjoy kale, spinach, broccoli, swiss chard, collards, mustard greens, cabbage, arugula, yellow bell peppers, winter squash, or yellow zucchini a couple of times a day.

OPT FOR MORE NATURAL
TOPICAL PRODUCTS

Aloe vera. Of the roughly 100 natural substances that have been researched to improve aging skin, aloe vera is possibly the most effective. (Visit http://www.greenmedinfo.com/disease/aging-skin for a comprehensive list.) In addition to its antiaging effects, this youth-enhancing plant has another 50 or so side benefits, ranging from topical application to heal wounds, treat burns, and promote dental health to treatment for many forms of cancer. Taken orally, aloe deeply soothes, hydrates, and increases the production of collagen. Aloe also decreases the gene activity that causes collagen production to decline in the first place. One study found that women who took aloe vera gel capsules had fewer wrinkles after 90 days. Moderate doses of about 1,200 milligrams will also improve skin's elasticity.[16]

You can take aloe vera gel capsules, but I always like to use products that are closest to the source—in this case, gel that comes straight from the aloe leaves. You don't need much aloe vera gel to see results.

Red ginseng has been dubbed a "beauty food" by a group of researchers in Korea, who were exploring the extract to measure how it diminishes wrinkles. They concluded that the herb had increased the synthesis of collagen in the skin.[17] Red ginseng is readily available as a tea, and you can drink it daily.

Pine-bark extract reduces unwanted pigmentation of age spots according to one Japanese study of more than 100 women. But its age-defying effects didn't stop there. The women also experienced greater skin elasticity and hydration, probably due to increased levels of hyaluronic acid, which is necessary for smooth and youthful skin. Pine bark also enhanced the expression genes that help produce new collagen. The study used a commercial extract known as Pycnogenol, which can be taken as a supplement. Doses as low as 40 milligrams were found to be effective.[18]

The Invisible Thorns
That Cause Joint Pain

Osteoarthritis is a degenerative joint disease characterized by out-of-control inflammation, chronic pain, and decreased mobility. We can take drugs to mask the pain, but we won't experience true relief unless we address the real causes. One of the most common causes of inflammation can be found on our dinner (and lunch and breakfast) plates. I'm speaking of lectins. Traditional ways of preparing foods, like cooking, sprouting, and fermenting, can help, but they do not remove them entirely. For instance, sprouted whole wheat may contain more wheat lectin (technically known as wheat germ agglutinin, or WGA) than regular bread, because the germ contains the largest amount and is removed in processed bread.

Consuming WGA lectins can lead to inflammation and joint pain—and for many people, that pain drives them to take NSAIDs or other drugs to relieve the symptoms. But NSAIDs can increase intestinal permeability, which allows the body to absorb even higher quantities of WGA and other problematic proteins found in wheat. Which means you'll have more symptoms and want to take more NSAIDs. To break the cycle, cut wheat and gluten-containing products out of your diet. This step can greatly relieve the pain of inflammatory arthritis. If you are sensitive to wheat lectin, you might need to remove other sources of lectins with similar binding properties as WGA (so-called "chitin-binding" lectins), such as potato,[19] barley, rye, tomato,[20] and even rice.[21] Because joint disease is often characterized by a deficiency of collagen, you can also take vitamin C and the amino acid lysine, both of which are required to produce collagen. Glucosamine is another option since it happens to have the exact same binding target as all the lectins mentioned above (namely, N-acetylglucosamine),[22] only they will bind to the supplement and not your tissues.

Of course, sometimes your joint pain will still flare up. You might not have the time to stop and wait for dietary changes to reveal their results. This may be a good opportunity to use a natural anti-inflammatory and antioxidant like black seed oil. Black seed is not well known in the United States, but it has a long and noble medicinal history that dates back to ancient times. A 2016 study, performed with volunteers in a nursing home in Iran, showed that when black seed oil is applied topically, it performs better than oral Tylenol for controlling the pain of osteoarthritis of the knee.[23]

What Is Black Seed Oil?

Black seed oil, known in ancient times as "the remedy for everything but death,"[24] is a complex food and spice—far more complex than most pharmaceuticals, which are often composed of single chemicals or simple combinations of single chemicals. Massage one milliliter (around one gram, which is a very small amount) of oil into the skin around your inflamed joint. Use your entire palm to massage around the front and the sides in a clockwise direction. Do this for about five minutes a day, three times a day. The Iranian study asked volunteers to use the oil for three weeks, which was enough time to produce measurable pain control.

NATURAL MENOPAUSE RELIEF

Women are often prescribed synthetic hormone replacement therapy (HRT) to mitigate the symptoms of menopause, including bone loss, cardiovascular risk, mood swings, and hot flashes. HRT contains estrogen and/or progesterone, which decreases in midlife as the ovaries naturally reduce their production. But HRT comes with clearly established dangers, including increasing the risk for breast and ovarian cancers, blood clots, and stroke.[25] While far safer, natural forms of HRT can still promote the physiological state of deficiency by sending a message to already poorly performing endocrine glands that they don't have to make more hormones. This also leads to a deepening dependency on external hormones and gland atrophy.

I suggest that you fortify your own regenerative stores during menopause by avoiding the Western Pattern Diet, especially these items:

- **Refined sugar and processed carbohydrates.**
  Many women worry about the weight gain that
  can come with menopause. These highly addictive
  foods can raise insulin levels, which in turn can
  lead to estrogen dominance, maladaptive patterns
  of fat deposition, and the physical symptoms the
  menopausal transition is notorious for.

- **Anything that's been treated with growth
  hormones.** Check your dairy and animal products to
  make sure they don't come from animals that were
  given recombinant bovine growth hormone (rBGH),
  also known as bovine somatotropin (BST), or any other
  growth- or weight-promoting hormones. To be safe, buy
  only pastured or grass-fed meat and dairy (if you must
  include dairy in your diet at all; it can be a good idea to
  remove it altogether for a few weeks and reintroduce to
  assess tolerance).

You can also add these hormone-regulating foods to your diet:

- **Fruits and vegetables.** They are rich in phytoestro-
  gens, a form of estrogen found in plants. They are
  adaptogens, adaptable to your body's estrogen level.
  If you need more estrogen activity, they increase it. If
  you've got too much, they help block it.

- **Flaxseed.** These incredibly therapeutic seeds can slow the growth of breast cancer.[26]

- **Blueberries.** They inhibit the development of cellular senescence (aging cells) in studies of animals that have had their ovaries removed.[27]

- **Ginger.** It reduces the loss of spatial memory in menopause.[28]

- **Soy.** It can improve bone health, decrease cardiovascular risk factors, and reduce hot flashes.[29]

- **Evening primrose oil.** This may decrease the severity of hot flashes, as well as improve measures of social activities, relationships with others, and sexuality in menopausal women.

- **Pomegranate.** Technically a berry and the fruiting ovary of a plant, it contains naturally occurring steroid hormones similar to the human ovary, such as estrogen and testosterone.

ANDROPAUSE

Women are not the only ones who experience hormonal changes in midlife. Men also undergo a transition called andropause, during which hormones such as testosterone and human growth hormone (HGH) are produced in lower quantities. Both testosterone and HGH are known as the virility hormones, and a robust industry plays on men's fears that they will become less virile—and, especially, less sexually potent—after age 50 or so. This industry sells more than $2 billion in testosterone drugs per year.[30] But there's a smarter way to think about the problem. This new approach might benefit far more than your sex life; it could address a condition underlying the primary cause of death in the modern world.

In men, impotence is often an early sign of endothelial dysfunction throughout the cardiovascular system. An erection depends on the free flow of blood to and from the penis, and that blood flow is made possible through a healthy endothelium, which fully relaxes and contracts in response to blood pressure fluctuations. Left unaddressed, endothelial dysfunction can lead to atherosclerosis. And *that* buildup of plaque in the blood vessel is what can eventually cause a stroke, heart attack, or coronary artery disease.

If you respond to erectile dysfunction by artificially amping up hormone production, you are throwing a Band-Aid on the problem, ignoring your body's cries for help while risking major side effects and even a heart attack. Keep in mind, not all causes of disease are physical. Beyond endothelial dysfunction, a deficiency of emotional intimacy and an unhealthy relationship dynamic can be just as important contributors to ED, both of which can be addressed with various forms of psychological and spiritual self-work.

The most direct way to address this early cardiovascular warning sign is through a radical transformation of your diet. Omit the grains and dairy products that our bodies do not recognize as sources of healing, renewing information. Focus on an ancestral diet rich in high-nutrient, low-carbohydrate vegetables, tubers, and fruits. Your diet should also include high-quality natural fats and protein sources that are consistent with our biological heritage. GreenMedInfo. com contains a database of over 100 natural substances[31] studied for reversing endothelial dysfunction, the top five being these: (1) arginine, (2) vitamin C, (3) flavonoids, (4) vitamin E, and (5) isoflavones. Exercise is also crucial. It powerfully improves vascular function within the cardiovascular system.[32] Conversely, inactivity has been demonstrated to contribute to erectile dysfunction.[33]

Another compelling approach may be to drink green tea. Preclinical research into the use of green tea for erectile dysfunction has shown extraordinary results, specifically diminished atherosclerotic plaque progression within the rodent corpus cavernosum, the erectile tissue forming the bulk of the penis, including increases in androgen hormones.[34] If you don't like green tea, you can enjoy other beverages that are rich in catechins, which are some of green tea's most active ingredients. Black tea is a good choice, but because it contains only about half the catechins of green tea, consider double-brewing your cup.

FATIGUE, DEPRESSION, ACHES, AND PAINS: SICKNESS SYNDROME

Sometimes what feels like old age is really something much more fundamental. Sickness Syndrome is a term that describes a cluster of symptoms: general fatigue, depression, low libido, aches and pains, suppressed appetite, and a desire for solitude. These symptoms fit our culture's stereotypes of old age, but they are not a normal, inevitable part of getting older. Nor are these symptoms limited to older people. A depressed mood, low energy, low libido, and a tendency toward isolation can happen at any time of life.

The aches, pains, depression, and other symptoms that we try to escape through various addictions are often related to a deficiency of our basic primal needs: water, light, exercise, interpersonal intimacy, and a felt sense of community. Without *all* these resources, we will feel fatigued and achy. In a scientific investigation known as the Rat Park study, researchers took rats that were addicted to morphine and sorted them into two groups. The first group was placed in a typical, crowded rat cage that was small and devoid of natural light. The second group was placed in what researchers called Rat Park, a kind of playground about 200 times larger. When the still-addicted rats were given access to either morphine-laced or tap water, only the conventionally caged rats preferred drug self-medicating as a response to their oppressive environment. The rats in Rat Park largely ignored the morphine, consuming 19 times less.[35] Their social environment was so healing that they no longer drugged themselves.

There are several lessons here, but I want to focus on this one: survival is contingent upon a healthy social and physical environment. Without it, we start showing signs of weariness and depression.

We lack motivation and want to crawl back under the covers almost as soon as we wake up.

What usually happens is that these behaviors are mistaken for the disease itself. The symptoms are pathologized. We try to medicate them away. This can happen in a formal setting—for example, a doctor might diagnose depression and prescribe antidepressants. My wife, holistic psychiatrist Kelly Brogan, M.D., has found that when many of her patients adopt lifestyle modifications and psychospiritual practices that foster deep levels of self-care, they're able to put into complete remission a range of "incurable" mental health disorders, and even autoimmune conditions such as lupus, without needing to stay on their psychiatric medications.[36] By redefining their suffering in such a way that they are able to extract meaning from it and perceive adversity as an opportunity for introspection and self-exploration, many are able to move through their illness into a greater state of empowerment and health.

Sickness Syndrome is an adaptive response to an unhealthy lifestyle, a compensatory coping mechanism designed for self-preservation. Your body may be telling you to shut down, withdraw, and redirect your energy toward rest, repair, and recovery as a last-ditch effort to survive in a world that fundamentally diverges from that which our physiology has evolved to recognize. It is therefore a self-protective, and even a regenerative, response, and we would be smart to tune in and honor it.

In the next part of this book, I'll help you put the Regenerate approach into practical action. Here you'll find a detox plan to help you begin to cleanse your body from the effects of the Western Pattern Diet and a lifestyle plan that will stimulate deep bodily renewal and rejuvenation.

PART THREE

REGENERATE RX

A FOUR-PHASE PROGRAM
FOR TRIGGERING
YOUR BODY'S
RADICAL RESILIENCE
MECHANISMS

PHASE 1

INDUCTION

Apples and Clean Water Mono Diet
(1–3 days)

PHASE 2

RE-ENTRY

Establishing Ancestral Diet Patterns
(2 weeks)

PHASE 3

SUPPLEMENTATION

Nourishing Your Regenerating Body
(2 weeks)

PHASE 4

MIND/BODY HEALING

Detox and Intentional Movement Techniques
(for life)

The Regenerate Rx program will help you take the information in this book and translate it into immediate action. My hope for you is that it will produce a direct experience of the profoundly regenerative forces that permeate not only your body but the entire universe. You're invited to take a quantum leap with me. You will eschew the automatic and mindless eating patterns of our age by eating *only organic apples*. This mono-diet (between one and three days) will jump-start your new life through a courageous act of radical simplification. This can release an incredible amount of psychic and physiological energy that you would otherwise subconsciously allocate, all day long, to planning, acquiring, preparing, eating, cleaning up, and digesting your normal meals. You'll also get a chance to utilize the untapped power of your body. You will learn to access nourishment both from a "cosmic source" (the quantum vacuum) and an earthly one (the incredible variety of foods and physical substances the Earth provides).

Until we have the experience of toggling between them, we won't know that we don't need to eat "three squares a day" every day of our lives to be healthy and happy. By experiencing a direct connection to a cosmic and limitless source of nourishment, you will know a type of lightness, joy, and vitality that was hitherto unknown.

The program is simple in design and principle. First, it focuses on removing and detoxifying the elements interfering with your body's immense capability for regeneration. Second, you will learn to eat, move, and think in a way that further activates and optimizes your ancient, built-in regenerative processes.

Phase 1 (Induction) of eating only apples lasts one to three days, depending on how long you can comfortably sustain it. Phase 2 (Re-entry) nourishes your body with the ancestral dietary template by removing the processed and toxic foods most of us have been eating since we were first introduced to solids. Once this new dietary pattern has been in place for two weeks, you can start Phase 3 (Supplementation) by adding core supplements. In Phase 4 (Mind/Body Healing), you will develop sustainable lifestyle practices for detoxification (inside and out), intentional movement, and emotional healing.

INDUCTION

Apples and Clean
Water Mono Diet
(1–3 days)

Evolutionarily, an apple is a perfect whole food, with all the nutrients and information you need to nourish, cleanse, and lighten your digestive burden while invigorating your microbiome. Apples also contain extremely rejuvenating plant stem cells and EZ water, dissolved oxygen, and other nutrients that don't require elaborate digestive processing to nourish you deeply. This seemingly radical move toward dietary simplicity will be a profound reset of your entire metabolism, helping your body to clean house while being deeply nourished. You'll find a similar reset and opening in other areas of your life, as you will have an abundant amount of time once dedicated to acquiring and preparing food that is now entirely yours to fill with new creative ventures.

For one to three days, you can eat any variety of organic apples; get rid of the seeds, but don't peel the skin, which contains astringent properties that cleanse your epithelial tissues for healthy oral, gut, and cardiovascular health.

Apples' structured biological water will nourish and infuse your tissues with both energy and information, and their pectin will enhance detoxification by drawing out bile and accumulated toxicants. Additionally, like all living foods, the apples have a complex and health-promoting microbiome that will reseed and reinvigorate your own microbiome. There are no restrictions on how many apples you can eat. Let your appetite (or lack thereof) be your guide. When you get hungry, just eat one. It's that simple. Drinking plenty of clean and pure water alongside the apples is equally essential. Spring water is best, but you can fortify purified filtered water with minerals, such as a pinch of Himalayan sea salt or trace minerals from the Great Salt Lake in Utah, to alkalize and restructure the water.

Water Is a Crucial Detox Factor

Since water makes up 99 percent of the molecules in your body, what you drink can be a major source of regeneration and enhanced detoxification. Aim for an ounce of water daily for every two pounds of body weight. But use your body's feedback when in doubt. If your pee is discolored, you could probably drink more. If it's clear, you should be good. Ideally, each day you should drink some EZ water, which has a molecular structure of H_3O_2. Water that comes from underground springs is a good source, and sunlight-infused water in a glass container will also be charged up. Avoid regular bottled water, and if you absolutely must drink municipal or city water that contains a highly toxic form of fluoride, try to use a reverse-osmosis filtration system.

While this phase of the diet omits protein and fat, your body will take what it needs by degrading its own less-than-healthy components and reusing what it can in a process known as "self-eating," or autophagy. Autophagy is your body's ancient system of cleaning house. In an elegant process, your body will disassemble poorly functioning, diseased, or worn-out cells and use what remains to make new cells.

Alcohol is not allowed in this phase, and coffee is not recommended. But for those who believe they have a physiological dependency, a cup of coffee (always organic) in the morning is allowed.

At first you will experience "hunger," but this sensation is oftentimes just a reaction to the body reorienting itself. This mono detox can have a laxative effect on some people but be binding to others. Remember to drink plenty of water, which can help the cleanse and provide an additional source of energy.

RE-ENTRY

Establishing Ancestral
Diet Patterns
(2 weeks)

The goal of Phase 2 is to strip your diet of the degenerative effects of the Western Pattern Diet and start rebooting your body with a naturally regenerative, ancestral diet of 100 percent organic and non-GMO foods, including fruit, vegetables, good fats, grass-fed or free-range meat and chicken, and wild fish. This Re-entry phase will restore your body's ideal operating system in a way that is perfectly matched to your biological hardware.

During and after the apple mono-diet, you will likely feel a little natural expansiveness or a lightness of being. From the Latin word *frui*, the word *fruit*, after all, literally means "enjoy." Phase 2 helps you to transition eventually back into a more standard diet of raw and cooked whole foods at your own pace, but take these two full weeks to establish this new pattern. Think about it in terms of the elimination of processed and evolutionarily incompatible industrial foods and replenishment with organic, whole, information-dense foods.

To transcend the Western Pattern Diet, you will need to eliminate the following:

- All gluten-containing products, including wheat, rye, barley, kamut, and spelt

- Cow dairy products

- Soy (unless organic, which is permissible in small amounts)

- Sugar, sugary products, and sugar-containing foods, including high-fructose corn syrup, or "fruit sugar"

- Mercury-laden fish, farm-raised fish, and shellfish

- Any synthetic or processed product containing man-made chemical ingredients or processed food isolates such as hydrolyzed yeast protein

- Food with additives, flavor enhancers, artificial colors, or preservatives (other than natural ones such as vitamin C)

- Microbiome-disrupting foods such as grain-fed meats, oxidized and genetically engineered vegetable oils, hybridized wheat, and glyphosate-laden food crops

Bottom line: When in doubt, don't!

For the Advanced Health Enthusiast

If you are an advanced health enthusiast, in Phase 2 you can move directly to *a grain-free diet, which excludes rice, oats, and corn.* Eliminating legumes and nightshades (tomatoes, eggplant, hot sauce, chili, peppers, tobacco) is also recommended. If desired, you can include some pseudograins, such as quinoa, amaranth, and millet; and remember, sweet potatoes can make for a wonderful, nourishment-packed alternative to other carbohydrate sources that is slow-burning and exceedingly rich in carotenoids and minerals.

The goal of the Re-entry phase is to move from the simplicity of apples to an ancestral diet of foods that preceded the industrialized food era. All processed, packaged, artificially enhanced or preserved, nonorganic foods and food ingredients are off the table. The natural consequence of this restriction is that you will be forced to eat a diet of whole and wholesome foods teeming with vital energy and information. Initially, you will remove gluten-containing grains and cow's-milk products (except butter, which is okay). Advanced health enthusiasts, or those working with serious disabilities and who want to accelerate their healing more rapidly, will remove all grains from the outset. You will be eating cooked food but should always have something raw with each meal, even if it's only a sprig of parsley, squeeze of lemon in your water, or slice of apple.

A major thrust of the Re-entry diet is to transition from nutrient-poor, starchy foods, which form the centerpiece of the agrarian, grain-based diet, to foods our ancestors would have consumed by foraging or hunting. You'll be adding in more high-quality fats, such as avocados, omega-3-rich flax, pasture-fed eggs, wild fish, and grass-fed meats. Increasing your consumption of good fats is the solution to end the vicious cycles of endless carbohydrate cravings caused by eating high-glycemic, insulin-releasing sugary and starchy foods. Keep in mind that as you remove the addictive foods you may have been eating to cover up difficult emotions, some of these feelings may come to the surface to be released. Embrace those challenging feelings and transform them by incorporating some of the lifestyle practices in Phase 4.

I'm sure you are wondering if, having moved from the Induction to the Re-entry phase, you can resume consuming coffee, caffeinated beverages, and alcohol. Coffee is okay, but only if it's organic and consumed in the morning. Caffeinated beverages like green and black tea are fine, but not in the late afternoon or evening. Alcohol is not allowed in the Re-entry phase but can be added in moderation (one to three drinks a week) after two full weeks of consistent ancestral-based eating. I ask, however, that beverages be gluten-free (which excludes most beers) and low-sugar (cocktails, if you must imbibe, should be crafted in accordance, without sweeteners) and that the wine be natural or organic (no sulfites added), with a preference for resveratrol-rich varieties like pinot noir. In this phase, I also encourage you to include homemade chicken broth, the perfect regenerative food, especially when you transition from eating raw fruit and vegetables to cooked food.

WHAT TO EAT

FRUITS, VEGETABLES, SEASONINGS, AND SWEETENERS

A foundational principle of Regenerate Rx is that raw plant foods contain regenerative stem cells (known as meristematic cells), which transmit immense vitality when consumed. Also, remember to add a raw fruit or vegetable to each meal. All fruits and vegetables should be USDA-certified organic and, when available, be of higher standard, meaning locally grown and biodynamic. For more information about biodynamic food, visit www.demeter-usa.org.

- All fruits, including but not limited to apricots, avocados, bananas, cherries, coconuts, dates, figs, grapefruit, grapes, guava, honeydew and cantaloupe melons, kiwis, lemons, limes, loquats, lychee nuts, mangoes, mangosteens, oranges, papayas, passion fruit, peaches, pears, pineapples, plums, pomegranates, raisins, star fruits, tomatoes, and watermelons—fresh, seasonal, and local fruit is preferable, but frozen is acceptable if it doesn't have added sugar

- All seasonal fresh or sugar-free frozen berries, including but not limited to blackberries, blueberries, cranberries, currants, elderberries, lingonberries, mulberries, raspberries, and strawberries

- All leafy green vegetables, including but not limited to arugula, chard, chicory, dandelion, endive, lettuce, spinach, watercress, and purslane

- All cruciferous vegetables, including but not limited to broccoli, bok choy, brussels sprouts, cabbage (red, purple, white, chinese, napa), cauliflower, collards, horseradish, kale, and mustard greens

- Olives (green and black) and capers

- All root vegetables, including but not limited to beets, carrots, daikon, radishes, parsnips, and turnips

- All dry or fresh legumes, including but not limited to adzuki beans, chickpeas (garbanzos), green and wax beans, lentils, mung beans, snap peas, snow peas, soybeans (in moderation, preferably fermented), and sugar peas

- All sprouts, including but not limited to alfalfa, broccoli, and mung beans

- Garlic and onions, including but not limited to chives, leeks, scallions, and shallots

- All members of the squash family, including but not limited to pumpkins and zucchini

- All other vegetables, including but not limited to artichokes, asparagus, bell (sweet) and chili peppers, celery, cucumbers, eggplant, plantains, prickly pear cactus, and rhubarb

- All tubers *except* white potatoes, including but not limited to sweet potatoes (all colors), taro, yams, and yucca (cassava)

- All mushrooms

- Dulse, kelp, nori, and other sea vegetables, preferably from the Atlantic Ocean, such as the Maine coast, which has less nuclear fallout than bodies of water such as the Sea of Japan and the Pacific Ocean

- All tree nuts, including but not limited to almonds, brazil nuts, macadamias, pecans, pine nuts, pistachios, and walnuts, as well as cashews (which are technically seeds) and peanuts (which are actually legumes)

- All edible seeds, including but not limited to black seed, chia, flaxseed, hemp, pumpkin (pepita), sesame, and sunflower

- All herbs, both fresh and dried, including but not limited to basil, bay leaf, cilantro, dill, marjoram, mint, oregano, parsley, peppermint, rosemary, sage, spearmint, tarragon, and thyme

- All spices, including but not limited to anise, black pepper, cardamom, cayenne, cinnamon, clove, cumin, fennel, fenugreek, ginger, saffron, turmeric, and curry powder mix

- Natural sweeteners, including but not limited to raw honey (and propolis and pollen), unprocessed maple syrup, unsulfured organic molasses, xylitol (if from birch trees), and stevia

- Pseudograins, including but not limited to amaranth, buckwheat, and quinoa

- Fermented foods, excluding cow's milk products (goat's milk is fine), and keeping in mind that none should be consumed with any added sugars; miso paste, natto, and other fermented soy products; kimchi, wasabi, coconut kefir, and beet kvass

- Seasonings, including but not limited to mustard (without sweeteners), real vanilla, tamarind, and vinegar (all kinds, preferably unpasteurized)

FATS AND OILS

All oils should be cold-pressed and organic. Varieties include the following:

- Avocado oil

- Extra-virgin coconut oil (to eat or to cook)

- Extra-virgin olive oil (for dressing, not cooking)

- Ghee (for cooking)

- Goat butter

- Macadamia nut oil

- Pumpkin seed oil

- Red palm oil (wild-harvested, ethical variety)

MEAT, POULTRY, AND EGGS

- All red meat and pork, which should be free-range (pastured) and/or grass-fed

- All poultry, which should be free-range (not just cage-free but organic and pasture-raised, if possible)

FISH AND SHELLFISH

- Only fatty fish (cold-water) and shellfish that are wild-caught and low on the food chain, including anchovies, sardines, herring, trout, Pacific and Alaskan salmon, oysters, and shrimp; see seafoodwatch.org for information on different fish species and what's safest to you and to the environment, and avoid all farmed and GMO fish, such as AquaBounty salmon

BEVERAGES

- Coconut milk

- Coconut water (organic)

- Coffee, organic and preferably sustainably grown (do not drink coffee in the afternoon)

- Green tea, black tea, herbal tea, rooibos, matcha

- Organic goat's milk

TREATS

- Cocoa/chocolate (72 percent cocoa or more only), organic and fair-trade

- Gluten-free grains such as black rice, wild rice, brown rice, basmati rice, rice bran, sorghum, millet, oats (in extreme moderation), and corn (non-GMO)

A Reminder on Food Quality

A basic premise of the Regenerate Rx program is that your microbiome is the primary driver of your health and well being. Since most cooked, preserved, and irradiated foods come from poor-quality soil and are not cultivated to support your microbiome, your best option for regenerative benefits is to eat locally sourced, organic, and/or fermented foods. Don't skimp on quality; you'll taste the difference and feel it in your body.

You are literally constructed from the things you eat, drink, and breathe. Of the three, you are in full control only over what you eat and drink. Eating quality food removes interference within your body and sends signals that turn gene expression on and off in just the right way that is appropriate for your individual constitution. Quality refers not just to taste and avoidance of chemicals but also to the kind of information conveyed: if food is produced from GMO seeds, sprayed with agrochemicals, grown in synthetic and factory-farmed, animal waste–amended soil, and then processed and irradiated, the biological information it contains will be distorted and will send harmful messages to your cells, interfering with your life energy and the optimal expression of your genome.

When to Eat and How Much

What you eat after you eliminate Western Pattern food staples is key, but equally important is timing of meals and portion size. If possible, have your last meal of the day before the sun goes down to remain in harmony with our natural ancestral cycle. If you must have a snack, the true test of whether you are truly hungry or just looking for a distraction is to eat an apple. Most of us eat habitually, but if you're not hungry for breakfast, which is *not* the most important meal of the day, skip it. Technically, the first meal of your day could be at 1 P.M. It can still be called breakfast because you are literally breaking the fast. There is no need to label this intermittent fasting when it could be termed "listening to your body."

Do have healthy snacks like a few almonds, a piece of grass-fed jerky, or a piece of fruit handy for when hunger strikes. Eat slowly, mindfully, and without the distractions of watching television or using other electronic devices. You'll notice that giving your full awareness and allowing for sensual enjoyment when you eat will nourish you and optimizes digestion far more deeply than when you eat mindlessly. Developing healthy eating practices and increasing your intake of fruits, vegetables, and healthy fats will deliver the biological information and energy needed to optimize cellular regeneration. And when you are no longer eating for hunger but as a source of distraction, entertainment, or self-medication, do eat less—those who do so live longer. Here are some daily eating practices to embrace:

1. Eat something raw with each meal. (It is worth repeating that only raw food contains plant stem cells known as meristematic cells, which powerfully contribute to your life energy and longevity.)

2. Be mindful and take joy in eating.

3. Remember: fat is your friend and the key to deeply satisfying your appetite and cravings for sweet things. Incorporate healthy oils for cooking and dressing vegetables. Add whole food sources of fat, such as coconut, avocado, olives, certain cold-water fish, nuts, and whole eggs with the yolks, to your diet.

4. Eat or drink something fermented daily to support the healthy bacteria in your microbiome.

5. Don't get overly fixated on eating three square meals a day. Replace at least one meal a day with delicious and highly therapeutic smoothies made from superfoods and regenerative plant extracts. You'll feel more deeply nourished and energized this way.

6. Increase your dietary fiber in the form of microbiota-accessible carbohydrates or prebiotics. Prebiotics are a special class of fiber that resists hydrolysis by gastric acidity and mammalian enzymes and is instead selectively fermented by the intestinal flora, augmenting the growth or activity of flora that confer a health benefit to the host. Prebiotics include Jerusalem artichokes, onions, garlic, leeks, asparagus, green bananas, cocoa, jicama, almonds, blueberries, carrots, cassava, pumpkin, and taro.

In this phase you are likely to experience a number of positive changes. First, the constant craving for quick-fix energy boosters, from caffeine to sugary or refined carbohydrate-rich snacks, will start to fall away. As your body becomes better fat-adapted, many of your past "comfort" foods will lose their addictive appeal. With this, your entire system will receive a signal of safety and deeper nourishment that it may not have experienced since back when you were a baby. When we rely on the neuroendocrine roller-coaster of high-glycemic foods followed by insulin releases and subsequent blood sugar crashes to power ourselves through the day, we are whipping our adrenals and following a fight-or-flight pattern that is deeply compromising to our health. As your general stress levels taper off, you may also notice your sleep improve, which can create an incredible enhancement in your regenerative capabilities. In addition, since many of the foods in the ancestral diet require you to acquire and prepare them yourself, you will be benefiting profoundly from the "medicine" of self-care. When you nourish yourself, your soul will heal just as much your body.

SUPPLEMENTATION

Nourishing Your Regenerating Body (2 weeks)

Even with a concerted effort to buy organic food, given the current universal problem of poor and declining food quality, it is often advisable to supplement your diet. While the Regenerate Rx philosophy prioritizes supplementing in culinary form rather than with a pill or tablet, in this phase, you will be encouraged to add a few core supplements to your regimen. Some of these supplements function as nutritional insurance against so many of the chronic diseases that inevitably proceed from the modern lifestyle. It is my belief that something as seemingly insignificant as a pinch of turmeric (or a capsule, when taken as a supplement) can contain biological information so indispensable for the health of your body that its regular use could profoundly alter your entire life's health destiny.

But the key is not to take excessive doses, nor dozens of different supplements. Research bears out that smaller doses are sometimes more therapeutic than larger ones! If you are trying something new, introduce it slowly, and don't add anything else for at least three days so your body has a chance to adjust. Your body is wise and knows what's good for it or not. You just have to listen carefully. My suggestion is to pick no more than two of the featured regenerative substances below to try over the next two weeks.

SPECIAL PLANT ALLIES/REGENERATORS

- **Turmeric**—A golden-hued spice and longtime culinary cornerstone of Chinese, Indian, Iranian, Malaysian, Polynesian, and Thai cultures, turmeric promotes tissue regeneration, targets cancer stem cells, and fights inflammation and tumor formation. Although turmeric can easily be incorporated into marinades, salad dressings, or smoothies, the lightly spiced drink known as "golden milk," prepared with warming spices such as cinnamon and ginger along with turmeric, coconut milk, and either raw honey or maple syrup to taste, has been revered since ancient times for its healing properties. Turmeric is a good spice for cooking, and a pinch of it can be added to a smoothie. The fat-soluble compound in turmeric known as alpha-turmerone has neural stem cell–regenerating properties,[1] which is why fat-based culinary applications using the whole root powder like curry are exceptionally beneficial for regeneration. When using it in culinary form, a teaspoon a few days a week is sufficient. If you are looking to get a more regular and consistent dose, I recommend using 500 mg daily of a broad-spectrum extract (containing all three water-, fat-, and alcohol-soluble forms).

- **Resveratrol**—The best sources of this incredibly regenerative compound can be found in a broad range of commonly consumed foods, including blueberries, cocoa, cranberries, grapes (organic and wild for higher concentrations), and peanuts, but you can use a 100–250 mg supplement daily to ensure you are receiving a consistent dose within a therapeutic range.

- **Black seed**—known in ancient Middle Eastern times as a veritable panacea, this versatile seed has been studied for its ability to kill MRSA, prevent chemical weapons toxicity, relieve joint pain, and stimulate regeneration in the beta cells of Type 1 diabetics. It can help soothe the nervous system and provides a natural anti-inflammatory alternative to NSAID drugs and aspirin. I prefer a teaspoon of cold-pressed oil taken in the evening before bedtime, as it has relaxing properties that can help you sleep.

- **Cannabidiol (from cannabis or hemp)** —CBD is the only supplement that has an entire body system (the endocannabinoid system) named after it. Hundreds of peer-reviewed studies show CBD's value in dozens of health conditions, most notably nervous system disorders. I take a liquid form containing 60 mg per serving in the evening before bed, in order to help me relax and take full advantage of the regenerative opportunity of a good night's sleep.

- **Flaxseed**—A mucilaginous seed similar in appearance to the mucus-secreting epithelial cells in the human digestive tract that it protects (a poetic example of "like cures like"), flaxseed has been found to be particularly effective at inhibiting the growth of breast and prostate cancers, which are also epithelial tissues in type.

  One of my favorite ways to use flaxseed is by adding a teaspoon or two to smoothies or putting a few pinches into cooked recipes, such as paleo pancakes. If you can eat at least a tablespoon a day, it also has a highly beneficial effect for elimination, as it is a natural laxative but can also provide bulk if the opposite is a problem.

- **Pomegranate**—Technically a berry and the fruiting ovary of the pomegranate plant, this extremely therapeutic food has the ability to support human hormone health by providing bioidentical steroid hormones (such as estrone and testosterone) normally found within the mammalian ovary. This translates into rejuvenating effects in women, including reducing complaints related to hormone insufficiency, as well as increasing bone strength and quality. It has powerful artery-cleaning and healing properties and potent anticancer and anti-infective activity. A glass of its juice a day can have transformative health effects. Remember that the whole food is always more therapeutic, so eat pomegranate seeds, which make a great snack or garnish for main dishes and green salads.

- **Fermented food**—Between the hard-and-fast dichotomies of cooked and raw and dead and alive is this beautiful category called fermented foods. These living foods contain a wide range of additional vitamins and therapeutic compounds that are a by-product of the amazing alchemical activities of the probiotic bacteria found within them. Whenever possible, consume fermented food like kimchi, sauerkraut, kombucha, and coconut yogurt daily as an ongoing support in restoring, regenerating, and maintaining your microbiome.

- **Ginger**—This widely used spice and folk medicine has a vast range of health benefits, particularly targeting cancer stem cell activity, reducing inflammation, and helping to address metabolic syndrome–related disorders and full-blown Type 2 diabetes. I like to include it as a culinary spice in curries, stir fries, and soups but will also add the fresh variety, grated, to a drink or a smoothie. A "shot" of several ounces a day boosts my circulation and energy levels, especially on the days I feel I need it. For convenience, a supplement containing 500–1,000 mg of organic ginger powder is an excellent way to take it (best in the middle of a meal with water).

- **Biomelanin (Chaga)** —Chaga mushroom is one of nature's best sources of the highly protective, dark melanin pigment, which has been used in traditional medicine to fight cancer. Biomelanin has unique properties and may help to protect against harmful electromagnetic radiation in the environment. As Chaga is neither commonly available nor regularly used in culinary practice, I prefer taking a supplement of 500 mg a day for general protection.

- **Chlorophyll-rich foods**—The plant pigment chlorophyll is essential for supercharging your mitochondria and enables them to extract sunlight energy from the environment similarly to plants. Choose foods that are replete with magnesium-based chlorophyll (therefore green), such as broccoli, chard, chlorella, collards, kale, and parsley. Sometimes I will take a supplement form (either pill or liquid extract) of chlorophyll concentrate containing 100 mg per serving, or chlorella tablets (500 mg a day) with broken cell walls in order to take advantage of their heavy metal–chelating properties.

- **Magnesium**—Fundamental to the function of thousands of biological pathways and hundreds of enzymes within the body, magnesium is essential to extracting energy from mitochondria in the form of magnesium-ATP chelate. Taking a supplement, such as magnesium glycinate (200–400 mg a day), can go a long way toward replenishing your stores. If you ingest too much, it will have a mild laxative effect, so you can taper down your dose. If the laxative effect is what you desire, take magnesium citrate or magnesium oxide, which are great stool softeners and laxatives.

- **Ginkgo biloba**—The only plant known to have survived the atomic blast at Hiroshima, ginkgo biloba is so ancient a species that it is described as "a living fossil." A growing body of research shows it may confer life-extending properties on those who take it, but make sure your supplement brand removes the naturally occurring antivitamin known as ginkgotoxin (4'-O-methylpyridoxine), which is structurally related to B_6, or make sure you have adequate B_6 in your diet or supplement regimen. I find a 60–120 mg dose range most therapeutic.

- **Aloe vera**—A succulent plant species originally from the Arabian Peninsula, aloe vera is now used throughout the world for dermal and digestive issues. It has a deeply soothing gel that can greatly increase hydration in your tissues, especially your skin. I prefer the Lakewood aloe gel, which comes in a glass jar and is preserved only with vitamin C, and take one to two ounces a day as a therapeutic dose.

- **Fish oil**—A high-quality fish oil consumed daily in a 1–3,000 mg dose will go a long way toward compensating for the widespread dietary deficiency of omega-3 rich fatty acids, particularly DHA and EPA. I prefer liquid forms in stored glass, preferably flushed with nitrogen to prevent rancidity (e.g., Carlson's cod liver oil).

- **Red and American wild-crafted ginseng—**
  A powerful longevity promoter, ginseng has been
  known since ancient times to enliven, invigorate, and
  extend life-span and quality of life. Wild-harvested
  and organically produced forms are best, with
  mountain-sourced forms being highest in life energy.
  A dose between 250 and 500 mg is well within the
  therapeutic range.

- **Olive leaf—**An incredibly rich source of vital
  antioxidant and genome-supercharging biomolecules,
  such as oleuropein and tyrosol, olive leaf captures
  many of the same benefits as high-quality olive
  oil, but you only need to take a small amount
  daily. It also doubles as a protective shield against
  opportunistic, pathogenic bacteria and viruses.
  There are manufacturers of broad-spectrum olive
  leaf extract, as well as capsule forms. In either case, a
  dose range of 500 mg will generally have a significant
  therapeutic impact.

- **Vitamin C—**One of the most compelling discoveries
  in modern nutritional science is that vitamin C can
  help to regenerate your steroid hormones,[2] as well
  as reduce the toxicity of hormone metabolites. All
  sources of vitamin C—which are most concentrated
  in fruits and vegetables—are optimal for your health,
  but if you feel you are not getting enough, you can
  add 1,000 mg a day from a food-extracted source,
  such as amla, camu camu, or a supplement from a
  whole-food vitamin manufacturer.

- **Sulforaphane-rich (cruciferous) foods—**Few
  foods carry as much detoxifying and regenerative
  power as cruciferous vegetables. These veggies, from
  cabbage to kale, but especially their sprouts, contain
  a sulfur-containing biomolecule that has over 100

evidence-based health benefits. They are most useful for the health of the liver (enhancing detoxification of fat-soluble toxicants), preventing cancer, and regenerating neural stem cells.[3] Broccoli sprouts are the most concentrated sources of sulforaphane known. For convenience, a supplement form can be used. A dose as low as 100 mg can have a potent therapeutic effect.

Note: for research on these regenerative compounds, visit the GreenMedInfo.com database, which contains thousands of studies supporting their benefits for hundreds of different conditions.

The list above is by no means exhaustive. There are an incredible number of plant and mineral allies you can work with on your healing path. Many of them are common foods and spices whose regenerative properties are seldom appreciated for their full power. Given all the amazing options, you might wonder how to find the ideal supplement to use specifically for you. You can start with your intuition and follow your senses by consuming more of what naturally appeals to you. If you are more left-brained, you can also use the accumulating body of research I've amassed on GreenMedInfo.com to find clues on how to best individualize your program. There you'll find about 2,000 natural substances that research has shown to have potential therapeutic value in over 3,000 conditions. If you are suffering from arthritis, for instance, you can view the arthritis topic page and see which of the 600 studies indexed on the topic appears most compelling. And keep in mind that the database also contains guidance for several hundred therapeutic actions, including yoga, energy work, and acupuncture, which provide "energetic" supplementation and which we'll discuss in greater depth next.

MIND/BODY HEALING

Detox and Intentional Movement Techniques (for life)

Once you've eliminated many of the degenerative ingredients and foods of the Western Pattern Diet, returned to the staples of the ancestral diet, and introduced supplements to fight inflammation, support cellular regeneration, and protect against initiation of chronic disease, you should be feeling an entirely new baseline of health emerge: one lighter, more energized, and with a growing sense of increased resilience at your core. Phase 4 is all about shifting your focus to sustaining and enhancing your newfound and newly felt sense of health and wellness by doing the following:

1. Establishing a detox routine for your body and home

2. Following intentional movement practices and connecting with nature's rhythms

3. Engaging in stress reduction and emotional healing techniques that will transform difficult emotions that underlie your food addictions and physical health issues

In Phase 4, you will learn to really enjoy your newfound bedrock of physical health by expanding on practices that encourage sustainable patterns of emotional wellness, enthusiasm, and resilience. The point is not simply to be physically fit and functional but to cultivate a sustained experience of feeling alive and well. Joseph Campbell once rightly said, "People say that what we're all seeking is a meaning for life. I don't think that's what we're really seeking. I think that what we're seeking is an experience of being alive, so that our life experiences on the purely physical plane will have resonances with our own innermost being and reality, so that we actually feel the rapture of being alive."[1]

Indeed, the word *health* is deeply connected etymologically with the words *whole* and *holy*—an indication that beyond the physical alone, true health integrates the psychospiritual and emotional dimensions as well.

Part 4 contains a range of techniques that will help you attain this spiritually integrated vision of health, which you can engage with one at a time or simultaneously, depending upon your priorities and challenges.

1. Establishing a Detox Routine

Detoxification need not involve elaborate protocols, laxatives, or a general comportment toward the body as being toxic and in need of purging. Detoxification is actually already occurring in every cell of your body, with every moment. We simply need to stop adding an excessive burden of biologically incompatible foods and toxic chemicals to it and gently support its ingeniously designed systems for eliminating wastes naturally, which include actions as simple as drinking enough water and moving daily, as you shall see.

HEALTHY BOWEL MOVEMENT

The body was designed, from the inside out, to move. The peristalsis (rhythmic contractions) of our intestines, which ensures the proper regularity and flow of our lymphatic system essential for detoxification, requires our daily movement. A change in our eating patterns can cause neurobiological rewiring, whereby habitual cravings and patterns of consumption will be neutralized and overridden by the world's most glorious inner pharmacopeia— your own brain and endocrine system. Daily movement will facilitate moving toxins and toxicants through and out of the body while breaking the cycle of addiction. The sensation of pleasure or stimulation from food will no longer act as a surrogate for deeper emotional needs or unresolved desires.

A simple bowel cleanse can kickstart the process. And that doesn't mean you will need to employ elaborate cleansing kits or heroic protocols; sometimes the best approach is simply selecting foods that have both nourishing and eliminating properties. These foods include most fruits and vegetables, nature's best cleansers and nourishers. In addition, eliminating wheat, dairy, corn, and soy, which are all used to produce industrial adhesives, will, in most cases, greatly reduce constipation.

You can also enhance elimination with the following:

- Magnesium citrate (100–200 mg a day and increasing by 200 mg a day until you have bowel tolerance, i.e., until you have regular, nonstraining bowel movements)

- Papaya (always choose organic because most conventional papaya is genetically modified and contains pesticide residues)

- Ground or milled flaxseed (three tablespoons a day)

- A bowel cleansing formula with psyllium in combination with plenty of additional water both during and after supplementation, as psyllium can absorb up to 100 times its weight in water

- Clean water (preferably spring water packaged in glass, but reverse osmosis filtered water with minerals added in will work)

- A good probiotic that was ensured to have been refrigerated while shipped to the store you are buying it from (heat can kill these strains) and/or fermented food

One of the most powerful testimonies to the power of bowel cleansing for tissue health is the book *Tissue Cleansing through Bowel Management* by Bernard Jensen. Ever since I was an infant, I struggled with constipation, and as a teen, I suffered from body-wide psoriasis. Jensen's work showed me that both linked conditions (constipation and psoriasis) can be placed into remission through the body's cleansing out of impacted stool, as well as accepting and releasing the pent-up emotions that sometimes come up. The concept is simple. Undigested processed-food components and toxic compounds, consumed over decades, accumulate and line the inside of our intestinal tracts. The use of psyllium, bentonite clay, and bowel-evacuation technologies like coffee enemas and Colema Boards help to dislodge and remove this highly toxic stool. These methods can help, as they did in my case, resolve psoriasis in a way that no medication can accomplish. I also felt that by making the effort to really take my healing into my own hands, I was able to confront and then release a layer of morbidity held in my gut, after which I felt an incredible sense of lightness and joy that I can still remember vividly 30 years later.

Additional Bowel Movement Support Mechanisms

- Daily run (use zero-drop shoes; i.e., the heel is the same height as the ball of the foot)

- Daily walk (especially after a meal, a walk can greatly facilitate digestion and elimination)

- Daily yoga (it's not just about the physical benefits; it's about learning to get comfortable with your discomfort, which has positive, wide-ranging effects in all other areas of your life)

- Sweating (e.g., through saunas in higher latitudes, infrared technologies, and consumption of fresh ginger)

- Skin brushing (a process of using a brush with stiff bristles to exfoliate dead skin cells and enhance blood flow)

A WEEKLY DIETARY DETOX THAT WORKS FOR YOU

Once a week, practice a form of caloric restriction, even if it is only skipping breakfast one morning. Don't do it if you are truly feeling hunger; rather, refrain from eating strictly out of habit. If you are intentional about it and you aren't feeling deprived by your own inner disciplinarian, it will enable your digestive organs to rest so your body can focus on cleaning house and regenerating internally.

If you like how you feel from the practice suggested above, you may want to work your way up from the one-day mono detox with apples to more advanced fasting techniques. If you don't feel like you are able to do an advanced fast, a mini-fast between dinner and lunch the next day will still be helpful.

Consider the concept of breakfast as "breaking the fast." Simply not eating for 12 hours, from dinner to breakfast, is a form of fasting, and breaking fast every morning is actually a normal part of our daily metabolic cycle. Since it was normal to experience cycles of feast followed by famine in ancestral times and life forms have adapted to the cycle of the seasons for millions of years, our bodies have likely evolved to benefit from occasional days without eating. And because our bodies have alternative sources of energy and matter available directly from the quantum vacuum, fasting can be defined as an act of intentional self-deprivation that reorients our bodily needs toward a source of sustenance that is invisible but no less real.

But fasting within the Regenerate Rx program is more than a way to simply obtain sustenance without food. It is a powerful source of transformation that produces extreme resilience. Scientists at the University of Southern California have found that after three days of water fasting, the body flips a regenerative switch. Stem cells begin to produce new white blood cells, thereby creating an entire new immune system.[2]

Fasting Progression

For an optimal fasting experience, start by practicing it one day per week, preferably on a weekend, and then, when you have confidence in your body's ability to maintain itself without food for a day, move to 2 or 3 days per week for a complete immune system regeneration. You can "fast" by avoiding food consumption for at least 8–12 hours a day, engaging in a one-day apple fast, a one- to three-day raw food fast, or a one- to three-day water fast.

Fasting is a time for deep rest. Reduce the activities and responsibilities in your schedule as much as possible within this window. This time without distractions will open you up for deep insight and a renewed sense of commitment to self-care. A deliberate fast is a way to engage intentionally and mindfully with the process of investing and caring for yourself in a way that will result in deeply reinvigorated physical and mental health.

Detox plans don't have to be brutal. Although a water fast can be a profoundly healing option for those who are ready for an advanced program, you do not need to go without food for long periods to experience detoxification's benefits. Below you'll find three detox plans. They range from short and simple to longer and more challenging. Choose the one that is right for you. When you're done with your detox, return to the ancestral diet to maintain your hard-won gains and to continue to experience their perpetual and ever-expanding dividends.

The Three-Day Raw Foods Detox

If you are ready to venture beyond the Apple and Clean Water Mono Diet, continue for another day with just apples, or proceed to a less restrictive diet by incorporating raw fruit and vegetables for three days. Graze on fresh fruit and vegetables in the amounts you desire. Fruits and vegetables with seeds are sometimes called "perfect foods" because they are designed by nature to be consumed by animals that have an ability to disperse their seeds. The flesh of the fruit and vegetables will provide essential biomolecular and informational support to your body, in addition to live enzymes, structured water, and bioactive phytonutrients, which gently modulate our gene expression and nudge our physiology toward homeostasis.

Shopping ahead is key. Stock your fridge so that you don't fall back on cooked options. If you are going to be away from home, take with you readily available raw snacks.

Temporary effects of this diet can include bloating and gas, which normally resolve within a day as your microbiome and elimination processes adjust. And as with the Apple and Clean Water Mono Diet, you can expect to feel joyful and light, and pain, inflammation, and extra pounds may melt away.

The Water Fast

Water fasts can be more intimidating than mono-diets. The idea of food deprivation, however short-lived, can inspire primal fear in some, but once you try it, you will realize that your body is incredibly resilient and healthy and revitalized when cut off from the often subpar and toxic foods we consume. That said, for those with chronic health conditions (especially if you are on medication), a water fast should only be done under the supervision of a health-care provider. Those without these constraints need only listen to their bodies (and their inner physicians) to embrace this challenge as a rich opportunity for resetting and regenerating their health.

To get the complete effects of a regenerated immune system, you will need to fast for three days. I highly recommend building up to a three-day water fast over three weeks. During the first week, take a one-day water fast. During the second week, fast for two days. By the third week, you'll be ready for the full three-day fast. During the buildup period, you'll gain experience navigating the break-the-fast phase. After a day (or two or three) of fasting, you should break the fast with a very simple raw food, such as berries or avocado. For lunch, move on to something basic but cooked, like a sweet potato or quinoa, including a pat of butter (goat butter is easiest to digest and least allergenic).

To help enable the successful completion of this fast, plan to do it on a weekend or during vacation, and recruit the support of a partner if you have other responsibilities, such as taking care of children.

Expect some listlessness and fatigue in the beginning stages. But after three days, your less-than-healthy tissues throughout your entire body will have undergone autophagy, and your immune system will be completely regenerated. You are likely to feel a renewed sense of lightness, and energy levels that well up from deep within the core of your being. You may experience a remarkable feeling of satiety and sustained energy, as well as a clear-headedness that comes from the fact that fasting can sometimes stabilize your insulin and blood sugar levels.

DETOX FROM CHEMICALS
IN TOPICAL AND CLEANING PRODUCTS
FOR YOUR BODY AND HOME

Our home and body products expose us to man-made toxicants that include over 80,000 chemicals registered with the EPA. I strongly recommend investing in home, cosmetics, and personal care products that do not contain petroleum derivatives. The first toxicants to target are frequently found in the following:

- Chemical cleaners and detergents

- Petrochemical-containing body care and cosmetics

- Over-the-counter drugs

- Fluoride-containing toothpastes

- Synthetic mattresses

Be especially aware of sunscreen, certain varieties of which can deliver an array of disruptive and degenerative chemicals directly into your body. To avoid sunburn, consider these topical and dietary protections:

- A petrochemical-free, nanoparticle-free titanium dioxide or zinc oxide–based sunscreen

- Coconut oil (SPF 7)

- Olive Oil (SPF 7.5)

- Castor oil (SPF 5.6)[3]

For the best sunburn remedy, apply the gel of the aloe vera plant, which, in addition to its healing role, is the best natural antiaging topical agent for your body. If you have access to an aloe plant, scrape the gel from the leaves and make sure to drain the red "latex," which can have a laxative effect. Or you can use a store-bought product such as Lakewood Organic Pure Aloe Gel.

2. Intentional Movement Practices and Connect with Nature's Rhythms

Sitting has been called "the new smoking" for a reason. Without daily exercise, metabolic waste products, toxins, and chemical toxicants can't move out of your body. Daily exercise will restore balance in your body and your nervous system and connect you to nature and its energetic rhythms and electromagnetic fields. That's the reason why Regenerate Rx posits that strenuous activity of at least 30 minutes every other day is essential to promoting radical resilience. A study published in *Advances in Experimental Medicine and Biology* showed that exercise induces a wave of gene-altering microRNAs, providing a molecular explanation for the incredible benefits of exercise for the heart.[4]

When you consider our sedentary lifestyles and the very limited, mechanistic, routine ways in which we engage in movement, it is no wonder that so many of us are left feeling tired, depressed, and powerless over our bodies and our destinies. Exercise affords an opportunity to retake the reins and move with intentionality and deliberation. It may be as simple as just setting a goal and striving in a very real, physical way toward accomplishing it. This is the spiritual heart of exercise and why it can generate a visceral sensation of deep empowerment and self-efficacy.

How I Learned to
Love Running

It took me a long time to begin a daily exercise program. As a child, I was far from athletic. Having struggled with severe respiratory challenges from asthma and a chronically inflamed hip and shortened right femur, I lacked vitality, had a limp, and was overweight. I had dabbled in various forms of athletics as a teenager and adult and eventually suffered a chronic back injury from lifting weights, which prevented me from doing strenuous forms of exercise requiring greater range of motion.

Finally, at the age of 44, I took up regular running. I found that jogging worked well for me, given that it only required I keep my back upright. Admittedly, it did not take me long to fall in love with this arduous but often joyous form of deliberate movement. I also discovered Christopher McDougall's *Born to Run*, which argues that our bodies are designed for and capable of running hundreds of miles, which our subsistence hunter ancestors had to do to catch their prey. The prey had to die of exhaustion before the human predator could eat!

I decided to try running longer distances and trusted that my body would support me. Now I am an avid half-marathon runner and completed a full marathon just for this book, in order to prove that it is possible to become fit at any age. The discomfort of a hard run is more than balanced by how good I feel afterward. In many ways, distance running has shown me that suffering and joy are two sides of the same coin. If you persist beyond what you thought your limitations were and succeed, you can build the confidence and resilience that is your birthright. What I love most about running is that it strengthens and enlivens both my spiritual and my physical hearts.

There are many forms of intentional movement that produce physical and mental benefits, and you should find what works for you. Engage in conscious movement of any kind, from high-intensity interval exercise to dancing to yoga. Intentional movement will help you retain muscle and keep lean, but even more crucially, it will help to clear out your lymphatic system. The lymphatic system doesn't have a pump and thus cannot detoxify without movement. Moving also enhances elimination (bowel movements), which is necessary for cleaning house. And sweating expels persistent accumulated toxins and chemicals that damage and kill cells. Saunas are not a substitute for exercise, but they also confer the deeply cleansing benefits of sweating.

In addition to more strenuous forms of exercise, remember to regularly connect with nature. Spending time outdoors is essential in supporting health. Air, sunshine, and grounding are intensely therapeutic and regenerative, especially when combined with an intentional movement practice. Exposing your body to the whole spectrum of light from sunrise to sunset helps to restore circadian rhythm. Practice natural photobiomodulation by being unencumbered by sunscreen, extensive clothing, and sunglasses (being careful not to overexpose yourself during the most intense midday hours). Consuming chlorophyll daily will provide you with sunscreen protection internally and will enable your body to harvest sunlight for enhanced mitochondrial function. Grounding will help to discharge electromagnetic flux within the body.

Intentional movement and contact with nature help to establish healthier sleeping habits. To support these benefits, minimize all contact with electronics after dusk. Wearing blue-blocking eyewear to shield against light pollution from self-luminous devices has been shown to improve sleep efficacy, sleep latency, and melatonin production.[5] Try to sleep in an electronic device–free, darkened room, preferably on a natural mattress. You can also use an eye mask if there is ambient light. Most people attain the best sleep by getting somewhere between seven and nine hours of it. When your body tells you it needs rest, it's wise to listen.

Lastly, develop a breathing practice or exercise involving significant exertion to pull in the energy (a.k.a. prana, chi, or shakti) of the environment and/or quantum vacuum. Early morning meditation or prayer is essential in setting up a baseline of stability within your nervous system that will carry you through the day with greater equanimity and resilience. Simply being aware of your breath will enable you to focus on being present. Sometimes a commitment of 10 minutes a day, divided between morning and night, helps to soothe and deescalate emotional distress. Setting a clear intention will help you to declutter your mind and realize your objectives and dreams with consistency. Meditation is also a form of psychic metabolism, without which life's many experiences, including the difficult ones, may never be digested and can manifest somatically as stomach and other bodily complaints.

3. MIND/BODY HEALING TECHNIQUES

As you move through this program, the emotions that may come up are the raw material for your alchemical transformation. Without anger, sadness, grief, fear, or anxiety surfacing, your self-reclamation of this transformative potential would have a low ceiling. The good news is that once they are released and metabolized, your autonomic nervous system will come back into balance. But without using the proper tools to identify, accept, and transform them, they will likely return to their subconscious expression.

Identifying and expressing emotion rather than suppressing it under the facade of positive thinking is an essential part of mind/body healing. Evolutionarily, emotions serve a purpose by helping you learn and survive. According to Candace Pert, it is not the emotions we should control but our response to them. "Anger, grief, fear—these emotional experiences are not negative in themselves," she wrote. "In fact, they are vital for our survival. We need anger to define boundaries, grief to deal with our losses, and fear to protect ourselves from danger."[6] Likewise, spiritual luminary Eckhart Tolle encourages us not to resist our pain: "Surrender to the grief, despair, fear, loneliness, or whatever form the suffering takes. Witness it without labeling it mentally. Allow it to be there. Embrace it. Then see how the miracle of surrender transmutes deep suffering into deep peace."[7]

It's so easy to fall headfirst, flailing and somersaulting down the bottomless abyss of self-pity. The reverberating chorus of "Why me?" can become a broken record player of negative self-talk, limiting beliefs, and a mind-set rooted in scarcity and what-ifs. To lose yourself under this weight is to become trapped, buried, and eventually broken.

However, allowing yourself to feel the tantrum, the tears, and the turmoil that are always buried beneath the surface of your ego's relatively limited awareness can help to heal and transform these crucially important parts of yourself. My wife, Kelly Brogan, M.D., wrote an entire book on this topic called *Own Your Self*, which I highly recommend. She shows you how the life-shattering, compass-changing, direction-altering magnitude of your experiences can be illuminated and how your maladaptive ruminations can be transformed into a cathartic release. But in order to do so, you have to pick yourself up, dust yourself off, and find the personal invitation and profound symbolism embedded within every symptom.

The robustness of this shift requires that we take radical responsibility for our well being and address all three of its pillars—mind, body, and health. To manage your mind-set and mitigate your stress, try out the following:

1. **Emotional Freedom Technique (EFT).** Sometimes described as a "psychological acupressure technique," EFT helps to manage the impact of difficult emotions through diaphragmatic breathing, mantras and affirmations, visualizations, and heart rate variability training tools. Also known as "tapping" and energy medicine, EFT is related to reiki and Eastern

traditions such as yoga, tai chi, qigong, and meditation, which can also provide relief.

2. **Aromatherapy.** Botanical agents provide a natural buffer to stress-induced pathophysiological changes and act as adaptogens that improve the body's ability to cope with and counteract stress. When organisms are confronted with stress, these substances enable them to avoid stressor-induced damage.[8] When used in concert with mindfulness techniques and an evolutionarily appropriate diet and lifestyle, adaptogens can course-correct our physiology and better contend with a barrage of never-ending stress. When inhaled, essential oils, such as patchouli, can reduce the activity of the sympathetic nervous system by up to 40 percent, and rose oil can reduce epinephrine (adrenaline) concentrations by up to 30 percent.[9] Orange and lavender oils have been found to significantly reduce anxiety and improve mood,[10] and aromatherapy with lavender, ylang-ylang, and bergamot has been found to significantly reduce psychological stress and serum cortisol, in addition to lowering blood pressure of people with essential hypertension.[11] Even the very brief exposure of five minutes to the aroma of lemongrass has been proven to mitigate tension and promote recovery from anxiety-provoking situations.[12]

3. **Therapeutic Massage and Deep Bodywork.** Therapeutic touch, including deep tissue massage, can go a long way in compensating for the inevitable stresses of modern living. For even deeper support, try myofascial release, Rolfing, and Amanae, which can help us work through deeper emotional blocks and triggers that are locked as stagnant and obstructed energy in our physical bodies. Sometimes chronic pain and immobility are symptoms of an

unexplored inner life calling out to be understood and loved. Deep childhood traumas, for instance, can manifest themselves in common medical complaints, as Louise Hay taught us many years ago in *You Can Heal Your Life.*

4. **Yoga and Meditation.** The ancient Indian practice of kundalini yoga balances your chakras and meridians by activating your energetic or ethereal body while also awakening the full potential of your physical body, including the nervous and glandular systems.[13] Sounds and chanting are believed to activate meridian points in your palate that connect to your hypothalamus and pituitary glands. Candace Pert has endorsed the ancient techniques of kundalini yoga as a means to restore a state of mind-body harmony.

   Meditation is another means of deriving immense mind-body benefits. An article in the journal *Psychiatry Research* showed that mindfulness techniques such as meditation are so powerful that they can even change the structure of the brain itself. Mindfulness-based stress reduction mitigates stress-induced pathophysiological changes by enhancing gray matter concentration within the hippocampus, the posterior cingulate cortex, the temporoparietal junction, and the cerebellum—the brain regions involved in memory, learning, emotional intelligence, perspective taking, and self-referential processing.[14] In addition, a meta-analysis published in *National Reviews in Neuroscience* found that mindfulness meditation consistently altered tissue morphology in six brain regions, including the anterior and posterior cingulate, amygdala, insula, prefrontal cortex, and striatum.[15] Meditation can also modify the parts of our neural circuitry that regulate self-awareness, emotional processing, and present-moment awareness.[16]

The Mindfulness/Resilience Connection

Mindfulness rituals improve the functioning of our nervous system, which coordinates our stress response and talks to our immune system in a lively two-way conversation. Meditation in all its incarnations—from a guided audio practice to yoga to tai chi to the flow state that comes from pursuing creative endeavors or our passions—quiets our "monkey mind" and optimizes bodily harmony. Through this natural technology, we can send top-down signals of safety throughout the body to allow for regeneration.

- **Journaling.** Sometimes simply putting pen to paper for five minutes each day, especially first thing in the morning or before bed in the evening, will help one identify feelings that were not fully conscious yet contributed to choices, experiences, and circumstances.

- **Homeopathy.** Under the guidance of a trained homeopath, this safe form of informational medicine uses exceedingly small doses of natural substances and can be customized to any individual's emotional and psychospiritual constitution.

- **Plant Medicine.** Under the guidance of a skilled and experienced medicine man, woman, or person, psychedelic agents such as psilocybin or ayahuasca can have lifesaving and transformative power. Denver, CO, and Sonoma County, CA, are some of the locations that have legalized the use of certain psychedelic plants for adults 21 and older.

- **Counseling.** Let's face it: without the help of others, none of us would be here today. A skilled, compassionate, professional counselor who can provide witness and support to your process will enable you to resolve some of your greatest challenges.

FINAL WORDS

The writing of this book was something of a journey (as I imagine has been the reading of it), and I want to sincerely thank you for joining me. When I look back at the path I've taken to get here, I am simply amazed at how much support I have received from sources known and unknown, delivering me through many physical and psychospiritual trials and tribulations to produce the book you are holding in your hands. From the regular, life-threatening asthma attacks I experienced as an infant to the lung-expanding marathon I ran last year, I am shown each and every day how profoundly resilient and regenerative is this miraculous technology called the human body, no matter how often we take it for granted.

We now find ourselves on the precipice of an amazing age of deep insight, where the full wisdom of the ancients, long encoded as remnants in myth and symbol, and leading-edge science in the New Biology and New Physics are coming into greater agreement and mutual validation of one another. I can only pray that by helping to uncover and share some of these insights that I have, in some small part, helped you find your way to a life of renewed vitality, insight, health, and joy so you can focus on what matters most in your life. At the very least, I hope you will walk away with greater confidence in just how amazing your body's immense regenerative potential and resilience really are. The best possible outcome I can imagine is that you will learn, as I have, to experience deeper awe and gratitude for what already is: this miracle of our incarnation and the planet that continually nourishes and supports everything in our lives.

ENDNOTES

INTRODUCTION

1. Scott R. Baier et al., "MicroRNAs Are Absorbed in Biologically Meaningful Amounts from Nutritionally Relevant Doses of Cow Milk and Affect Gene Expression in Peripheral Blood Mononuclear Cells, HEK-293 Kidney Cell Cultures, and Mouse Livers," *The Journal of Nutrition* 144, no. 10 (October 2014): 1495–500, https://doi.org/10.3945/jn.114.196436.

2. S. Byars, S. Stearns, J. Boomsma, "Association of Long-Term Risk of Respiratory, Allergic, and Infectious Diseases With Removal of Adenoids and Tonsils in Childhood," *JAMA Otolaryngolgy Head Neck Surgery* 144, 7 (2018): 594–603, https://doi.org/10.1001/jamaoto.2018.0614.

PART ONE

CHAPTER I

1. "Chronic Disease: A Significant Public Health Threat," Centers for Disease Control, November 21, 2017, https://www.cdc.gov/nccdphp/dch/about/index.htm.

2. Carlton Gyles, "Skeptical of Medical Science Reports?," *Canadian Veterinary Journal*, 56, no. 10 (October 2015): 1011–1012, https://www.ncbi.nlm.nih.gov/pmc/articles/PMC4572812/.

3. Gyles, "Skeptical of Medical Science Reports?,"1011–1012.

4. Florence T. Bourgeois, Srinivas Murthy, and Kenneth D. Mandl, "Outcome Reporting among Drug Trials Registered in ClinicalTrials.gov," *Annals of Internal Medicine* 153, no. 3 (2010): 158–66, https://doi.org/10.7326/0003-4819-153-3-201008030-00006.

5. Erick H. Turner et al., "Selective Publication of Antidepressant Trials and Its Influence on Apparent Efficacy," *New England Journal of Medicine* 358, no. 3 (2008): 252–60, https://doi.org/10.1056/NEJMsa065779.

6. John P. A. Ioannidis, "Why Most Published Research Findings Are False," *PLoS Medicine* 2, no. 8 (2005): e124, https://doi.org/10.1371/journal.pmed.0020124; and Alex Hern and Pamela Duncan, "Predatory Publishers: The Journals That Churn Out Fake Science," *The Guardian*, August 10, 2018, https://www.theguardian.com/technology/2018/aug/10/predatory-publishers-the-journals-who-churn-out-fake-science.

7. Jessica J. Liu et al., "Payments by US Pharmaceutical and Medical Device Manufacturers to US Medical Journal Editors: Retrospective Observational Study," *BMJ* 359 (October 26, 2017): j4619, https://doi.org/10.1136/bmj.j4619.

8. Eric G. Campbell et al., "A National Survey of Physician-Industry Relationships," *New England Journal of Medicine* 356, no. 17 (2007):1742–50, https://doi.org/10.1056/NEJMsa064508.

9. Freek Fickweiler, Ward Fickweiler, and Ewout Urbach, "Interactions Between Physicians and the Pharmaceutical Industry Generally and Sales Representatives Specifically and Their Association With Physicians' Attitudes and Prescribing Habits: A Systematic Review," *BMJ Open* 7, no. 9 (2017): e016408, https://doi.org/10.1136/bmjopen-2017-016408.

10. Iakes Ezkurdia et al., "Multiple Evidence Strands Suggest That There May Be as Few as 19,000 Human Protein-Coding Genes," *Human Molecular Genetics* 23, no. 22 (2014): 5866–78, https://doi.org/10.1093/hmg/ddu309.

11. Bob Weinhold, "Epigenetics: The Science of Change," *Environmental Health Perspectives* 114, no. 3 (2006): A160–67, https://doi.org/10.1289/ehp.114-a160.

12. Nevilde Maria Riselo Sales, Patrícia Barbosa Pelegrini, and Maria Clara da Silva Goersch, "Nutrigenomics: Definitions and Advances of This New Science," *Journal of Nutrition and Metabolism* (2014): 202759, https://doi.org/10.1155/2014/202759.

13. Christopher Paul Wild, "The Exposome: From Concept to Utility," *International Journal of Epidemiology* 41, no. 1 (February 2012): 24–32, https://doi.org/10.1093/ije/dyr236.

14. Stephen M. Rappaport, "Genetic Factors Are Not the Major Causes of Chronic Diseases," *PLOS ONE* 11, no. 4 (2016): e0154387, https://doi.org/10.1371/journal.pone.0154387.

15. Weinhold, "Epigenetics: The Science of Change," A160–67.

16. Weinhold, "Epigenetics: The Science of Change," A160–67.

17. Matthew D. Anway et al., "Epigenetic Transgenerational Actions of Endocrine Disruptors and Male Fertility," *Science* 308, 5727 (2005): 1466–69, https://doi.org/10.1126/science.1108190.

18. Brian G. Dias and Kerry J. Ressler, "Parental Olfactory Experience Influences Behavior and Neural Structure in Subsequent Generations," *Nature Neuroscience* 17, no. 1 (2014): 89–98, https://doi.org/10.1038/nn.3594.

19. Aryeh Stein et al., "Maternal Exposure to the Dutch Famine Before Conception and During Pregnancy: Quality of Life and Depressive Symptoms in Adult Offspring," *Epidemiology* 20, no. 6 (2009): 909–15, https://doi.org/10.1097/EDE.0b013e3181b5f227.

20. Amit Shrira, Ravit Menashe, and Moshe Bensimon, "Filial Anxiety and Sense of Obligation among Offspring of Holocaust Survivors," *Aging & Mental Health* 23, 6 (2018): 752–761, https://www.doi.org/10.1080/13607863.2018 .1448970.

21. K. M. Radke et al., "Transgenerational Impact of Intimate Partner Violence on Methylation in the Promoter of the Glucocorticoid Receptor," *Translational Psychiatry* 1 (2011): e21, https://doi.org/10.1038/tp.2011.21.

22. Anoek Zomer, et al., "Exosomes: Fit to deliver Deliver small Small RNA," *Communicative and & Integrative Biology* 3, no. 5 (2010): 447–450, https://doi .org/10.4161/cib.3.5.12339.

23. Christina Cossetti et al., "Soma-to-Germline Transmission of RNA in Mice Xenografted with Human Tumour Cells: Possible Transport by Exosomes," *PLOS ONE* 9, no. 7 (2014): e101629, https://doi.org/10.1371/journal.pone .0101629.

24. Jana P. Lim and Anne Brunet, "Bridging the Transgenerational Gap with Epigenetic Memory," *Trends in Genetics* 29, no. 3 (2013): 176–86, https://doi.org/10.1016/j.tig.2012.12.008.

25. Weinhold, "Epigenetics: The Science of Change," A160–67.

26. "The Ghost in Your Genes," BBC, September 24, 2014, http://www.bbc.co .uk/sn/tvradio/programmes/horizon/ghostgenes.shtml.

27. Alan C. Logan, Martin A. Katzman, and Vicent Balanzá-Martínez, "Natural Environments, Ancestral Diets, and Microbial Ecology: Is There a Modern 'Paleo-Deficit Disorder'? Part I," *Journal of Physiological Anthropology* 34, no. 1 (2015), https://doi.org/10.1186/s40101-015-0041-y.

28. Alan C. Logan, Martin A. Katzman, and Vicent Balanzá-Martínez, "Natural Environments, Ancestral Diets, and Microbial Ecology: Is There a Modern 'Paleo-Deficit Disorder'? Part II," *Journal of Physiological Anthropology* 34, no. 9 (2015), https://doi.org/10.1186/s40101-014-0040-4.

29. Stephanie E. Chiuve et al., "Healthy Lifestyle Factors in the Primary Prevention of Coronary Heart Disease Among Men: Benefits Among Users and Nonusers of Lipid-Lowering and Antihypertensive Medications," *Circulation* 114, no. 2 (2006): 160–67, https://doi.org/10.1161/circulationaha .106.621417.

30. Roshan Karki et al., "Defining 'Mutation' and 'Polymorphism' in the Era of Personal Genomics," *BMC Medical Genomics* 8, no. 37 (2015), https://doi.org/10.1186/s12920-015-0115-z.

31. Sandro Eridani, "Sickle Cell Protection from Malaria: A Review," *Hematology Reports* 3, no. 3 (2011): e24, 72–77, https://doi.org/10.4081/hr.2011.e24.

32. Associated Press, "Clue to Why Cystic Fibrosis Has Survived," *The New York Times*, October 7, 1994, https://www.nytimes.com/1994/10/07/us/clue-to -why-cystic-fibrosis-has-survived.html.

33. Prashant Singh et al., "Global Prevalence of Celiac Disease: Systematic Review and Meta-Analysis," *Clinical Gastroenterology and Hepatology* 16, no. 6 (June 2018): 823–36, https://doi.org/10.1016/j.cgh.2017.06.037.

34. Ludvig M. Sollid and Bana Jabri, "Triggers and Drivers of Autoimmunity: Lessons from Coeliac Disease," *Nature Reviews Immunology* 13, no. 4 (2013): 294–302, https://doi.org/10.1038/nri3407.

35. Ellen R. Copson et al., "Germline BRCA Mutation and Outcome in Young-Onset Breast Cancer (POSH): A Prospective Cohort Study," *The Lancet Oncology* 19, no. 2 (2018): 169–80, https://doi.org/10.1016/ S1470-2045(17)30891-4.

36. Renguang Pei et al., "Association of BRCA1 K1183R Polymorphism with Survival in BRCA1/2-Negative Chinese Familial Breast Cancer," *Clinical Laboratory* 60, no. 1 (2014): 47–53, https://doi.org/10.7754/Clin.Lab .2013.121130.

37. Recep Ozgur Taskent et al., "Variation and Functional Impact of Neanderthal Ancestry in Western Asia," *Genome Biology and Evolution* 9, no. 12 (December 2017): 3516–24, https://doi.org/10.1093/gbe/evx216.

38. Matthew D. Neal et al., "Intestinal Stem Cells and Their Roles During Mucosal Injury and Repair," *Journal of Surgical Research* 167, no. 1 (2011): 1–8, https://doi.org/10.1016/j.jss.2010.04.037.

39. Maranke I. Koster, "Making an Epidermis," *Annals of the New York Academy of Sciences* 1170, no. 1 (2009): 7–10, https://doi.org/10.1111/j.1749-6632.2009.04363.x.

40. Matthew L. Steinhauser and Richard T. Lee, "Regeneration of the Heart," *EMBO Molecular Medicine* 3, no. 12 (2011): 701–12, https://doi.org/10.1002/ emmm.201100175.

41. Olle Lindvall and Ron McKay, "Brain Repair by Cell Replacement and Regeneration," *Proceedings of the National Academy of Sciences of the United States of America* 100, no. 13 (2003): 7430–31, https://doi.org/10.1073/ pnas.1332673100.

42. Lin Zhang et al., "Exogenous Plant MIR168a Specifically Targets Mammalian LDLRAP1: Evidence of Cross-Kingdom Regulation by MicroRNA," *Cell Research* 22 (2012): 107–26, https://doi.org/10.1038/cr.2011.158.

43. Sergey I. Ivashuta et al., "Endogenous Small RNAs in Grain: Semi- Quantification and Sequence Homology to Human and Animal Genes," *Food and Chemical Toxicology* 47, no. 2 (February 2009): 353–60, https://doi.org/10.1016/j.fct.2008.11.025.

44. Leon A. Terry, Gemma A. Chope, and Jordi Giné Bordonaba, "Effect of Water Deficit Irrigation and Inoculation with *Botrytis cinerea* on Strawberry (*Fragaria x ananassa*) Fruit Quality," *Journal of Agricultural and Food Chemistry* 55, no. 26 (2007): 10812–19, https://doi.org/10.1021/jf072101n.

45. Deepak M. Kasote et al., "Significance of Antioxidant Potential of Plants and Its Relevance to Therapeutic Applications," *International Journal of Biological Sciences* 11, no. 8 (2015): 982–91, https://doi.org/10.7150/ijbs.12096.

46. Anna Vallverdú-Queralt et al., "Evaluation of a Method to Characterize the Phenolic Profile of Organic and Conventional Tomatoes," *Journal of Agricultural and Food Chemistry* 60, no. 13 (2012): 3373–80, https://doi.org/10.1021/jf204702f.

47. Universidad de Barcelona, "Organic Tomatoes Contain Higher Levels of Antioxidants Than Conventional Tomatoes, Study Suggests," ScienceDaily, July 3, 2012, https://www.sciencedaily.com/releases/2012/07/120703120630.htm.

48. Konrad T. Howitz and David A. Sinclair, "Xenohormesis: Sensing the Chemical Cues of Other Species," *Cell* 133, no. 3 (2008): 387–91, https://doi.org/10.1016/j.cell.2008.04.019.

49. Joseph A. Baur and David A. Sinclair, "What Is Xenohormesis?," *American Journal of Pharmacology and Toxicology* 3, no. 1 (2008): 152–59, https://doi.org/10.3844/ajptsp.2008.152.159.

50. Bob Allkin et al., "Useful Plants—Medicines," in *State of the World's Plants 2017*, report, ed. K. J. Willis (London: Royal Botanic Gardens, Kew), 22–29, https://stateoftheworldsplants.org/2017/report/SOTWP_2017_4_useful_plants_medicines.pdf.

51. David Newman and G. Cragg. "Natural Products from Marine Invertebrates and Microbes as Modulators of Antitumor Targets." *Current Drug Targets* 7 (April 1, 2006): 279–304. https://doi.org/10.2174/138945006776054960.

52. Arnold Ehret, *Rational Fasting* (Pomeroy, WA: Health Research,1996), 11.

53. Michael Lutter and Eric J. Nestler, "Homeostatic and Hedonic Signals Interact in the Regulation of Food Intake," *The Journal of Nutrition* 139, no. 3 (March 2009): 629–32, https://doi.org/10.3945/jn.108.097618.

54. Bodo C. Melnik and Gerd Schmitz, "MicroRNAs: Milk's Epigenetic Regulators," *Best Practice & Research: Clinical Endocrinology & Metabolism* 31, no. 4 (August 2017): 427–42, https://doi.org/10.1016/j.beem.2017.10.003.

55. Barbara O. Rennard et al., "Chicken Soup Inhibits Neutrophil Chemotaxis *In Vitro*," *CHEST* 118, no. 4 (October 2000): 1150–57, https://doi.org/10.1378/chest.118.4.1150.

56. Kiumars Saketkhoo, Adolph Januszkiewicz, and Marvin A. Sackner, "Effects of Drinking Hot Water, Cold Water, and Chicken Soup on Nasal Mucus Velocity and Nasal Airflow Resistance," *CHEST* 74, no. 4 (October 1978): 408–10, https://doi.org/10.1016/S0012-3692(15)37387-6.

57. Norie Nagatsuka et al., "Measurement of the Radical Scavenging Activity of Chicken Jelly Soup, a Part of the Medicated Diet, 'Yakuzen', Made from Gelatin Gel Food 'Nikogori', Using Chemiluminescence and Electron Spin Resonance Methods," *International Journal of Molecular Medicine* 18, no. 1 (July 2006): 107–11, https://doi.org/10.3892/ijmm.18.1.107.

58. Farzad Zehsaz, Negin Farhangi, and Lamia Mirheidari. "The Effect of Zingiber Officinale R. Rhizomes (Ginger) on Plasma pro-Inflammatory Cytokine Levels in Well-Trained Male Endurance Runners," *Central-European Journal of Immunology* 39, no. 2 (2014): 174–80, https://doi.org/10.5114/ceji.2014.43719.

59. Seunghae Kim et al., "Ginger Extract Ameliorates Obesity and Inflammation via Regulating MicroRNA-21/132 Expression and AMPK Activation in White Adipose Tissue," *Nutrients* 10, 11 (October 2018): 1567, https://doi.org/10.3390/nu10111567.; Yun Teng et al., "Plant-Derived Exosomal MicroRNAs Shape the Gut Microbiota," *Cell Host & Microbe* 24, 5 (November 2018): 637–652, https://doi.org/10.1016/j.chom.2018.10.001.

60. Guoyao Wu et al., "Proline and Hydroxyproline Metabolism: Implications for Animal and Human Nutrition," *Amino Acids* 40, no. 4 (April 2011): 1053–63, https://doi.org/10.1007/s00726-010-0715-z.

CHAPTER 2

1. Mahmood Najafian et al., "Phloridzin Reduces Blood Glucose Levels and Improves Lipids Metabolism in Streptozotocin-Induced Diabetic Rats," *Molecular Biology Reports* 39, no. 5 (May 2012): 5299–306, https://doi.org/10.1007/s11033-011-1328-7.

2. Shu-Kun Lin, "The Fourth Phase of Water: Beyond Solid, Liquid, and Vapor. By Gerald H. Pollack (Ebner & Sons Publishers, 2013)," *Water* 5, no. 2: 638–639. https://doi.org/10.3390/w5020638.

3. "80 Adverse Effects Associated with Isolated Fructose," GreenMedInfo, accessed December 12, 2019, https://www.greenmedinfo.health/toxic-ingredient/fructose.

4. Zhen Zhou et al., "Honeysuckle-Encoded Atypical MicroRNA2911 Directly Targets Influenza A Viruses," *Cell Research* 25, no. 1 (2015): 39–49, https://doi.org/10.1038/cr.2014.130.

5. Mihaela Pertea, "The Human Transcriptome: An Unfinished Story," *Genes* 3, no. 3 (2012): 344–60, https://doi.org/10.3390/genes3030344.

6. Mark G. Caprara and Timothey W. Nilsen, "RNA: Versatility in Form and Function," *Nature Structural & Molecular Biology* 7, no. 10 (2000): 831–33, https://doi.org/10.1038/82816.

7. Laure Jobert and Hilde Nilsen, "Regulatory Mechanisms of RNA Function: Emerging Roles of DNA Repair Enzymes," *Cellular and Molecular Life Sciences* 71, no. 13 (July 2014): 2451–65, https://doi.org/10.1007/s00018-014-1562-y.

8. Zomer et al., "Exosomes: Fit to Deliver," 447–50.

9. Songwen Ju et al., "Grape Exosome-Like Nanoparticles Induce Intestinal Stem Cells and Protect Mice from DSS-Induced Colitis," *Molecular Therapy* 21, no. 7 (2013): 1345–57, https://doi.org/10.1038/mt.2013.64.

10. Ju et al., "Grape Exosome-Like Nanoparticles," 1345–57.

11. Dominique L. Ouellet et al., "MicroRNAs in Gene Regulation: When the Smallest Governs It All," *Journal of Biomedicine and Biotechnology* 2006, no. 4 (2006): 69616, https://doi.org/10.1155/JBB/2006/69616.

12. Ju et al., "Grape Exosome-Like Nanoparticles," 1345–57.

13. Ju et al., "Grape Exosome-Like Nanoparticles," 1345–57.

14. Zhang, "Exogenous Plant MIR168a," 107–26.

15. Yu-Chen Liu et al., "Plant MiRNAs Found in Human Circulating System Provide Evidences of Cross Kingdom RNAi," *BMC Genomics* 18, suppl. 2 (2017): 112, https://doi.org/10.1186/s12864-017-3502-3.

16. Ju et al., "Grape Exosome-Like Nanoparticles," 1345–57.

17. Ju et al., "Grape Exosome-Like Nanoparticles," 1345–57.

18. Ju et al., "Grape Exosome-Like Nanoparticles," 1345–57.

19. Hervé Groux and Françoise Cottrez, "The Complex Role of Interleukin-10 in Autoimmunity," *Journal of Autoimmunity* 20, no. 4 (June 2003): 281–85, https://doi.org/10.1016/S0896-8411(03)00044-1.

20. Andrew R. Chin et al., "Cross-Kingdom Inhibition of Breast Cancer Growth by Plant MiR159," *Cell Research* 26, no. 2 (2016): 217–28, https://doi.org/10.1038/cr.2016.13.

21. Groux and Cottrez, "Complex Role of Interleukin-10," 281–85.

22. Farrukh Aqil et al., "Exosomal Delivery of Berry Anthocyanidins for the Management of Ovarian Cancer," *Food & Function* 8, no. 11 (2017): 4100–7, https://doi.org/10.1039/c7fo00882a.

23. Farrukh Aqil et al., "Exosomal Delivery of Berry Anthocyanidins," 4100–7.

24. Sai Manasa Jandhyala et al., "Role of the Normal Gut Microbiota," *World Journal of Gastroenterology* 21, no. 29 (2015): 8787–803, https://doi.org/10.3748/wjg.v21.i29.8787.

25. Kenji Oishi et al., "Effect of Probiotics, Bifidobacterium Breve and Lactobacillus Casei, on Bisphenol A Exposure in Rats." *Bioscience, Biotechnology, and Biochemistry* 72, no. 6 (June 23, 2008): 1409–15. https://doi.org/10.1271/bbb.70672; and Hayato Yamanaka et al., "Degradation of Bisphenol A by Bacillus Pumilus Isolated from Kimchi, a Traditionally Fermented Food." *Applied Biochemistry and Biotechnology* 136 (February 1, 2007): 39–51. https://doi.org/10.1007/BF02685937.

26. Raish Oozeer et al., "Intestinal Microbiology in Early Life: Specific Prebiotics Can Have Similar Functionalities as Human-Milk Oligosaccharides," *The American Journal of Clinical Nutrition* 98, no. 2 (August 2013): 561S–71S, https://doi.org/10.3945/ajcn.112.038893.

27. Megan Clapp et al., "Gut Microbiota's Effect on Mental Health: The Gut-Brain Axis," *Clinics and Practice* 7, no. 4 (2017): 987, https://doi.org/10.4081/cp.2017.987.

28. M. Nazmul Huda et al., "Stool Microbiota and Vaccine Responses of Infants," *Pediatrics* 134, no. 2 (2014): e362–72, https://doi.org/10.1542/peds.2013-3937.

29. Jan-Hendrik Hehemann et al., "Transfer of Carbohydrate-Active Enzymes from Marine Bacteria to Japanese Gut Microbiota," *Nature* 464 (2010): 908–12, https://doi.org/10.1038/nature08937.

30. Tanudeep Bhattacharya, Tarini Shankar Ghosh, and Sharmila S. Mande, "Global Profiling of Carbohydrate Active Enzymes in Human Gut Microbiome," *PLOS ONE* 10, no. 11 (2015): e0142038, https://doi.org/10.1371/journal.pone.0142038.

31. Anastasia Balakireva and Andrey Zamyatnin Jr., "Properties of Gluten Intolerance: Gluten Structure, Evolution, Pathogenicity and Detoxification Capabilities," *Nutrients* 8, no. 10 (2016): 644, https://doi.org/10.3390/nu8100644.

32. Klaas Vandepoele and Yves Van de Peer, "Exploring the Plant Transcriptome through Phylogenetic Profiling," *Plant Physiology* 137, no. 1 (January 2005): 31–42, https://doi.org/10.1104/pp.104.054700.

33. Alberto Caminero et al., "Diversity of the Cultivable Human Gut Microbiome Involved in Gluten Metabolism: Isolation of Microorganisms with Potential Interest for Coeliac Disease," *FEMS Microbiology Ecology* 88, no. 2 (May 2014): 309–19, https://doi.org/10.1111/1574-6941.12295.

34. Elizabeth Thursby and Nathalie Juge, "Introduction to the Human Gut Microbiota," *Biochemical Journal* 474, no. 11 (June 2017): 1823–36, https://doi.org/10.1042/BCJ20160510.

35. Liyong Chen et al., "Sources and Intake of Resistant Starch in the Chinese Diet," *Asia Pacific Journal of Clinical Nutrition* 19, no. 2 (2010): 274–82.

36. Joanne Slavin, "Fiber and Prebiotics: Mechanisms and Health Benefits," *Nutrients* 5, no. 4 (2013):1417–35, https://doi.org/10.3390/nu5041417.

37. David J. Griffiths, "Endogenous Retroviruses in the Human Genome Sequence," *Genome* Biology 2, no. 6 (2001): reviews1017.1–17.5, https://doi.org/10.1186/gb-2001-2-6-reviews1017.

38. Jennifer Schwamm Willis, *A Lifetime of Peace: Essential Writings by and about Thich Nhat Hanh* (New York: Marlowe & Company, 2003), 141.

39. Joanne Bradbury, "Docosahexaenoic Acid (DHA): An Ancient Nutrient for the Modern Human Brain," *Nutrients* 3, no. 5 (2011): 529–54, https://doi.org/10.3390/nu3050529.

40. Alejandra Vásquez et al., "Symbionts as Major Modulators of Insect Health: Lactic Acid Bacteria and Honeybees," *PLoS ONE* 7, no. 3 (March 2012): e33188, https://doi.org/10.1371/journal.pone.0033188.

41. Ling-Nan Bu et al., "*Lactobacillus casei rhamnosus* Lcr35 in Children with Chronic Constipation," *Pediatrics International* 49, no. 4 (August 2007): 485–90, https://doi.org/10.1111/j.1442-200X.2007.02397.x.

42. Svante Twetman and Christina Stecksén-Blicks, "Probiotics and Oral Health Effects in Children," *International Journal of Paediatric Dentistry* 18, no. 1 (January 2008): 3–10, https://doi.org/10.1111/j.1365-263X.2007.00885.x.

43. Kristin Wickens et al., "A Differential Effect of 2 Probiotics in the Prevention of Eczema and Atopy: A Double-Blind, Randomized, Placebo-Controlled Trial," *The Journal of Allergy and Clinical Immunology* 122, no. 4 (October 2008): 788–94, https://doi.org/10.1016/j.jaci.2008.07.011.

44. E. Bruzzese et al., "Randomised Clinical Trial: A Lactobacillus GG and Micronutrient-Containing Mixture is Effective in Reducing Nosocomial Infections in Children, vs. Placebo," *Alimentary Pharmacology and Therapeutics* 44, no. 6 (September 2016): 568–75, https://doi.org/10.1111/apt.13740.

45. Susumu Eguchi et al., "Perioperative Synbiotic Treatment to Prevent Infectious Complications in Patients after Elective Living Donor Liver Transplantation: A Prospective Randomized Study," *The American Journal of Surgery* 201, no. 4 (April 2011): 498–502, https://doi.org/10.1016/j.amjsurg.2010.02.013.

46. E Guillemard et al., "Consumption of a Fermented Dairy Product Containing the Probiotic Lactobacillus casei DN-114 001 Reduces the Duration of Respiratory Infections in the Elderly in a Randomised Controlled Trial," *British Journal of Nutrition* 103, no. 1 (2010): 58–68, https://doi.org/10.1017/S0007114509991395.

47. K. Kajander et al., "Clinical Trial: Multispecies Probiotic Supplementation Alleviates the Symptoms of Irritable Bowel Syndrome and Stabilizes Intestinal Microbiota," *Alimentary Pharmacology & Therapeutics* 27 (2008): 48–57, https://doi.org/10.1111/j.1365-2036.2007.03542.x.

48. Hung-Chih Lin et al., "Oral Probiotics Reduce the Incidence and Severity of Necrotizing Enterocolitis in Very Low Birth Weight Infants," *Pediatrics* 115, no. 1 (January 2005): 1–4, https://doi.org/10.1542/peds.2004-1463.

49. Fady F. Abd El-Malek, Amany S. Yousef, and Samy A. El-Assar, "Hydrogel Film Loaded with New Formula from Manuka Honey for Treatment of Chronic Wound Infections," *Journal of Global Antimicrobial Resistance* 11 (2017): 171–76, https://doi.org/10.1016/j.jgar.2017.08.007.

50. Kamran Ishaque Malik, M. A. Nasir Malik, and Azhar Aslam, "Honey Compared with Silver Sulphadiazine in the Treatment of Superficial Partial-Thickness Burns," *International Wound Journal* 7, no. 5 (October 2010): 413–17, https://doi.org/10.1111/j.1742-481X.2010.00717.x.

51. Hamid Rasad et al., "The Effect of Honey Consumption Compared with Sucrose on Lipid Profile in Young Healthy Subjects (Randomized Clinical Trial)," *Clinical Nutrition ESPEN* 26 (August 2018): 8–12, https://doi.org/10.1016/j.clnesp.2018.04.016.

52. Renata Alleva et al., "Organic Honey Supplementation Reverses Pesticide-Induced Genotoxicity by Modulating DNA Damage Response," *Molecular Nutrition & Food Research* 60, no. 10 (October 2016): 2243–55, https://doi.org/10.1002/mnfr.201600005.

53. Prathibha A. Nayak, Ullal A. Nayak, and R. Mythili, "Effect of Manuka Honey, Chlorhexidine Gluconate and Xylitol on the Clinical Levels of Dental Plaque," *Contemporary Clinical Dentistry* 1, no. 4 (October–December 2010): 214–17, https://www.ncbi.nlm.nih.gov/pubmed/22114423.

54. Ian M. Paul et al., "Effect of Honey, Dextromethorphan, and No Treatment on Nocturnal Cough and Sleep Quality for Coughing Children and Their Parents," *Archives of Pediatric Adolescent Medicine* 161, no. 12 (2007): 1140–46, https://doi.org/10.1001/archpedi.161.12.1140.

55. Georgina Gethin and Seamus Cowman, "Retracted: Manuka Honey vs. Hydrogel—a Prospective, Open Label, Multicentre, Randomised Controlled Trial to Compare Desloughing Efficacy and Healing Outcomes in Venous Ulcers," *Journal of Clinical Nursing* 18, no. 3 (February 2009): 466–74, https://doi.org/10.1111/j.1365-2702.2008.02558.x.

56. Mabrouka Bouacha, Hayette Ayed, and Nedjoud Grara, "Honey Bee as Alternative Medicine to Treat Eleven Multidrug-Resistant Bacteria Causing Urinary Tract Infection during Pregnancy," *Scientia Pharmaceutica* 86, no. 2 (2018): 14, https://doi.org/10.3390/scipharm86020014.

57. Georgina Gethin and Seamus Cowman, "Bacteriological Changes in Sloughy Venous Leg Ulcers Treated with Manuka Honey or Hydrogel: An RCT," *Journal of Wound Care* 17, no. 6 (2008): 241–47, https://doi.org/10.12968/jowc.2008.17.6.29583.

CHAPTER 3

1. Martin H. Fischer and Gertrude Moore, "On the Swelling of Fibrin," *American Journal of Physiology* 20, no. 2 (November 1907): 330–42, https://doi.org/10.1152/ajplegacy.1907.20.2.330.

2. Gerald H. Pollack, *The Fourth Phase of Water: Beyond Solid, Liquid, and Vapor* (Seattle: Ebner & Sons, 2013).

3. Mario G. Bianchetti, Giacomo D. Simonetti, and Alberto Bettinelli, "Body Fluids and Salt Metabolism—Part I," *Italian Journal of Pediatrics* 35, no. 36 (2009): https://doi.org/10.1186/1824-7288-35-36.

4. Francesca Fassioli et al., "Photosynthetic Light Harvesting: Excitons and Coherence," *Journal of the Royal Society Interface* 11, no. 92 (2014), https://doi.org/10.1098/rsif.2013.0901.

5. Pollack, *The Fourth Phase of Water;* and Mina Rohani and Gerald H. Pollack, "Flow through Horizontal Tubes Submerged in Water in the Absence of a Pressure Gradient: Mechanistic Considerations," *Langmuir* 29, no. 22 (2013): 6556–61, https://doi.org/10.1021/la4001945.

6. Gerald H. Pollack, *Cells, Gels and the Engines of Life: A New, Unifying Approach to Cell Function* (Seattle: Ebner & Sons, 2001).

7. Stanislaw Karpiński and Szechyńska-Hebda, "Secret Life of Plants: From Memory to Intelligence," *Plant Signaling & Behavior* 5, no. 11 (2010): 1391–94, https://doi.org/10.4161/psb.5.11.13243.

8. João Pimenta, Roberto Soldá, and Carlos Britto Pereira, "Tachycardia Mediated by an AV Universal (DDD) Pacemaker Triggered by a Ventricular Depolarization," *Pacing and Clinical Electrophysiology* 9, no. 1 (January 1986): 107–7, https://doi.org/10.1111/j.1540-8159.1986.tb05366.x.

9. Nancy A. Moran and Tyler Jarvik, "Lateral Transfer of Genes from Fungi Underlies Carotenoid Production in Aphids, " *Science* 328, no. 5978 (April 30, 2010): 624–27, https://doi.org/10.1126/science.1187113.

10. C. Xu et al., "Light-harvesting Chlorophyll Pigments Enable Mammalian Mitochondria to Capture Photonic Energy and Produce ATP," *Journal of Cell Science*, no. 127 (January 2014): 388–99, https://doi.org/10.1242/jcs.134262.

11. Jeffrey Walch et al., "The Effect of Sunlight on Postoperative Analgesic Medication Use: A Prospective Study of Patients Undergoing Spinal Surgery," *Psychosomatic Medicine* 67, no. 1 (January–February 2005): 156–63, https://doi.org/10.1097/01.psy.0000149258.42508.70.

12. Mirjam Münch et al., "Effects of Prior Light Exposure on Early Evening Performance, Subjective Sleepiness, and Hormonal Secretion," *Behavioral Neuroscience* 126, no. 1 (February 2012): 196–203, https://doi.org/10.1037/a0026702.

13. Walter E. Lowell and George E. Davis Jr., "The Effect of Solar Cycles on Human Lifespan in the 50 United States: Variation in Light Affects the Human Genome," *Medical Hypotheses* 75, no. 1 (July 2010): 17–25, https://doi.org/10.1016/j.mehy.2010.01.015.

14. Chen Xu et al., "Light-Harvesting Chlorophyll Pigments Enable Mammalian Mitochondria to Capture Photonic Energy and Produce ATP," *Journal of Cell Science* 127, no. 2 (2014): 388–99, https://doi.org/10.1242/jcs.134262.

15. Albertus B. Mostert et al., "Role of Semiconductivity and Ion Transport in the Electrical Conduction of Melanin," *Proceedings of the National Academy of Sciences* 109, no. 23 (2012): 8943–47, https://doi.org/10.1073/pnas.1119948109.

16. Motohiro Takeda et al., "Biophoton Detection as a Novel Technique for Cancer Imaging," *Cancer Science* 95, no. 8 (August 2004): 656–https://doi.org/10.1111/j.1349-7006.2004.tb03325.x.

17. Arturo S. Herrera et al., "Beyond Mitochondria, What Would Be the Energy Source of the Cell?," *Central Nervous System Agents in Medicinal Chemistry* 15, no. 1 (2015): 32–41, https://doi.org/10.2174/1871524915666150203093656.

18. Geoffrey Goodman and Dani Bercovich, "Melanin Directly Converts Light for Vertebrate Metabolic Use: Heuristic Thoughts on Birds, Icarus and Dark Human Skin," *Medical Hypotheses* 71, no. 2 (August 2008): 190–202, https://doi.org/10.1016/j.mehy.2008.03.038.

19. Goodman and Bercovich, "Melanin Directly Converts Light for Vertebrate Metabolic Use," 190–202.

20. Sheng Meng and Efthimios Kaxiras. "Mechanisms for Ultrafast Nonradiative Relaxation in Electronically Excited Eumelanin Constituents," *Biophysics Journal* 95, no. 9 (2008): 4396–402, https://doi.org/10.1529/biophysj.108.135756.

21. Iain Mathewson, "Did Human Hairlessness Allow Natural Photobiomodulation 2 Million Years Ago and Enable Photobiomodulation Therapy Today? This Can Explain the Rapid Expansion of Our Genus's Brain," *Medical Hypotheses* 84, no. 5 (May 2015): 421–28, https://doi.org/10.1016/j.mehy.2015.01.032.

22. Gerald H. Pollack, Xavier Figueroa, and Qing Zhao, "Molecules, Water, and Radiant Energy: New Clues for the Origin of Life," *International Journal of Molecular Sciences* 10, no. 4 (April 2009): 2009 Apr; 10(4): 1419–1429, https://doi.org/10.3390/ijms10041419.

23. Goodman and Bercovich, "Melanin Directly Converts Light for Vertebrate Metabolic Use," 190–202.

24. V. Vember and N. Zhdanova, "Peculiarities of Linear Growth of the Melanin-Containing Fungi *Cladosporium sphaerospermum* Penz. and *Alternaria alternata* (Fr.) Keissler" [in Russian], *Mikrobiolohichnyĭ Zhurnal* 63, no. 3 (May–June 2001): 3–12.

25. Lora Mangum Shields, L. W. Durrell, and Arnold H. Sparrow, "Preliminary Observations on Radiosensitivity of Algae and Fungi from Soils of the Nevada Test Site," *Ecology* 42, no. 2 (April 1961): 440–41, https://doi.org/10.2307/1932103.

26. Charles E. Turick et al., "In Situ Uranium Stabilization by Microbial Metabolites," *Journal of Environmental Radioactivity* 99, no. 6 (June 2008): 890–99, https://doi.org/10.1016/j.jenvrad.2007.11.020.

27. Ekaterina Dadachova and Arturo Casadevall, "Ionizing Radiation: How Fungi Cope, Adapt, and Exploit with the Help of Melanin," *Current Opinion in Microbiology* 11, no. 6 (December 2008): 525–31, https://doi.org/10.1016/j.mib.2008.09.013.

28. Ekaterina Dadachova et al., "Ionizing Radiation Changes the Electronic Properties of Melanin and Enhances the Growth of Melanized Fungi," *PLoS ONE* 2, no. 5 (2007): e457, https://doi.org/10.1371/journal.pone.0000457.

29. Ekaterina Revskaya et al., "Compton Scattering by Internal Shields Based on Melanin-Containing Mushrooms Provides Protection of Gastrointestinal Tract from Ionizing Radiation," *Cancer Biotherapy and Radiopharmaceuticals* 27, no. 9 (November 2012): 570–76, https://doi.org/10.1089/cbr.2012.1318.

30. Charles E. Turick et al., "Gamma Radiation Interacts with Melanin to Alter Its Oxidation-Reduction Potential and Results in Electric Current Production," *Bioelectrochemistry* 82, no. 1 (August 2011): 69–73, https://doi.org/10.1016/j.bioelechem.2011.04.009.

31. A. Kunwar et al., "Melanin, a Promising Radioprotector: Mechanisms of Actions in a Mice Model," *Toxicology and Applied Pharmacology* 264, no. 2 (2012): 202–11, https://doi.org/10.1016/j.taap.2012.08.002.

32. Kenneth Maiese, "Moving to the Rhythm with Clock (Circadian) Genes, Autophagy, mTOR, and SIRT1 in Degenerative Disease and Cancer," *Current Neurovascular Research* 14, no. 3 (2017): 299–304, https://doi.org/10.2174 /1567202614666170718092010; and Roberto Paganelli, Claudia Petrarca, and Mario Di Gioacchino, "Biological Clocks: Their Relevance to Immune-Allergic Diseases," Clinical and Molecular Allergy 16, no. 1 (January 10, 2018), https://doi.org/10.1186/s12948-018-0080-0.

33. Alan C. Logan, Martin A. Katzman, and Vicent Balanzá-Martínez, "Natural Environments, Ancestral Diets, and Microbial Ecology: Is There a Modern 'Paleo-Deficit Disorder'? Part II," *Journal of Physiological Anthropology* 34, no. 9 (2015), https://doi.org/10.1186/s40101-014-0040-4.

34. Marianne Berwick, "Can UV Exposure Reduce Mortality?," *Cancer Epidemiology, Biomarkers & Prevention* 20, no. 4 (April 2011): 582–84, https://doi.org/10.1158/1055-9965.EPI-10-1255.

35. Masahiko Ayaki et al., "Protective Effect of Blue-Light Shield Eyewear for Adults against Light Pollution from Self-Luminous Devices Used at Night," *Chronobiology International* 33, no. 1 (January 2, 2016): 134–39, https://doi.org/10.3109/07420528.2015.1119158.

36. Roger Applewhite, "The Effectiveness of a Conductive Patch and a Conductive Bed Pad in Reducing Induced Human Body Voltage via the Application of Earth Ground," *European Biology and Bioelectromagnetics* 1 (2005): 23–40.

37. Gaétan Chevalier et al., "Earthing: Health Implications of Reconnecting the Human Body to the Earth's Surface Electrons," *Journal of Environmental and Public Health* 2012 (2012): 291541, https://doi.org/10.1155/2012/291541.

38. Chevalier et al., "Earthing: Health Implications," 291541.

39. Chevalier et al., "Earthing: Health Implications," 291541.

40. Maurice Ghaly and Dale Teplitz, "The Biologic Effects of Grounding the Human Body during Sleep as Measured by Cortisol Levels and Subjective Reporting of Sleep, Pain, and Stress," *The Journal of Alternative and Complementary Medicine* 10, no. 5 (October 2004): 767–76, https://doi.org/10.1089/acm.2004.10.767.

41. A. Clinton Ober, "Grounding the Human Body to Neutralize Bioelectrical Stress from Static Electricity and EMFs," *ESD Journal*, accessed October 14, 2019, http://www.esdjournal.com/articles/cober/ground.htm.

42. James L. Oschman, "Charge Transfer in the Living Matrix," *Journal of Bodywork and Movement Therapies* 13, no. 3 (July 2009): 215–28, https://doi.org/10.1016/j.jbmt.2008.06.005.

43. Gaétan Chevalier et al., "Earthing (Grounding) the Human Body Reduces Blood Viscosity—a Major Factor in Cardiovascular Disease," *The Journal of Alternative and Complementary Medicine* 19, no. 2 (February 2013): 102–10, https://doi.org/10.1089/acm.2011.0820.

44. Gaétan Chevalier, "Changes in Pulse Rate, Respiratory Rate, Blood Oxygenation, Perfusion Index, Skin Conductance, and Their Variability Induced During and After Grounding Human Subjects for 40 Minutes," *The Journal of Alternative and Complementary Medicine* 16, no. 1 (January 2010): 81–87, https://doi.org/10.1089/acm.2009.0278.

45. Claudio Franceschi et al., "Inflamm-aging: An Evolutionary Perspective on Immunosenescence," *Annals of the New York Academy of Sciences* 908, no. 1 (June 2000): 244–54, https://doi.org/10.1111/j.1749-6632.2000.tb06651.x.

46. Chevalier et al., "Earthing: Health Implications," 291541.

47. James L. Oschman, Gaétan Chevalier, and Richard Brown, "The Effects of Grounding (Earthing) on Inflammation, the Immune Response, Wound Healing, and Prevention and Treatment of Chronic Inflammatory and Autoimmune Diseases," *Journal of Inflammation Research* 2015, no. 8 (March 24, 2015): 83–96, https://doi.org/10.2147/JIR.S69656.

48. Katherine M. Tyner, Raoul Kopelman, and Martin A. Philbert, "'Nanosized Voltmeter' Enables Cellular-Wide Electric Field Mapping," *Biophysical Journal* 93, no. 4 (August 15, 2007): 1163–74, https://doi.org/10.1529/biophysj.106.092452.

49. Nick Lane and William Martin, "The Energetics of Genome Complexity," *Nature* 467, no. 7318 (2010): 929–34, https://doi.org/10.1038/nature09486.

50. H. B. G. Casimir and D. Polder, "The Influence of Retardation on the London-van Der Waals Forces," *Physical Review* 73, no. 4 (February 1948): 360–72, https://doi.org/10.1103/PhysRev.73.360.

51. Michael Grothaus, "These Gloves Let You Climb Walls Like Spider-Man," *Fast Company*, January 28, 2016, https://www.fastcompany.com/3056023/these-gloves-let-you-climb-walls-like-spider-man.

52. Elliot W Hawkes et al., "Human Climbing with Efficiently Scaled Gecko-Inspired Dry Adhesives," *Journal of The Royal Society Interface* 12, no. 102 (January 6, 2015): 20140675, https://doi.org/10.1098/rsif.2014.0675.

53. Austin Booth and W. Ford Doolittle, "Eukaryogenesis, How Special Really?," *Proceedings of the National Academy of Sciences of the United States of America* 112, no. 33 (August 18, 2015): 10278–85, https://doi.org/10.1073/pnas.1421376112.

54. Douglas Wallace, "KCU - University Lecture Series - Dr. Douglas Wallace," YouTube video, 1:14:46, Kansas City University of Medicine and Biosciences, May 3, 2016, 24:30, https://www.youtube.com/watch?v=ahlDLjf8c90.

55. R. Sherr, K. T. Bainbridge, and H. H. Anderson, "Transmutation of Mercury by Fast Neutrons," *Physical Review* 60, no. 7 (October 1941): 473–79, https://doi.org/10.1103/PhysRev.60.473.

56. Jean-Paul Biberian, "Biological Transmutations: Historical Perspective," *The Journal of Condensed Matter Nuclear Science* 7 (January 2012): 11–25.

57. Robert A. Nelson, *Adept Alchemy* (self-pub., 2000), 101.

58. Jöns Jacob Berzelius, *Treatise on Mineral, Plant & Animal Chemistry* (Paris, 1849), cited in Nelson, "Biological Transmutations," part II, chap. 8 in *Adept Alchemy* (self-pub., 2000).

59. Hideo Kozima, "The TNCF Model—a Phenomelogical Model for the Cold Fusion Phenomenon," *Cold Fusion* 23, 18 (1997): 43–47.

60. Miklós Müller et al., "Biochemistry and Evolution of Anaerobic Energy Metabolism in Eukaryotes," *Microbiology and Molecular Biology Reviews* 76, no. 2 (June 2012): 444–95, https://doi.org/10.1128/mmbr.05024-11.

61. S. Goldfein, "Energy Development from Elemental Transmutations in Biological Systems: Final Report December 1977–April 1978," Army Mobility Equipment Research and Development Center, Fort Belvoir, VA, January 1, 1978.

62. Christopher Earls Brennen, *Cavitation and Bubble Dynamics* (New York: Oxford University Press, 1995).

63. Max Fomitchev-Zamilov, "Cavitation-Induced Fusion: Proof of Concept," Quantum Potential Corporation, September 9, 2012.

64. Claudia Eberlein, "Sonoluminescence as Quantum Vacuum Radiation," *Physical Review Letters* 76, 20 (1996): 3842–3845, https://doi.org/10.1103/PhysRevLett.76.3842.

PART II

CHAPTER 4

1. "National Cancer Act of 1971," National Cancer Institute, February 16, 2016, https://www.cancer.gov/about-nci/legislative/history/national-cancer-act-1971.

2. Douglas Hanahan, "Rethinking the War on Cancer," *The Lancet* 383, no. 9916 (2014): 558–63, https://doi.org/10.1016/S0140-6736(13)62226-6.

3. Bryan Oronsky et al., "The War on Cancer: A Military Perspective," *Frontiers in Oncology* 4, no. 387 (January 2015): https://doi.org/10.3389/fonc.2014.00387.

4. Kimberly Leonard, "Global Cancer Spending Reaches $100B," *U.S. News & World Report*, May 5, 2015, https://www.usnews.com/news/blogs/data-mine/2015/05/05/global-cancer-spending-reaches-100b.

5. "Cancer Fact Sheets," Cancer Today, accessed October 14, 2019, http://gco.iarc.fr/today/fact-sheets-cancers?cancer=29&type=0&sex=0.

6. "Leading Causes of Death," CDC/National Center for Health Statistics, last modified March 17, 2017, https://www.cdc.gov/nchs/fastats/leading-causes-of-death.htm.

7. Paolo Vineis and Christopher P. Wild, "Global Cancer Patterns: Causes and Prevention," *The Lancet* 383, no. 9916 (2014): 549–57, https://doi.org/10.1016/S0140-6736(13)62224-2.

8. Ian Haines, "The War on Cancer: Time for a New Terminology," *The Lancet* 383, no. 9932 (2014): 1883, https://doi.org/10.1016/S0140-6736(14)60907-7.

9. Robert A. Gatenby, Robert J. Gillies, and Joel S. Brown, "Of Cancer and Cave Fish," *Nature Reviews Cancer* 11, no. 4 (2011): 237–38, https://doi.org/10.1038/nrc3036.

10. Herui Yao et al., "Adrenaline Induces Chemoresistance in HT-29 Colon Adenocarcinoma Cells," *Cancer Genetics and Cytogenetics* 190, no. 2 (April 15, 2009): 81–87, https://doi.org/10.1016/j.cancergencyto.2008.12.009.

11. Mauricio Burotto et al., "The MAPK Pathway across Different Malignancies: A New Perspective," *Cancer* 120, no. 22 (November 15, 2014): 3446–56, https://doi.org/10.1002/cncr.28864.

12. Caryn Mei Hsien Chan et al., "Course and Predictors of Post-Traumatic Stress Disorder in a Cohort of Psychologically Distressed Patients with Cancer: A 4-Year Follow-Up Study," *Cancer* 124, no. 2 (January 15, 2018): 406–16, https://doi.org/10.1002/cncr.30980.

13. Fang Fang et al., "Suicide and Cardiovascular Death after a Cancer Diagnosis," *New England Journal of Medicine* 366, no. 14 (April 5, 2012): 1310–18, https://doi.org/10.1056/NEJMoa1110307.

14. Fang et al., "Suicide and Cardiovascular Death," 1310–18.

15. Laura J. Esserman, Ian M. Thompson Jr., and Brian Reid, "Overdiagnosis and Overtreatment in Cancer: An Opportunity for Improvement," *JAMA* 310, no. 8 (August 28, 2013): 797–98, https://doi.org/10.1001/jama.2013.108415.

16. H. Gilbert Welch and William C. Black, "Overdiagnosis in Cancer," *JNCI: Journal of the National Cancer Institute* 102, no. 9 (May 5, 2010): 605–13, https://doi.org/10.1093/jnci/djq099.

17. Vinay Prasad, Jeanne Lenzer, and David H. Newman, "Why Cancer Screening Has Never Been Shown to 'Save Lives'—and What We Can Do about It," *BMJ* 352, no. 8039 (January 6, 2016): h6080, https://doi.org/10.1136/bmj.h6080.

18. Welch, H. Gilbert, and William C. Black, "Overdiagnosis in Cancer." *JNCI: Journal of the National Cancer Institute* 102, no. 9 (May 5, 2010): 605–13. https://doi.org/10.1093/jnci/djq099.

19. William C. Black, David A. Haggstrom, and H. Gilbert Welch, "All-Cause Mortality in Randomized Trials of Cancer Screening," *JNCI: Journal of the National Cancer Institute* 94, no. 3 (February 6, 2002): 167–73, https://doi.org/10.1093/jnci/94.3.167.

20. Nazmus Saquib, Juliann Saquib, and John P. A. Ioannidis, "Does Screening for Disease Save Lives in Asymptomatic Adults? Systematic Review of Meta-Analyses and Randomized Trials," *International Journal of Epidemiology* 44, no. 1 (February 2015): 264–77, https://doi.org/10.1093/ije/dyu140.

21. Peter C. Gøtzsche and Karsten Juhl Jørgensen, "Screening for Breast Cancer with Mammography (Review)," *Cochrane Database of Systematic Reviews*, no. 6 (2013), https://doi.org/10.1002/14651858.CD001877.pub5.

22. Gianfranco Domenighetti et al., "Women's Perception of the Benefits of Mammography Screening: Population-Based Survey in Four Countries," *International Journal of Epidemiology* 32, no. 5 (October 2003): 816–21, https://doi.org/10.1093/ije/dyg257.

23. Welch and Black, "Overdiagnosis in Cancer," 605–13.

24. Welch and Black, "Overdiagnosis in Cancer," 605–13.

25. Jingbo Zhang et al., "Distribution of Renal Tumor Growth Rates Determined by Using Serial Volumetric CT Measurements," *Radiology* 250, no. 1 (January 2009): 137–44, https://doi.org/10.1148/radiol.2501071712.

26. Gloria Y. F. Ho et al., "Risk Factors for Persistent Cervical Intraepithelial Neoplasia Grades 1 and 2: Managed by Watchful Waiting," *Journal of Lower Genital Tract Disease* 15, no. 4 (2011), https://doi.org/10.1097/LGT.0b013e3182216fef.

27. K. Yamamoto et al., "Spontaneous Regression of Localized Neuroblastoma Detected by Mass Screening," *Journal of Clinical Oncology* 16, no. 4 (April 1998): 1265–69, https://doi.org/10.1200/JCO.1998.16.4.1265.

28. Welch and Black, "Overdiagnosis in Cancer," 605–13

29. Esserman, Thompson Jr, and Reid, "Overdiagnosis and Overtreatment in Cancer," 797–98.

30. Stephen W. Duffy et al., "Correcting for Lead Time and Length Bias in Estimating the Effect of Screen Detection on Cancer Survival," *American Journal of Epidemiology* 168, no. 1 (May 25, 2008): 98–104, https://doi.org/10.1093/aje/kwn120.

31. Domenighetti et al., "Women's Perception of the Benefits of Mammography Screening" 816–21.

32. Nikola Biller-Andorno and Peter Jüni, "Abolishing Mammography Screening Programs? A View from the Swiss Medical Board," *New England Journal of Medicine* 370, no. 21 (April 16, 2014): 1965–67, https://doi.org/10.1056/NEJMp1401875.

33. Prasad, Lenzer, and Newman, "Never Been Shown to 'Save Lives'," h6080.

34. Archie Bleyer and H. Gilbert Welch, "Effect of Three Decades of Screening Mammography on Breast-Cancer Incidence," *New England Journal of Medicine* 367, no. 21 (November 21, 2012): 1998–2005, https://doi.org/10.1056/NEJMoa1206809.

35. H. Gilbert Welch and William C. Black. "Overdiagnosis in Cancer." *JNCI: Journal of the National Cancer Institute* 102, no. 9 (May 5, 2010): 605–13. https://doi.org/10.1093/jnci/djq099.

36. Lydia E. Pace and Nancy L. Keating, "A Systematic Assessment of Benefits and Risks to Guide Breast Cancer Screening Decisions," *JAMA* 311, no. 13 (April 2, 2014): 1327–35, https://doi.org/10.1001/jama.2014.1398.

37. John Brodersen and Volkert Dirk Siersma, "Long-Term Psychosocial Consequences of False-Positive Screening Mammography," *Annals of Family Medicine* 11, no. 2 (March/April 2013): 106–15, https://doi.org/10.1370/afm.1466.

38. G. J. Heyes, A. J. Mill, and M. W. Charles, "Enhanced Biological Effectiveness of Low Energy X-Rays and Implications for the UK Breast Screening Programme," *BJR* 79, no. 939 (March 2006): 195–200, https://doi.org/10.1259/bjr/21958628.

39. Heyes, Mill, and Charles, "Low Energy X-Rays," 195–200.

40. Anouk Pijpe et al., "Exposure to Diagnostic Radiation and Risk of Breast Cancer among Carriers of BRCA1/2 Mutations: Retrospective Cohort Study (GENE-RAD-RISK)," *BMJ (Clinical Research Ed.)* 345, no. 7878 (October 13, 2012): e5660, https://doi.org/10.1136/bmj.e5660.

41. Cheryl Lin et al., "The Case against BRCA 1 and 2 Testing," *Surgery* 149, no. 6 (June 2011): 731–34, https://doi.org/10.1016/j.surg.2010.11.009.

42. Alexandra J. van den Broek et al., "Worse Breast Cancer Prognosis of *BRCA1/BRCA2* Mutation Carriers: What's the Evidence? A Systematic Review with Meta-Analysis," *PLOS ONE* 10, no. 3 (March 27, 2015): e0120189, https://doi.org/10.1371/journal.pone.0120189.

43. Bleyer and Welch, "Three Decades of Screening Mammography," 1998–2005.

44. Andrea Veronesi et al., "Familial Breast Cancer: Characteristics and Outcome of BRCA 1–2 Positive and Negative Cases," *BMC Cancer* 5, no. 70 (2005), https://doi.org/10.1186/1471-2407-5-70.

45. Mary-Claire King, Joan H. Marks, and Jessica B. Mandell, "Breast and Ovarian Cancer Risks Due to Inherited Mutations in BRCA1 and BRCA2," *Science* 302, no. 5645 (October 24, 2003): 643–46, https://doi.org/10.1126/science.1088759.

46. van den Broek et al., "Worse Breast Cancer Prognosis," e0120189.

47. Fritz H. Schröder et al., "Screening and Prostate-Cancer Mortality in a Randomized European Study," *New England Journal of Medicine* 360, no. 13 (March 26, 2009): 1320–28, https://doi.org/10.1056/NEJMoa0810084.

48. Esserman, Thompson Jr, and Reid, "Overdiagnosis and Overtreatment in Cancer," 797–98.

49. Gerrit Draisma et al., "Lead Times and Overdetection Due to Prostate-Specific Antigen Screening: Estimates from the European Randomized Study of Screening for Prostate Cancer," *JNCI: Journal of the National Cancer Institute* 95, no. 12 (June 18, 2003): 868–78, https://doi.org/10.1093/jnci/95.12.868.

50. Stacy Loeb et al., "Overdiagnosis and Overtreatment of Prostate Cancer," *European Urology* 65, no. 6 (June 2014): 1046–55, https://doi.org/10.1016/j.eururo.2013.12.062.

51. Bridget Bickers and Claire Aukim-Hastie, "New Molecular Biomarkers for the Prognosis and Management of Prostate Cancer—the Post PSA Era," *Anticancer Research* 29, no. 8 (August 2009): 3289–98, http://ar.iiarjournals.org/content/29/8/3289.abstract.

52. Bickers and Aukim-Hastie, "New Molecular Biomarkers," 3289–98.

53. Shahrokh F. Shariat et al., "Beyond Prostate-Specific Antigen: New Serologic Biomarkers for Improved Diagnosis and Management of Prostate Cancer," *Reviews in Urology* 6, no. 2 (2004): 58–72, https://www.ncbi.nlm.nih.gov/pubmed/16985579.

54. Bickers and Aukim-Hastie, "New Molecular Biomarkers," 3289–98.

55. Gerald L. Andriole et al., "Mortality Results from a Randomized Prostate-Cancer Screening Trial," *New England Journal of Medicine* 360, no. 13 (March 26, 2009): 1310–19, https://doi.org/10.1056/NEJMoa0810696.

56. Andriole et al., "Randomized Prostate-Cancer Screening Trial," 1310–19.

57. Schröder et al., "Screening and Prostate-Cancer Mortality," 1320–28.

58. Schröder et al., "Screening and Prostate-Cancer Mortality," 1320–28.

59. Gilbert H. Welch and Peter C. Albertsen. "Prostate Cancer Diagnosis and Treatment after the Introduction of Prostate-Specific Antigen Screening: 1986–2005." *Journal of the National Cancer Institute* 101, no. 19 (October 7, 2009): 1325–29. https://doi.org/10.1093/jnci/djp278.

60. Arnold Rice Rich, "On the Frequency of Occurrence of Occult Carcinoma of the Prostrate," *International Journal of Epidemiology* 36, no. 2 (April 2007): 274–77, https://doi.org/10.1093/ije/dym050.

61. "Stanford Researcher Declares 'PSA Era is Over' in Predicting Prostate Cancer Risk," Stanford Medicine News Center, September 10, 2004, https://med.stanford.edu/news/all-news/2004/stanford-researcher-declares-psa-era-is-over-in-predicting-prostate-cancer-risk.html.

62. Ronald E. Wheeler, "Is It Necessary to Cure Prostate Cancer When It Is Possible? (Understanding the Role of Prostate Inflammation Resolution to Prostate Cancer Evolution)," *Clinical Interventions in Aging* 2, no. 1 (2007): 153–61, https://www.ncbi.nlm.nih.gov/pubmed/18044088.

63. Bickers and Aukim-Hastie, "New Molecular Biomarkers," 3289–98.

64. Schröder et al., "Screening and Prostate-Cancer Mortality," 1320–28.

65. Girish Sardana, Barry Dowell, and Eleftherios P. Diamandis, "Emerging Biomarkers for the Diagnosis and Prognosis of Prostate Cancer," *Clinical Chemistry* 54, no. 12 (December 2008): 1951–60, https://doi.org/10.1373/clinchem.2008.110668.

66. Anna Bill-Axelson et al., "Radical Prostatectomy versus Watchful Waiting in Localized Prostate Cancer: The Scandinavian Prostate Cancer Group-4 Randomized Trial," *JNCI: Journal of the National Cancer Institute* 100, no. 16 (August 20, 2008): 1144–54, https://doi.org/10.1093/jnci/djn255.

67. Arnold L. Potosky et al., "Quality of Life following Localized Prostate Cancer Treated Initially with Androgen Deprivation Therapy or No Therapy," *JNCI: Journal of the National Cancer Institute* 94, no. 6 (March 20, 2002): 430–37, https://doi.org/10.1093/jnci/94.6.430.

68. Grace L. Lu-Yao et al., "Survival following Primary Androgen Deprivation Therapy among Men with Localized Prostate Cancer," *JAMA* 300, no. 2 (July 9, 2008): 173–81, https://doi.org/10.1001/jama.300.2.173.

69. Kay-Tee Khaw et al., "Endogenous Testosterone and Mortality Due to All Causes, Cardiovascular Disease, and Cancer in Men," *Circulation* 116, no. 23 (December 4, 2007): 2694–701, https://doi.org/10.1161/CIRCULATIONAHA.107.719005.

70. S. E. Oliver, D. Gunnell, and J. L. Donovan, "Comparison of Trends in Prostate-Cancer Mortality in England and Wales and the USA," *The Lancet* 355, no. 9217 (2000): 1788–89, https://doi.org/10.1016/S0140-6736(00)02269-8.

71. Dragan Ilic et al., "Screening for Prostate Cancer," *Cochrane Database of Systematic Reviews*, no. 1 (2013): CD004720, https://doi.org/10.1002/14651858.CD004720.pub3.

72. Fang et al., "Suicide and Cardiovascular Death," 1310–18.

73. "PSA Era is Over," Stanford Medicine News Center, 2004.

74. "PSA Era is Over," Stanford Medicine News Center, 2004.

75. E. Kesse et al., "Dairy Products, Calcium and Phosphorus Intake, and the Risk of Prostate Cancer: Results of the French Prospective SU.VI.MAX (Supplémentation en Vitamines et Minéraux Antioxydants) Study," *British Journal of Nutrition* 95, no. 3 (2006): 539–45, https://doi.org/10.1079/BJN20051670.

76. Wendy Demark-Wahnefried et al., "Flaxseed Supplementation (Not Dietary Fat Restriction) Reduces Prostate Cancer Proliferation Rates in Men Presurgery," *Cancer Epidemiology Biomarkers & Prevention* 17, no. 12 (December 2008): 3577–87, https://doi.org/10.1158/1055-9965.EPI-08-0008.

77. Wheeler, "Is It Necessary to Cure Prostate Cancer?," 153–61.

78. Denise R. Aberle et al., "Reduced Lung-Cancer Mortality with Low-Dose Computed Tomographic Screening," *New England Journal of Medicine* 365, no. 5 (August 4, 2011): 395–409, https://doi.org/10.1056/NEJMoa1102873.

79. Edward F. Patz Jr. et al., "Overdiagnosis in Low-Dose Computed Tomography Screening for Lung Cancer," *JAMA Internal Medicine* 174, no. 2 (February 2014): 269–74, https://doi.org/10.1001/jamainternmed.2013.12738.

80. David Brenner and Eric Hall, "Computed Tomography—An Increasing Source of Radiation Exposure," *New England Journal of Medicine* 357, 22 (2007): 2277–84, https://www.doi.org/10.1056/NEJMra072149.

81. Juan P. Brito et al., "Papillary Lesions of Indolent Course: Reducing the Overdiagnosis of Indolent Papillary Thyroid Cancer and Unnecessary

Treatment," *Future Oncology* 10, no. 1 (December 11, 2013): 1–4, https://doi.org/10.2217/fon.13.240.

82. Lola Rahib et al., "Projecting Cancer Incidence and Deaths to 2030: The Unexpected Burden of Thyroid, Liver, and Pancreas Cancers in the United States," *Cancer Research* 74, no. 11 (June 2014): 2913–21, https://doi.org/10.1158/0008-5472.CAN-14-0155.

83. Sabrina Jegerlehner et al., "Overdiagnosis and Overtreatment of Thyroid Cancer: A Population-Based Temporal Trend Study," *PLOS ONE* 12, no. 6 (June 14, 2017): e0179387, https://doi.org/10.1371/journal.pone.0179387.

84. Jegerlehner et al., "Overdiagnosis and Overtreatment of Thyroid Cancer," e0179387.

85. Brito et al., "Papillary Lesions of Indolent Course," 1–4.

86. Brito et al., "Papillary Lesions of Indolent Course," 1–4.

87. Brito et al., "Papillary Lesions of Indolent Course," 1–4.

88. H. Rubén Harach, Kaarle O. Franssila, and Veli-Matti Wasenius, "Occult Papillary Carcinoma of the Thyroid. A 'normal' Finding in Finland. A Systematic Autopsy Study," *Cancer* 56, no. 3 (August 1985): 531–38, https://doi.org/10.1002/1097-0142(19850801)56:3<531::aid-cn-cr2820560321>3.0.co;2-3.

89. Jegerlehner et al., "Overdiagnosis and Overtreatment of Thyroid Cancer," e0179387.

90. Jegerlehner et al., "Overdiagnosis and Overtreatment of Thyroid Cancer," e0179387.

91. Sun-Seog Kweon et al., "Thyroid Cancer Is the Most Common Cancer in Women, Based on the Data from Population-Based Cancer Registries, South Korea," *Japanese Journal of Clinical Oncology* 43, no. 10 (July 25, 2013): 1039–46, https://doi.org/10.1093/jjco/hyt102.

92. Jegerlehner et al., "Overdiagnosis and Overtreatment of Thyroid Cancer," e0179387.

93. Jegerlehner et al., "Overdiagnosis and Overtreatment of Thyroid Cancer," e0179387.

94. Jegerlehner et al., "Overdiagnosis and Overtreatment of Thyroid Cancer," e0179387.

95. Brito et al., "Papillary Lesions of Indolent Course," 1–4.

96. N. Gopalakrishna Iyer et al., "Rising Incidence of Second Cancers in Patients with Low-Risk (T1N0) Thyroid Cancer Who Receive Radioactive Iodine Therapy," *Cancer* 117, no. 19 (October 1, 2011): 4439–46, https://doi.org/10.1002/cncr.26070.

97. Yuri E. Nikiforov et al., "Nomenclature Revision for Encapsulated Follicular Variant of Papillary Thyroid Carcinoma: A Paradigm Shift to Reduce Overtreatment of Indolent Tumors," *JAMA Oncology* 2, no. 8 (August 2016): 1023–29, https://doi.org/10.1001/jamaoncol.2016.0386.

98. Zoë Slote Morris, Steven Wooding, and Jonathan Grant, "The Answer Is 17 Years, What Is the Question: Understanding Time Lags in Translational Research," *Journal of the Royal Society of Medicine* 104, no. 12 (December 2011): 510–20, https://doi.org/10.1258/jrsm.2011.110180.

99. J. D. Nabarro, "Nitrogen Mustard Therapy in Reticuloses," *British Journal of Radiology* 24 (1951): 507–10.

100. Tao Wang et al., "Cancer Stem Cell Targeted Therapy: Progress amid Controversies," *Oncotarget* 6, no. 42 (2015): 44191–206, https://doi.org/10.18632/oncotarget.6176.

101. Wang et al., "Cancer Stem Cell Targeted Therapy," 44191–206.

102. Geum-Soog Kim et al., "Muricoreacin and Murihexocin C, Mono-Tetrahydrofuran Acetogenins, from the Leaves of Annona Muricata in Honour of Professor G. H. Neil Towers 75th Birthday," *Phytochemistry* 49, no. 2 (1998): 565–71, https://doi.org/10.1016/S0031-9422(98)00172-1.

103. Chih-Chuang Liaw et al., "New Cytotoxic Monotetrahydrofuran Annonaceous Acetogenins from Annona Muricata," *Journal of Natural Products* 65, no. 4 (April 2002): 470–75, https://doi.org/10.1021/np0105578.

104. Yumin Dai et al., "Selective Growth Inhibition of Human Breast Cancer Cells by Graviola Fruit Extract In Vitro and In Vivo Involving Downregulation of EGFR Expression," *Nutrition and Cancer* 63, no. 5 (July 2011): 795–801, https://doi.org/10.1080/01635581.2011.563027.

105. Carol Ann Huff et al., "The Paradox of Response and Survival in Cancer Therapeutics," *Blood* 107, no. 2 (January 15, 2006): 431–34, https://doi.org/10.1182/blood-2005-06-2517.

106. Huff et al., "Paradox of Response and Survival," 431–34.

107. Graeme Morgan, Robyn Ward, and Michael Barton, "The Contribution of Cytotoxic Chemotherapy to 5-Year Survival in Adult Malignancies," *Clinical Oncology* 16, no. 8 (December 2004): 549–60, https://doi.org/10.1016/j.clon.2004.06.007.

108. U. Abel, "Chemotherapy of Advanced Epithelial Cancer - a Critical Review," *Biomedicine & Pharmacotherapy* 46, no. 10 (1992): 439–52, https://doi.org/10.1016/0753-3322(92)90002-O.

109. Huff et al., "Paradox of Response and Survival," 431–34.

110. Huff et al., "Paradox of Response and Survival," 431–34.

111. Qin Feng et al., "An Epigenomic Approach to Therapy for Tamoxifen-Resistant Breast Cancer," *Cell Research* 24, no. 7 (2014): 809–19, https://doi.org/10.1038/cr.2014.71.

112. Rubí Viedma-Rodríguez et al., "Mechanisms Associated with Resistance to Tamoxifen in Estrogen Receptor-Positive Breast Cancer (Review)," *Oncology Reports* 32, no. 1 (2014): 3–15, https://doi.org/10.3892/or.2014.3190.

113. Dan Yao et al., "Synthesis and Reactivity of Potential Toxic Metabolites of Tamoxifen Analogues: Droloxifene and Toremifene o-Quinones," *Chemical Research in Toxicology* 14, no. 12 (December 2001): 1643–53, https://doi.org/10.1021/tx010137i.

114. Giovanni Pagano et al., "The Role of Oxidative Stress in Developmental and Reproductive Toxicity of Tamoxifen," *Life Sciences* 68, no. 15 (2001): 1735–49, https://doi.org/10.1016/S0024-3205(01)00969-9.

115. Bernard Fisher et al., "Endometrial Cancer in Tamoxifen-Treated Breast Cancer Patients: Findings from the National Surgical Adjuvant Breast and Bowel Project (NSABP) B-14," *JNCI: Journal of the National Cancer Institute* 86, no. 7 (April 6, 1994): 527–37, https://doi.org/10.1093/jnci/86.7.527.

116. Y. Matsuyama et al., "Second Cancers after Adjuvant Tamoxifen Therapy for Breast Cancer in Japan," *Annals of Oncology* 11, no. 12 (December 2000): 1537–43, https://doi.org/10.1093/oxfordjournals.annonc.a010406.

117. Lars E. Rutqvist et al., "Adjuvant Tamoxifen Therapy for Early Stage Breast Cancer and Second Primary Malignancies," *JNCI: Journal of the National Cancer Institute* 87, no. 9 (May 3, 1995): 645–51, https://doi.org/10.1093/jnci/87.9.645.

118. S. Yalçin et al., "Acute Leukaemia during Tamoxifen Therapy," *Medical Oncology* 14, no. 1 (1997): 61–62, https://doi.org/10.1007/BF02990948.

119. Hervé Mignotte et al., "Iatrogenic Risks of Endometrial Carcinoma after Treatment for Breast Cancer in a Large French Case-Control Study." *International Journal of Cancer* 76, no. 3 (May 4, 1998): 325–30, https://doi.org/10.1002/(SICI)1097-0215(19980504)76:3<325::AID-IJC7>3.0.CO;2-X.

120. Annlia Paganini-Hill and Linda J. Clark, "Preliminary Assessment of Cognitive Function in Breast Cancer Patients Treated with Tamoxifen," *Breast Cancer Research and Treatment* 64, no. 2 (November 1, 2000): 165–76, https://doi.org/10.1023/A:1006426132338.

121. Paganini-Hill and Clark, "Preliminary Assessment of Cognitive Function," 165–76.

122. Yoshihisa Nemoto, et al., "Tamoxifen-Induced Nonalcoholic Steatohepatitis in Breast Cancer Patients Treated with Adjuvant Tamoxifen," *Internal Medicine* 41, no. 5 (2002): 345–50, https://doi.org/10.2169/internalmedicine.41.345.

123. Annlia Paganini-Hill and Linda J Clark, "Eye Problems in Breast Cancer Patients Treated With Tamoxifen." *Breast Cancer Research and Treatment* 60, no. 2 (March 2000): 167–172, https://doi.org/10.1023/a:1006342300291.

124. Lin, Hsien-Feng Lin et al., "Correlation of the Tamoxifen Use with the Increased Risk of Deep Vein Thrombosis and Pulmonary Embolism in Elderly Women with Breast Cancer: A Case-Control Study," *Medicine* 97, no. 51 (December 2018): e12842–e12842, https://doi.org/10.1097/MD.0000000000012842.

125. Christina Davies et al., "Long-Term Effects of Continuing Adjuvant Tamoxifen to 10 Years versus Stopping at 5 Years after Diagnosis of Oestrogen Receptor-Positive Breast Cancer: ATLAS, a Randomised Trial,"

The Lancet 381, no. 9869 (March 9, 2013): 805–16.
https://doi.org/10.1016/S0140-6736(12)61963-1.

126. Lauren M. F. Merlo et al., "Cancer as an Evolutionary and Ecological Process," *Nature Reviews Cancer* 6, no. 12 (2006): 924–35, https://doi.org/10.1038/nrc2013.

127. Paul C. W. Davies and Charles H. Lineweaver, "Cancer Tumors as Metazoa 1.0: Tapping Genes of Ancient Ancestors," *Physical Biology* 8, no. 1 (February 2011): 15001, https://doi.org/10.1088/1478-3975/8/1/015001.

128. Naoyo Nishida et al., "Angiogenesis in Cancer," *Vascular Health and Risk Management* 2, no. 3 (2006): 213–19, https://doi.org/10.2147/vhrm.2006.2.3.213.

129. Davies and Lineweaver, "Cancer Tumors as Metazoa 1.0," 15001.

130. Davies and Lineweaver, "Cancer Tumors as Metazoa 1.0," 15001.

131. Davies and Lineweaver, "Cancer Tumors as Metazoa 1.0," 15001.

132. Davies and Lineweaver, "Cancer Tumors as Metazoa 1.0," 15001.

133. Davies and Lineweaver, "Cancer Tumors as Metazoa 1.0," 15001.

134. Huff et al., "Paradox of Response and Survival," 431–34.

135. Tao Wang et al., "Cancer Stem Cell Targeted Therapy: Progress amid Controversies," *Oncotarget* 6, no. 42 (2015): 44191–206, https://doi.org/10.18632/oncotarget.6176.

136. Huff et al., "Paradox of Response and Survival," 431–34.

137. Emmanuelle Charafe-Jauffret et al., "Aldehyde Dehydrogenase 1–Positive Cancer Stem Cells Mediate Metastasis and Poor Clinical Outcome in Inflammatory Breast Cancer," *Clinical Cancer Research* 16, no. 1 (January 2010): 45–55, https://doi.org/10.1158/1078-0432.CCR-09-1630; and Paola Marcato et al., "Aldehyde Dehydrogenase Activity of Breast Cancer Stem Cells Is Primarily Due to Isoform ALDH1A3 and Its Expression Is Predictive of Metastasis," *Stem Cells* 29, no. 1 (January 2011): 32–45, https://doi.org/10.1002/stem.563.

138. Huff et al., "Paradox of Response and Survival," 431–34.

139. Chann Lagadec et al., "Radiation-Induced Reprogramming of Breast Cancer Cells," *Stem Cells* 30, no. 5 (May 2012): 833–44, https://doi.org/10.1002/stem.1058.

140. Anasuya Ray, Smreti Vasudevan, and Suparna Sengupta, "6-Shogaol Inhibits Breast Cancer Cells and Stem Cell-Like Spheroids by Modulation of Notch Signaling Pathway and Induction of Autophagic Cell Death," *PLOS ONE* 10, no. 9 (September 10, 2015): e0137614, https://doi.org/10.1371/journal.pone.0137614.

141. Dominique Bonnet and John E. Dick, "Human Acute Myeloid Leukemia Is Organized as a Hierarchy That Originates from a Primitive Hematopoietic Cell," *Nature Medicine* 3, no. 7 (1997): 730–37, https://doi.org/10.1038/nm0797-730.

142. Jim Moselhy et al., "Natural Products That Target Cancer Stem Cells," *Anticancer Research* 35, no. 11 (November 2015): 5773–88, http://ar.iiarjournals.org/content/35/11/5773.abstract.

143. Lagadec et al., "Radiation-Induced Reprogramming of Breast Cancer Cells," 833–44.

144. Tsing Tsao et al., "Cancer Stem Cells in Prostate Cancer Radioresistance." *Cancer Letters* 465 (November 28, 2019): 94–104. https://doi.org/10.1016/j.canlet.2019.08.020.

145. Moselhy et al., "Natural Products That Target Cancer Stem Cells," 5773–88.

146. Colin A. Ross, "The Trophoblast Model of Cancer," *Nutrition and Cancer* 67, no. 1 (January 2, 2015): 61–67, https://doi.org/10.1080/01635581.2014.956257.

147. Nicholas J. Gonzalez, *Conquering Cancer: Volume One—50 Pancreatic and Breast Cancer Patients on the Gonzalez Nutritional Protocol* (New York: New Spring Press, 2016).

148. Ross, "The Trophoblast Model of Cancer," 61–67.

149. Ross, "The Trophoblast Model of Cancer," 61–67.

150. Ross, "The Trophoblast Model of Cancer," 61–67.

151. Nicholas J. Gonzalez, "The History of the Enzyme Treatment of Cancer," *Alternative Therapies in Health and Medicine* 20, suppl. 2 (October 2014): 30–44, https://www.ncbi.nlm.nih.gov/pubmed/25362215.

152. Ross, "The Trophoblast Model of Cancer," 61–67.

153. Gonzalez, "History of the Enzyme Treatment of Cancer," 61–67.

154. Ross, "The Trophoblast Model of Cancer," 61–67.

155. Gonzalez, "History of the Enzyme Treatment of Cancer," 61–67.

156. Ross, "The Trophoblast Model of Cancer," 61–67.

157. Gonzalez, "History of the Enzyme Treatment of Cancer," 61–67.

158. Ross, "The Trophoblast Model of Cancer," 61–67.

159. John Beard, *The Enzyme Treatment of Cancer* (London: Chatto & Windus, 1911).

160. Vladimir Vinnitsky, "Oncogerminative Hypothesis of Tumor-Formation," *Medical Hypotheses* 40, 1 (January 1993):19–27, https://doi.org/10.1016/0306-9877(93)90191-r.

161. Davies and Lineweaver, "Cancer Tumors as Metazoa 1.0," 15001.

162. Markus Hartl et. al., "Stem Cell-Specific Activation of an Ancestral Myc Protooncogene with Conserved Basic Functions in the Early Metazoan Hydra." *Proceedings of the National Academy of Sciences of the United States of America* 107, no. 9 (March 2, 2010): 4051–56. https://doi.org/10.1073/pnas.0911060107.

163. H. Land, L. Parada, and R. Weinberg, "Cellular Oncogenes and Multistep Carcinogenesis." *Science* 222, no. 4625 (November 18, 1983): 771. https://doi.org/10.1126/science.6356358.

164. Davies and Lineweaver, "Cancer Tumors as Metazoa 1.0," 15001.

165. Davies and Lineweaver, "Cancer Tumors as Metazoa 1.0," 15001.

166. Brian K. Hall, "Developmental Mechanisms Underlying the Atavisms," *Biological Reviews*, 59: 89–124, https://doi.org/10.1111/j.1469-185X.1984.tb00402.x.

167. Davies and Lineweaver, "Cancer Tumors as Metazoa 1.0," 15001.

168. Davies and Lineweaver, "Cancer Tumors as Metazoa 1.0," 15001.

169. Salam Ranabir and K. Reetu, "Stress and Hormones," *Indian Journal of Endocrinology and Metabolism* 15, no. 1 (January 2011): 18–22, https://doi.org/10.4103/2230-8210.77573.

170. James P. Herman et al., "Central Mechanisms of Stress Integration: Hierarchical Circuitry Controlling Hypothalamo–Pituitary–Adrenocortical Responsiveness," *Frontiers in Neuroendocrinology* 24, no. 3 (2003): 151–80, https://doi.org/https://doi.org/10.1016/j.yfrne.2003.07.001.

171. Kristin Tessmar-Raible et al., "Conserved Sensory-Neurosecretory Cell Types in Annelid and Fish Forebrain: Insights into Hypothalamus Evolution," *Cell* 129, no. 7 (June 29, 2007): 1389–1400, https://doi.org/10.1016/j.cell.2007.04.041.

172. Margaret E. Kemeny and Manfred Schedlowski, "Understanding the Interaction between Psychosocial Stress and Immune-Related Diseases: A Stepwise Progression," *Brain, Behavior, and Immunity* 21, no. 8 (November 2007): 1009–18, https://doi.org/10.1016/j.bbi.2007.07.010.

173. Kemeny and Schedlowski, "Interaction between Psychosocial Stress and Immune-Related Diseases," 1009–18.

174. Kemeny and Schedlowski, "Interaction between Psychosocial Stress and Immune-Related Diseases," 1009–18.

175. Isaac M. Chiu, Christian A. von Hehn, and Clifford J. Woolf, "Neurogenic Inflammation and the Peripheral Nervous System in Host Defense and Immunopathology," *Nature Neuroscience* 15, no. 8 (July 26, 2012): 1063–67, https://doi.org/10.1038/nn.3144.

176. Eric S. Wohleb et al., "Monocyte Trafficking to the Brain with Stress and Inflammation: A Novel Axis of Immune-to-Brain Communication That Influences Mood and Behavior," *Frontiers in Neuroscience* 8 (January 2015): 447, https://doi.org/10.3389/fnins.2014.00447.

177. Yao et al., "Adrenaline Induces Chemoresistance in HT-29 Colon Adenocarcinoma Cells," *Cancer Genetics* 190, no. 2 (April 15, 2009): 81–87, https://doi.org/10.1016/j.cancergencyto.2008.12.009.

178. "Crops Are Drenched with Roundup Pesticide Right before Harvest," *Washington's Blog*, November 17, 2014, http://washingtonsblog. com/2014/11/roundup-dumped-crops-right-harvest.html.

179. "262 Abstracts with Glyphosate Research," GreenMedInfo.com, accessed October 14, 2019, http://www.greenmedinfo.com/toxic-ingredient/glyphosate.

180. "Breast Cancer Hormone Receptor Status," American Cancer Society, last modified September 20, 2019, https://www.cancer.org/cancer/breast-cancer/under- standing-a-breast-cancer-diagnosis/breast-cancer-hormone-receptor- status.html.

181. Siriporn Thongprakaisang et al., "Glyphosate Induces Human Breast Cancer Cells Growth via Estrogen Receptors," *Food and Chemical Toxicology* 59 (September 2013): 129–36, https://doi.org/10.1016/j.fct.2013.05.057.

182. Feng-chih Chang, Matt F. Simcik, and Paul D. Capel, "Occurrence and Fate of the Herbicide Glyphosate and Its Degradate Aminomethylphosphonic Acid in the Atmosphere," *Environmental Toxicology and Chemistry* 30, no. 3 (March 2011): 548–55, https://doi.org/10.1002/etc.431.

183. Josep Sanchís et al., "Determination of Glyphosate in Groundwater Samples Using an Ultrasensitive Immunoassay and Confirmation by On-Line Solid- Phase Extraction Followed by Liquid Chromatography Coupled to Tandem Mass Spectrometry," *Analytical and Bioanalytical Chemistry* 402, no. 7 (March 2012): 2335–45, https://doi.org/10.1007/s00216-011-5541-y.

184. Christopher Exley et al., "Aluminium in Human Breast Tissue," *Journal of Inorganic Biochemistry* 101, no. 9 (September 2007): 1344–46, https:// doi.org/10.1016/j.jinorgbio.2007.06.005; and P. D. Darbre, "Aluminium, Antiperspirants and Breast Cancer," *Journal of Inorganic Biochemistry* 99, no. 9 (September 2005): 1912–19, https://doi.org/10.1016/j.jinorgbio.2005.06.001.

185. I. R. Wanless and W. R. Geddie, "Mineral Oil Lipogranulomata in Liver and Spleen. A Study of 465 Autopsies," *Archives of Pathology & Laboratory Medicine* 109, no. 3 (March 1985): 283–86, https://www.ncbi.nlm.nih.gov/ pubmed/3838459.

186. Øistein Svanes et al., "Cleaning at Home and at Work in Relation to Lung Function Decline and Airway Obstruction," *American Journal of Respiratory and Critical Care Medicine* 197, no. 9 (February 16, 2018): 1157–63, https://doi.org/10.1164/rccm.201706-1311OC.

187. Anna Liza C. Agero and Vermén M. Verallo-Rowell, "A Randomized Double-Blind Controlled Trial Comparing Extra Virgin Coconut Oil with Mineral Oil as a Moisturizer for Mild to Moderate Xerosis," *Dermatitis* 15, no. 3 (2004): 109–16, https://www.ncbi.nlm.nih.gov/pubmed/15724344; and S. B. Ruetsch et al., "Secondary Ion Mass Spectrometric Investigation of Penetration of Coconut and Mineral Oils into Human Hair Fibers: Relevance to Hair Damage," *Journal of the Society of Cosmetic Chemists* 52, no. 3 (May–June 2001): 169–84, https://www.ncbi.nlm.nih.gov/pubmed/11413497.

CHAPTER 5

1. Erum Naqvi, "Alzheimer's Disease Statistics," *Alzheimer's News Today*, accessed October 14, 2019, https://alzheimersnewstoday.com/alzheimers-disease-statistics/.

2. Tom Foster et al., "Normal Intracranial Calcifications," Radiopaedia, accessed October 14, 2019, https://radiopaedia.org/articles/normal-intracranial-calcifications.

3. Luisa-Sophie Liebrich et al., "Morphology and Function: MR Pineal Volume and Melatonin Level in Human Saliva Are Correlated," *Journal of Magnetic Resonance Imaging* 40, no. 4 (October 2014): 966–71, https://doi.org/10.1002/jmri.24449.

4. Rong-Yu Liu et al., "Decreased Melatonin Levels in Postmortem Cerebrospinal Fluid in Relation to Aging, Alzheimer's Disease, and Apolipoprotein E-ε4/4 Genotype1," *The Journal of Clinical Endocrinology & Metabolism* 84, no. 1 (January 1999): 323–27, https://doi.org/10.1210/jcem.84.1.5394.

5. Debra J. Skene and Dick F. Swaab, "Melatonin Rhythmicity: Effect of Age and Alzheimer's Disease," *Experimental Gerontology* 38, no. 1–2 (January 2003): 199–206, https://doi.org/10.1016/S0531-5565(02)00198-5.

6. Fèlix Grases, Antònia Costa-Bauzà, and Rafael M. Prieto, "A Potential Role for Crystallization Inhibitors in Treatment of Alzheimer's Disease," *Medical Hypotheses* 74, no. 1 (January 2010): 118–19, https://doi.org/10.1016/j.mehy.2009.07.029.

7. Owen Dyer, "Is Alzheimer's Really Just Type III Diabetes?: A Lack of Insulin May Cause AD, but Statins Could Keep It in Check," *National Review of Medicine* 2, no. 21, December 15, 2005, https://www.nationalreviewofmedicine.com/issue/2005/12_15/2_advances_medicine01_21.html.

8. T. Ohara et al., "Glucose Tolerance Status and Risk of Dementia in the Community," *Neurology* 77, no. 12 (September 20, 2011): 1126–34, https://doi.org/10.1212/WNL.0b013e31822f0435.

9. Suzanne M. de la Monte and Jack R. Wands, "Alzheimer's Disease Is Type 3 Diabetes—Evidence Reviewed," *Journal of Diabetes Science and Technology* 2, no. 6 (November 2008): 1101–13, https://doi.org/10.1177/193229680800200619.

10. Rudy J. Castellani et al., "Reexamining Alzheimer's Disease: Evidence for a Protective Role for Amyloid-Beta Protein Precursor and Amyloid-Beta," *Journal of Alzheimer's Disease* 18, no. 2 (2009): 447–52, https://doi.org/10.3233/JAD-2009-1151; Stephanie Plummer et al., "The Neuroprotective Properties of the Amyloid Precursor Protein Following Traumatic Brain Injury," *Aging and Disease* 7, no. 2 (March 15, 2016): 163–79, https://doi.org/10.14336/AD.2015.0907; and Deepak Kumar Vijaya Kumar et al., "Amyloid-β Peptide Protects against Microbial Infection in Mouse and Worm Models of Alzheimer's Disease," *Science Translational Medicine* 8, no. 340 (May 25, 2016): 340ra72, https://doi.org/10.1126/scitranslmed.aaf1059.

11. Jack Rubinstein, Feras Aloka, and George S. Abela, "Statin Therapy Decreases Myocardial Function as Evaluated via Strain Imaging," *Clinical Cardiology* 32, no. 12 (December 2009): 684–89, https://doi.org/10.1002/clc.20644.

12. Ryo Nakazato et al., "Statins Use and Coronary Artery Plaque Composition: Results from the International Multicenter CONFIRM Registry," *Atherosclerosis* 225, no. 1 (November 2012): 148–53, https://doi.org10.1016/j.atherosclerosis.2012.08.002.

13. Arjan van der Tol et al., "Statin Use and the Presence of Microalbuminuria. Results from the ERICABEL Trial: A Non-Interventional Epidemiological Cohort Study," *PLoS ONE* 7, no. 2 (2012): e31639, https://doi.org/10.1371/journal.pone.0031639.

14. "546 Abstracts with Statin Drugs Research," GreenMedInfo.com, accessed October 14, 2019, https://www.greenmedinfo.com/toxic-ingredient/statin-drugs.

15. "10 Abstracts with Statin Drugs & Carcinogenic Research," GreenMedInfo.com, accessed October 14, 2019, https://www.greenmedinfo.com/toxic-ingredient/statin-drugs?ed=35415.

16. "FDA Drug Safety Communication: Important Safety Label Changes to Cholesterol-Lowering Statin Drugs," U.S. Food & Drug Administration, February 28, 2012, https://www.fda.gov/drugs/drug-safety-and-availability/fda-drug-safety-communication-important-safety-label-changes-cholesterol-lowering-statin-drugs.

17. Adam D. M. Briggs, Anja Mizdrak, and Peter Scarborough, "A Statin a Day Keeps the Doctor Away: Comparative Proverb Assessment Modelling Study," *BMJ* 347, no. 7938 (2013): f7267, https://doi.org/10.1136/bmj.f7267.

18. Andrew J. Gawron et al., "Brand Name and Generic Proton Pump Inhibitor Prescriptions in the United States: Insights from the National Ambulatory Medical Care Survey (2006–2010)," *Gastroenterology Research and Practice* 2015 (2015): 689531, https://doi.org/10.1155/2015/689531.

19. "92 Abstracts with Acid Blockers Research," GreenMedInfo.com, accessed October 14, 2019, https://www.greenmedinfo.com/toxic-ingredient/acid-blockers.

20. Nigam H. Shah et al., "Proton Pump Inhibitor Usage and the Risk of Myocardial Infarction in the General Population," *PLOS ONE* 10, no. 6 (June 10, 2015): e0124653, https://doi.org/10.1371/journal.pone.0124653.

21. George Karamanolis et al., "A Glass of Water Immediately Increases Gastric pH in Healthy Subjects," *Digestive Diseases and Sciences* 53, no. 12 (December 2008): 3128–32, https://doi.org/10.1007/s10620-008-0301-3.

22. Fèlix Grases, Antònia Costa-Bauzà, and Rafael M. Prieto, "A Potential Role for Crystallization Inhibitors in Treatment of Alzheimer's Disease," *Medical Hypotheses* 74, no. 1 (January 2010): 118–19, https://doi.org/10.1016/j.mehy.2009.07.029.

23. Martha E. Payne et al., "Elevated Brain Lesion Volumes in Older Adults Who Use Calcium Supplements: A Cross-Sectional Clinical Observational Study," *The British Journal of Nutrition* 112, no. 2 (July 28, 2014): 220–27, https://doi.org/10.1017/S0007114514000828.

24. N. Bhala et al., "Vascular and Upper Gastrointestinal Effects of Non-Steroidal Anti-Inflammatory Drugs: Meta-Analyses of Individual Participant Data from Randomised Trials," *The Lancet* 382, no. 9894 (August 31, 2013): 769–79, https://doi.org/10.1016/S0140-6736(13)60900-9.

25. Geoffrey R .O. Durso, Andrew Luttrell, and Baldwin M. Way, "Over-the-Counter Relief from Pains and Pleasures Alike: Acetaminophen Blunts Evaluation Sensitivity to Both Negative and Positive Stimuli," *Psychological Science* 26, no. 6 (June 2015): 750–58, https://doi.org/10.1177/0956797615570366.

26. William Parker, "Tylenol Damages the Brains of Children, Research Reveals," GreenMedInfo.com, December 22, 2018, https://www.greenmedinfo.com/blog/tylenol-damages-brains-children-research-reveals.

27. Evie Stergiakouli et al., "Association of Acetaminophen Use during Pregnancy with Behavioral Problems in Childhood: Evidence Against Confounding," *JAMA Pediatrics* 170, no. 10 (October 2016): 964–70, https://doi.org/10.1001/jamapediatrics.2016.1775; and Magdalena Janecka et al., "Association of Autism Spectrum Disorder With Prenatal Exposure to Medication Affecting Neurotransmitter Systems," *JAMA Psychiatry* 75, no. 12 (2018): 1217–24, https://doi.org/10.1001/jamapsychiatry.2018.2728.

28. Paul Connett, "50 Reasons to Oppose Fluoridation," Fluoride Alert, last modified September 2012, accessed June 6, 2018, http://fluoridealert.org/articles/50-reasons/.

29. "The Extent of Water Fluoridation," 3rd. ed., *One in a Million: The Facts about Water Fluoridation*, British Fluoridation Society, May 2012, PDF.

30. "5 Abstracts with Fluoride & Childhood Cognitive Disorders Research," GreenMedInfo.com, accessed October 14, 2019, https://www.greenmedinfo.com/toxic-ingredient/fluoride?ed=24862.

31. Q. Tang et al., "Fluoride and Children's Intelligence: A Meta-Analysis," *Biological Trace Element Research* 126, no. 1–3 (2008): 115–200, https://doi.org/10.1007/s12011-008-8204-x.

32. "169 Abstracts with Gluten Research," GreenMedInfo.com, accessed October 14, 2019, http://www.greenmedinfo.com/toxic-ingredient/gluten.

33. "59 Abstracts with Cow Milk Research," GreenMedInfo.com, accessed October 14, 2019, http://www.greenmedinfo.com/toxic-ingredient/cow-milk.

34. Andreas Stefferl et al., "Butyrophilin, a Milk Protein, Modulates the Encephalitogenic T Cell Response to Myelin Oligodendrocyte Glycoprotein in Experimental Autoimmune Encephalomyelitis," *The Journal of Immunology* 165, no. 5 (September 2000): 2859–2865, https://doi.org/10.4049/jimmunol.165.5.2859.

35. K.-L. Reichelt and D. Jensen, "IgA Antibodies against Gliadin and Gluten in Multiple Sclerosis," Acta Neurologica Scandinavica 110, no. 4 (October 2004): 239–41, https://doi.org/10.1111/j.1600-0404.2004.00303.x.

36. Laura de Magistris et al., "Antibodies against Food Antigens in Patients with Autistic Spectrum Disorders," *BioMed Research International* 2013 (2013): 729349, https://doi.org/10.1155/2013/729349.

37. Vincent T. Ramaekers et al., "A Milk-Free Diet Downregulates Folate Receptor Autoimmunity in Cerebral Folate Deficiency Syndrome," *Developmental Medicine and Child Neurology* 50, no. 5 (May 2008): 346–52, https://doi.org/10.1111/j.1469-8749.2008.02053.x.

38. Kate S. Collison et al., "Prediabetic Changes in Gene Expression Induced by Aspartame and Monosodium Glutamate in Trans Fat-Fed C57Bl/6 J Mice," *Nutrition & Metabolism* 10, no. 55 (2013), https://doi.org/10.1186/1743-7075-10-44.

39. "Focused Research Topics Aspartame & Neurotoxic," GreenMedInfo.com, accessed October 15, 2019, https://www.greenmedinfo.com/greenmed/topic/52533/focus/35335/page; "Focused Research Topics Aspartame & Carcinogenic," GreenMedInfo.com, accessed October 15, 2019, https://www.greenmedinfo.com/greenmed/topic/52533/focus/35415/page; and Morando Soffritti et al., "The Carcinogenic Effects of Aspartame: The Urgent Need for Regulatory Re-evaluation," *American Journal of Industrial Medicine* 57, no. 4 (April 2014): 383–97, https://doi.org/10.1002/ajim.22296.

40. "75 Abstracts with Aspartame Research," GreenMedInfo.com, accessed October 15, 2019, http://www.greenmedinfo.com/toxic-ingredient/aspartame.

41. Ashok Iyyaswamy and Sheeladevi Rathinasamy, "Effect of Chronic E xposure to Aspartame on Oxidative Stress in the Brain Discrete Regions of Albino Rats," *Journal of Biosciences* 37, no. 4 (September 2012): 679–88, https://doi.org/10.1007/s12038-012-9236-0.

42. Susan S. Schiffman and Kristina I. Rother, "Sucralose, a Synthetic Organochlorine Sweetener: Overview of Biological Issues," *Journal of Toxicology and Environmental Health*, Part B 16, no. 7 (2013): 399–451, https://doi.org/10.1080/10937404.2013.842523.

43. Sayer Ji, "Top Five Reasons Never to Use Splenda," GreenMedInfo. com, accessed July 23, 2018, http://www.greenmedinfo.com/blog/top-5-reasons-never-use-splenda.

44. C. Y. Chang, D. S. Ke, and J. Y. Chen, "Essential Fatty Acids and Human Brain," *Acta Neurologica Taiwanica* 18, no. 4 (December 2009): 231–41, https://www.ncbi.nlm.nih.gov/pubmed/20329590.

45. "537 Abstracts with Omega-3 Fatty Acids Research," GreenMedInfo.com, accessed October 15, 2019, https://www.greenmedinfo.com/substance/omega-3-fatty-acids.

46. Ya-xing Gui et al., "Glyphosate Induced Cell Death through Apoptotic and Autophagic Mechanisms," *Neurotoxicology and Teratology* 34, no. 3 (2012): 344–49, https://doi.org/10.1016/j.ntt.2012.03.005.

47. "16 Abstracts with Aerotoxic Syndrome Research," GreenMedInfo.com, accessed October 15, 2019, https://www.greenmedinfo.com/disease/aerotoxic-syndrome.

48. Jim Gold, "Boeing Suit Settlement Stirs Jetliner Air Safety Debate," *NBC News*, October 6, 2011, http://www.nbcnews.com/id/44777304/ns/travel-news/t/boeing-suit-settlement-stirs-jetliner-air-safety-debate/#.XbsuxEVKgUE.

49. Suzanne Roggeveen et al., "EEG Changes Due to Experimentally Induced 3G Mobile Phone Radiation," *PLOS ONE* 10, no. 6 (June 8, 2015): e0129496, https://doi.org/10.1371/journal.pone.0129496.

50. Laura Zheng et al., "Curcuminoids Enhance Amyloid-Beta Uptake by Macrophages of Alzheimer's Disease Patients," *Journal of Alzheimer's Disease* 10, no. 1, (2006): 1–7, https://doi.org/10.3233/JAD-2006-10101.

51. Ava Masoumi et al., "1α,25-dihydroxyvitamin D3 Interacts with Curcuminoids to Stimulate Amyloid-β Clearance by Macrophages of Alzheimer's Disease Patients," *Journal of Alzheimer's Disease* 17, no. 3 (2009): 703–17, https://doi.org/10.3233/JAD-2009-1080.

52. Hongying Liu et al., "The Inhibitory Effects of Different Curcuminoids on β-Amyloid Protein, β-Amyloid Precursor Protein and β-Site Amyloid Precursor Protein Cleaving Enzyme 1 in swAPP HEK293 Cells," *Neuroscience Letters* 485, no. 2 (November 19, 2010): 83–88, https://doi.org/10.1016/j.neulet.2010.08.035; Shilpa Mishra et al., "Tetrahydrocurcumin Confers Protection against Amyloid β-Induced Toxicity," *NeuroReport* 22, no. 1 (January 5, 2011): 23–27, https://doi.org/10.1097/WNR.0b013e328341e141; and Xiao-Yan Qin, Yong Cheng, and Long-Chuan Yu, "Potential Protection of Curcumin against Intracellular Amyloid β-Induced Toxicity in Cultured Rat Prefrontal Cortical Neurons," *Neuroscience Letters* 480, no. 1 (August 9, 2010): 21–24, https://doi.org/10.1016/j.neulet.2010.05.062.

53. "303 Abstracts with Ginger Research," GreenMedInfo.com, accessed July 22, 2018, https://www.greenmedinfo.com/substance/ginger.

54. Maya Mathew and Sarada Subramanian, "In Vitro Evaluation of Anti-Alzheimer Effects of Dry Ginger (Zingiber officinale Roscoe) Extract," *Indian Journal of Experimental Biology* 52, no. 6 (June 2014): 606–12, https://www.ncbi.nlm.nih.gov/pubmed/24956891/.

55. "303 Abstracts with Ginger Research," GreenMedInfo.com.

56. Xingyi Chen, You Zhou, and Jiujiu Yu, "Exosome-like Nanoparticles from Ginger Rhizomes Inhibited NLRP3 Inflammasome Activation," *Molecular Pharmaceutics* 16, no. 6, (2019): 2690–99, https://doi.org/10.1021/acs.molpharmaceut.9b00246.

57. "303 Abstracts with Ginger Research," GreenMedInfo.com.

58. Andrew Pengelly et al., "Short-Term Study on the Effects of Rosemary on Cognitive Function in an Elderly Population," *Journal of Medicinal Food* 15, no. 1 (August 30, 2011): 10–17, https://doi.org/10.1089/jmf.2011.0005.

59. Lei Wu, Dali Sun, and Yao He. "Coffee Intake and the Incident Risk of Cognitive Disorders: A Dose–Response Meta-Analysis of Nine Prospective Cohort Studies," Clinical Nutrition 36, no. 3 (June 2017): 730–736, https://doi.org/10.1016/j.clnu.2016.05.015.

60. Lei Wu, Dali Sun, and Yao He, "Coffee Intake and the Incident Risk of Cognitive Disorders: A Dose–Response Meta-Analysis of Nine Prospective Cohort Studies." Clinical Nutrition 36, no. 3 (June 1, 2017): 730–36. https://doi.org/10.1016/j.clnu.2016.05.015.

61. Ashley May, "Coffee Linked to Longer Life in Latest Study, Suggesting It's Part of a Healthy Diet," USA Today, July 3, 2018, https://www.usatoday.com/story/news/nation-now/2018/07/03/coffee-linked-longer-life-jama-study/753894002/.

62. Keiko Unno et al., "Daily Ingestion of Green Tea Catechins from Adulthood Suppressed Brain Dysfunction in Aged Mice," BioFactors 34, no. 4 (2008): 263–71, https://doi.org/10.1002/biof.5520340402; and Keiko Unno et al., "Daily Consumption of Green Tea Catechin Delays Memory Regression in Aged Mice," Biogerontology 8, no. 2 (April 2007): 89–95, https://doi.org/10.1007/s10522-006-9036-8.

63. Shinichi Kuriyama et al., "Green Tea Consumption and Cognitive Function: A Cross-Sectional Study from the Tsurugaya Project," The American Journal of Clinical Nutrition 83, no. 2 (February 2006): 355–61, https://doi.org/10.1093/ajcn/83.2.355.

64. Usha Gundimeda et al., "Green Tea Catechins Potentiate the Neuritogenic Action of Brain-Derived Neurotrophic Factor: Role of 67-KDa Laminin Receptor and Hydrogen Peroxide," Biochemical and Biophysical Research Communications 445, no. 1 (2014): 218–24, https://doi.org/10.1016 j.bbrc.2014.01.166.

65. Keiko Unno et al., "Stress-Reducing Function of Matcha Green Tea in Animal Experiments and Clinical Trials," Nutrients 10, no. 10 (October 2018): 1468, https://doi.org/10.3390/nu10101468.

66. Peter Pribis et al., "Effects of Walnut Consumption on Cognitive Performance in Young Adults," British Journal of Nutrition 107, no. 9 (2012): 1393–1401, https://doi.org/10.1017/S0007114511004302; and Cheng-Chen Zhang et al., "Chemical Constituents from Hericium Erinaceus Promote Neuronal Survival and Potentiate Neurite Outgrowth via the TrkA/Erk1/2 Pathway," International Journal of Molecular Sciences 18, no. 8 (July 30, 2017): 1659, https://doi.org/10.3390/ijms18081659.

67. Blanka Klimova et al., "Role of Nut Consumption in the Management of Cognitive Decline—a Mini-Review," Current Alzheimer Research 15, no. 9 (2018): 877–82, https://doi.org/10.2174/1567205015666180202100721.

68. "Ginkgo biloba & Cognitive Decline/Dysfunction," GreenMedInfo.com, https://www.greenmedinfo.health/greenmed/topic/18529/focus/6380/page.

69. "230 Abstracts With Ginkgo Biloba Research," GreenMedInfo.com, https://www.greenmedinfo.health/substance/ginkgo-biloba.

70. Xiang Yang Zhang et al., "Brain-Derived Neurotrophic Factor Levels and Its Val66Met Gene Polymorphism Predict Tardive Dyskinesia Treatment Response to Ginkgo Biloba." *Biological Psychiatry* 72, no. 8 (October 15, 2012): 700–706, https://doi.org/10.1016/j.biopsych.2012.04.032.

71. Lisa M. Eubanks et al., "A Molecular Link between the Active Component of Marijuana and Alzheimer's Disease Pathology," *Molecular Pharmaceutics* 3, no. 6 (2006): 773–77, https://doi.org/10.1021/mp060066m; and "657 Abstracts with Cannabidiol Research," GreenMedInfo.com, accessed October 15, 2019, https://www.greenmedinfo.com/substance/cannabidiol?ed=5423.

72. Thorne Research, "Medium Chain Triglycerides," *Alternative Medicine Review* 7, no. 5 (2002): 418–20.

73. W. Fernando et al., "The Role of Dietary Coconut for the Prevention and Treatment of Alzheimer's Disease: Potential Mechanisms of Action," *British Journal of Nutrition* 144, no. 1, (July 14, 2015): 1–14, https://doi.org/10.1017/S0007114515001452.

74. Lulu Xie, Lulu et al., "Sleep Drives Metabolite Clearance from the Adult Brain," *Science* 342, no. 6156 (October 18, 2013): 373, https://doi.org/10.1126/science.1241224.

75. Brendan P. Lucey and Randall J. Bateman, "Amyloid-β Diurnal Pattern: Possible Role of Sleep in Alzheimer's Disease Pathogenesis," *Neurobiology of Aging* 35, suppl. 2 (September 2014): S29–34, https://doi.org/10.1016/j.neurobiolaging.2014.03.035.

76. Miguel A. Pappolla et al., "The Neuroprotective Activities of Melatonin against the Alzheimer β-Protein Are Not Mediated by Melatonin Membrane Receptors," *Journal of Pineal Research* 32, no. 3 (April 2002): 135–42, https://doi.org/10.1034/j.1600-079x.2002.1o838.x.

77. Daniel M. Johnstone et al., "Turning On Lights to Stop Neurodegeneration: The Potential of Near Infrared Light Therapy in Alzheimer's and Parkinson's Disease," *Frontiers in Neuroscience* 9 (January 11, 2016): 500, https://doi.org/10.3389/fnins.2015.00500.

78. Rui-xia Jia et al., "Effects of Physical Activity and Exercise on the Cognitive Function of Patients with Alzheimer Disease: a Meta-analysis," *BMC Geriatrics* 19, no. 1 (July 2019): 181, https://doi.org/10.1186/s12877-019-1175-2.

79. Nicole L. Spartano et al., "Midlife Exercise Blood Pressure, Heart Rate, and Fitness Relate to Brain Volume 2 Decades Later," *Neurology* 86, no. 14 (April 5, 2016): 1313–19, https://doi.org/10.1212/WNL.0000000000002415.

80. Michael P. Bancks et al., "Cardiovascular Health in Young Adulthood and Structural Brain MRI in Midlife: The CARDIA Study," *Neurology* 89, no. 7 (August 15, 2017): 680–86, https://doi.org/10.1212/WNL.0000000000004222.

81. Nicole L. Spartano and Tiia Ngandu, "Fitness and Dementia Risk," *Neurology* 90, no. 15 (April 10, 2018): 675–76, https://doi.org/10.1212/WNL.0000000000005282.

82. J. Eric Ahlskog, "Does Vigorous Exercise Have a Neuroprotective Effect in Parkinson Disease?," *Neurology* 77, no. 3 (July 19, 2011): 288–94, https://doi.org/10.1212/WNL.0b013e318225ab66.

83. Kathrin Rehfeld et al., "Dancing or Fitness Sport? The Effects of Two Training Programs on Hippocampal Plasticity and Balance Abilities in Healthy Seniors," *Frontiers in Human Neuroscience* 11 (June 15, 2017): 305, https://www.ncbi.nlm.nih.gov/pubmed/28674488.

84. Josif Milin, "Stress-Reactive Response of the Gerbil Pineal Gland: Concretion Genesis," *General and Comparative Endocrinology* 110, no. 3 (June 1998): 237–51, https://doi.org/10.1006/gcen.1998.7069.

85. Sarah Lazar, "Meditation Can Reshape the Brain: TEDx Cambridge 2011," YouTube video, 8:33, Tedx Talks, January 23, 2012, https://www.youtube.com/watch?v=m8rRzTtP7Tc.

86. Kim E. Innes et al., "Meditation and Music Improve Memory and Cognitive Function in Adults with Subjective Cognitive Decline: A Pilot Randomized Controlled Trial," *Journal of Alzheimer's Disease* 56, no. 3 (2017): 899–916, https://doi.org/10.3233/jad-160867.

87. Hajime Fukui and Kumiko Toyoshima, "Music Facilitate the Neurogenesis, Regeneration and Repair of Neurons," *Medical Hypotheses* 71, 5 (November 2008): 765–769, https://doi.org/10.1016/j.mehy.2008.06.019.

88. Hajime Fukui and Kumiko Toyoshima, "Music Facilitate the Neurogenesis, Regeneration and Repair of Neurons," *Medical Hypotheses* 71, no. 5 (2008): 765–69, https://doi.org/10.1016/j.mehy.2008.06.019.

89. Michael H. Thaut, Martina Demartin, and Jerome N. Sanes, "Brain Networks for Integrative Rhythm Formation," *PLoS ONE* 3, no. 5 (May 2008): e2312, https://doi.org/10.1371/journal.pone.0002312; and Michael H. Thaut et al., "Neurologic Music Therapy Improves Executive Function and Emotional Adjustment in Traumatic Brain Injury Rehabilitation," *Annals of the New York Academy of Sciences* 1169, no. 1 (July 2009): 406–16, https://doi.org/10.1111/j.1749-6632.2009.04585.x.

CHAPTER 6

1. Antonio P. Beltrami et al., "Evidence That Human Cardiac Myocytes Divide after Myocardial Infarction," *New England Journal of Medicine* 344, no. 23 (June 7, 2001): 1750–57, https://doi.org/10.1056/NEJM200106073442303.

2. Matthew L. Steinhauser and Richard T. Lee, "Regeneration of the Heart," *EMBO Molecular Medicine* 3, no. 12 (December 2011): 701–12, https://doi.org/10.1002/emmm.201100175.

3. Annelieke M. Roest et al., "Anxiety and Risk of Incident Coronary Heart Disease: A Meta-Analysis," *Journal of the American College of Cardiology* 56, no. 1 (June 29, 2010): 38–46, https://doi.org/10.1016/j.jacc.2010.03.034.

4. P. J. Tully et al., "Panic Disorder and Incident Coronary Heart Disease: A Systematic Review and Meta-Regression in 1,131,612 Persons and 58,111 Cardiac Events," *Psychological Medicine* 45, no. 14 (2015): 2909–20, https://doi.org/10.1017/S0033291715000963.

5. Andrew Steptoe and Mika Kivimaki, "Stress and Cardiovascular Disease," *Nature Reviews Cardiology* 9 (2012): 360–70, https://doi.org/10.1038/nrcardio.2012.45.

6. Nobutaka Inoue, "Stress and Atherosclerotic Cardiovascular Disease," *Journal of Atherosclerosis and Thrombosis* 21, no. 5 (2014): 391–401, https://doi.org/10.5551/jat.21709.

7. Steptoe and Kivimaki, "Stress and Cardiovascular Disease," 360–70.

8. Alain Tedgui and Ziad Mallat, "Cytokines in Atherosclerosis: Pathogenic and Regulatory Pathways," *Physiological Reviews* 86 (May 2006): 515–81, https://doi.org/10.1152/physrev.00024.2005.

9. Tedgui and Mallat, "Cytokines in Atherosclerosis," 515–81.

10. Ka He et al., "Magnesium Intake and the Metabolic Syndrome: Epidemiologic Evidence to Date," *Journal of the CardioMetabolic Syndrome* 1, no. 5 (September 2006): 351–55, https://doi.org/10.1111/j.1559-4564.2006.05702.x.

11. Robert J. Chilton, "Pathophysiology of Coronary Heart Disease: A Brief Review," *The Journal of the American Osteopathic Association* 104, no. 9, suppl. 7 (September 2004): S5–8.

12. Chilton, "Pathophysiology of Coronary Heart Disease," S5–8.

13. Manfredi Rizzo and Kaspar Berneis, "Small, Dense Low-Density-Lipoproteins and the Metabolic Syndrome," *Diabetes/Metabolism Research and Reviews* 23, no. 1 (January 2007): 14–20, https://doi.org/10.1002/dmrr.694; and G. Pichler et al., "LDL Particle Size and Composition and Incident Cardiovascular Disease in a South-European Population: The Hortega-Liposcale Follow-Up Study," *International Journal of Cardiology* 264 (March 1, 2018): 172–78, https://doi.org/10.1016/j.ijcard.2018.03.128.

14. Kathiresan Sekar et al., "Increased Small Low-Density Lipoprotein Particle Number," *Circulation* 113, no. 1 (January 3, 2006): 20–29, https://doi.org/10.1161/CIRCULATIONAHA.105.567107.

15. Emil Ginter, Igo Kajaba, and Marián Šauša, "Addition of Statins into the Public Water Supply? Risks of Side Effects and Low Cholesterol Levels" [in Czech], *Cas Lek Cesk* 151, no. 5 (2012): 243–47, https://www.ncbi.nlm.nih.gov/pubmed/22779765.

16. Amit Sachdeva et al., "Lipid Levels in Patients Hospitalized with Coronary Artery Disease: An Analysis of 136,905 Hospitalizations in Get With The Guidelines," *American Heart Journal* 157, no. 1 (January 2009): 111–17.e2, https://doi.org/10.1016/j.ahj.2008.08.010.

17. Pavel Otruba, Petr Kanovsky, and Petr Hlustik, "Treatment with Statins and Peripheral Neuropathy: Results of 36-Months a Prospective Clinical and Neurophysiological Follow-Up," *Neuro Endocrinology Letters* 32, no. 5 (September 14, 2011): 688–90.

18. Charles Harper and Terry Jacobson, "The Broad Spectrum of Statin Myopathy: From Myalgia to Rhabdomyolysis," *Current Opinion in Lipidology* 18, no. 4 (August 2007): 401–8, https://doi.org/10.1097/ MOL.0b013e32825a6773.

19. Einar Björnsson, Elin I. Jacobsen, and Evangelos Kalaitzakis, "Hepatotoxicity Associated with Statins: Reports of Idiosyncratic Liver Injury Post-Marketing," *Journal of Hepatology* 56, no. 2 (February 2012): 374–80, https:// doi.org/10.1016/j.jhep.2011.07.023.

20. Robin J. Edison and Maximilian Muenke, "Central Nervous System and Limb Anomalies in Case Reports of First-Trimester Statin Exposure," *New England Journal of Medicine* 350, no. 15 (April 8, 2004): 1579–82, https://doi.org/10.1056/NEJM200404083501524.

21. Markku T. Hyyppä et al., "Does Simvastatin Affect Mood and Steroid Hormone Levels in Hypercholesterolemic Men? A Randomized Double-Blind Trial," *Psychoneuroendocrinology* 28, no. 2 (February 2003): 181–94, https://doi.org/10.1016/S0306-4530(02)00014-8.

22. Leslie R. Wagstaff et al., "Statin-Associated Memory Loss: Analysis of 60 Case Reports and Review of the Literature," *Pharmacotherapy: The Journal of Human Pharmacology and Drug Therapy* 23, no. 7 (July 2003): 871–80, https://doi.org/10.1592/phco.23.7.871.32720.

23. David Preiss et al., "Risk of Incident Diabetes With Intensive-Dose Compared with Moderate-Dose Statin Therapy: A Meta-Analysis," *JAMA* 305, no. 24 (June 22, 2011): 2556–64, https://doi.org/10.1001/jama.2011.860.

24. Ian Hamilton-Craig et al., "At Sea with SEAS: The First Clinical Endpoint Trial for Ezetimibe, Treatment of Patients with Mild to Moderate Aortic Stenosis, Ends with Mixed Results and More Controversy," *Heart, Lung and Circulation* 18, no. 5 (October 2009): 343–46, https://doi.org/10.1016/j. hlc.2009.02.007.

25. Aramesh Saremi et al., "Progression of Vascular Calcification Is Increased with Statin Use in the Veterans Affairs Diabetes Trial (VADT)," *Diabetes Care* 35, no. 11 (November 2012): 2390–92, https://doi.org/10.2337/dc12-0464.

26. E. J. Mills et al., "Efficacy and Safety of Statin Treatment for Cardiovascular Disease: A Network Meta-Analysis of 170 255 Patients from 76 Randomized Trials," *QJM: Monthly Journal of the Association of Physicians* 104, no. 2 (February 2011): 109–24, https://doi.org/10.1093/qjmed/hcq165.

27. Michel de Lorgeril et al., "Lipid-Lowering Drugs and Essential Omega-6 and Omega-3 Fatty Acids in Patients with Coronary Heart Disease," *Nutrition, Metabolism & Cardiovascular Diseases* 15, no. 1 (February 2005): 36–41, https://doi.org/10.1016/j.numecd.2004.09.001.

28. Majid Ghayour-Mobarhan et al., "Effect of Statin Therapy on Serum Trace Element Status in Dyslipidaemic Subjects," *Second International Symposium on Trace Elements and Minerals in Medicine and Biology* 19, no. 1 (September 19, 2005): 61–67, https://doi.org/10.1016/j.jtemb.2005.06.003.

29. Bernd Moosmann and Christian Behl, "Selenoprotein Synthesis and Side-Effects of Statins," *The Lancet* 363, no. 9412 (April 2004): 892–94, https://doi.org/10.1016/S0140-6736(04)15739-5.

30. Francesco Galli and Luigi Iuliano, "Do Statins Cause Myopathy by Lowering Vitamin E Levels?," *Medical Hypotheses* 74, no. 4 (April 2010): 707–9, https://doi.org/10.1016/j.mehy.2009.10.031.

31. "546 Abstracts with Statin Drugs Research," GreenMedInfo.com.

32. Aidan Ryan, Simon Heath, and Paul Cook, "Primary Prevention with Statins for Older Adults," *BMJ* 362, no. 8166 (2018): k3695, https://doi.org/10.1136/bmj.k3695.

33. Halfdan Petursson et al., "Is the Use of Cholesterol in Mortality Risk Algorithms in Clinical Guidelines Valid? Ten Years Prospective Data from the Norwegian HUNT 2 Study," *Journal of Evaluation in Clinical Practice* 18 (February 2012): 159–68, https://doi.org/10.1111/j.1365-2753.2011.01767.x; and Dariush Mozaffarian and David S. Ludwig, "The 2015 US Dietary Guidelines: Lifting the Ban on Total Dietary Fat," *JAMA* 313, no. 24 (June 23, 2015): 2421–22, https://doi.org/10.1001/jama.2015.5941.

34. Christopher E. Ramsden et al., "Re-evaluation of the Traditional Diet-Heart Hypothesis: Analysis of Recovered Data from Minnesota Coronary Experiment (1968–73)," *BMJ* 353, no. 8053 (2016): i1246, https://doi.org/10.1136/bmj.i1246.

35. Patty Siri-Tarino et al., "Meta-Analysis of Prospective Cohort Studies Evaluating the Association of Saturated Fat with Cardiovascular Disease," *The American Journal of Clinical Nutrition* 91, no. 3 (March 2010): 535–46, https://doi.org/10.3945/ajcn.2009.27725.

36. Russell J. de Souza et al., "Intake of Saturated and Trans Unsaturated Fatty Acids and Risk of All Cause Mortality, Cardiovascular Disease, and Type 2 Diabetes: Systematic Review and Meta-Analysis of Observational Studies," *BMJ* 351 (2015): h3978, https://doi.org/10.1136/bmj.h3978.

37. F. L. Santos et al., "Systematic Review and Meta-Analysis of Clinical Trials of the Effects of Low Carbohydrate Diets on Cardiovascular Risk Factors," *Obesity Reviews* 13, no. 11 (November 2012): 1048–66, https://doi.org/10.1111/j.1467-789X.2012.01021.x.

38. B. Burlingame et al., "Fats and Fatty Acids in Human Nutrition: Introduction," *Annals of Nutrition & Metabolism* 55, no. 1–3 (2009): 5–7, https://doi.org/10.1159/000228993.

39. Bruce A. Griffin et al., "APOE4 Genotype Exerts Greater Benefit in Lowering Plasma Cholesterol and Apolipoprotein B than Wild Type (E3/E3), after Replacement of Dietary Saturated Fats with Low Glycaemic Index Carbohydrates," *Nutrients* 10, no. 10 (October 17, 2018): 1524, https://doi.org/10.3390/nu10101524.

40. Venkatesh Mani, James H. Hollis, and Nicholas K. Gabler, "Dietary Oil Composition Differentially Modulates Intestinal Endotoxin Transport and Postprandial Endotoxemia," *Nutrition & Metabolism* 10, no. 1 (January 10, 2013): 6, https://doi.org/10.1186/1743-7075-10-6.

41. Paul B. Nolan et al., "Prevalence of Metabolic Syndrome and Metabolic Syndrome Components in Young Adults: A Pooled Analysis," *Preventive Medicine Reports* 7 (July 19, 2017): 211–15, https://doi.org/10.1016 j.pmedr.2017.07.004.

42. "Third Report of the National Cholesterol Education Program (NCEP) Expert Panel on Detection, Evaluation, and Treatment of High Blood Cholesterol in Adults (Adult Treatment Panel III) Final Report," *Circulation* 106, no. 25 (December 17, 2002): 3143, https://doi.org/10.1161/circ.106.25.3143.

43. Scott M. Grundy et al., "Diagnosis and Management of the Metabolic Syndrome," *Circulation* 112, no. 17 (October 25, 2005): 2735–52, https://doi.org/10.1161/CIRCULATIONAHA.105.169404.

44. Mark Houston, "Nutrition and Nutraceutical Supplements for the Treatment of Hypertension: Part II," *The Journal of Clinical Hypertension* 15, no. 11 (November 2013): 845–51, https://doi.org/10.1111/jch.12212.

45. Houston, "Nutrition and Nutraceutical Supplements," 845–51.

46. Grundy et al., "Diagnosis and Management of the Metabolic Syndrome," 2735–52.

47. Darcy B. Carr et al., "Intra-Abdominal Fat Is a Major Determinant of the National Cholesterol Education Program Adult Treatment Panel III Criteria for the Metabolic Syndrome," *Diabetes* 53, no. 8 (August 2004): 2087–94, https://doi.org/10.2337/diabetes.53.8.2087.

48. Markku Laakso, "Hyperglycemia as a Risk Factor for Cardiovascular Disease in Type 2 Diabetes," *Primary Care: Clinics in Office Practice* 26, no. 4 (December 1999): 829–39, https://doi.org/10.1016/S0095-4543(05)70133-0.

49. Tongjian You et al., "Abdominal Adipose Tissue Cytokine Gene Expression: Relationship to Obesity and Metabolic Risk Factors," *American Journal of Physiology-Endocrinology and Metabolism* 288, no. 4 (April 2005): E741–47, https://doi.org/10.1152/ajpendo.00419.2004; and Jeffrey D. Browning et al., "Prevalence of Hepatic Steatosis in an Urban Population in the United States: Impact of Ethnicity," *Hepatology* 40, no. 6 (December 2004): 1387–95, https://doi.org/10.1002/hep.20466.

50. Gianluca Perseghin et al., "Metabolic Defects in Lean Nondiabetic Offspring of NIDDM Parents: A Cross-Sectional Study," *Diabetes* 46, no. 6 (June 1997): 1001–9, https://doi.org/10.2337/diab.46.6.1001.

51. Grundy et al., "Diagnosis and Management of the Metabolic Syndrome," 2735–52.

52. Hannele Yki-Järvinen, "Nutritional Modulation of Non-alcoholic Fatty Liver Disease and Insulin Resistance," *Nutrients* 7, no. 11 (November 5, 2015): 9127–38, https://doi.org/10.3390/nu7115454.

53. E. Corpeleijn, W. H. M. Saris, and E. E. Blaak, "Metabolic Flexibility in the Development of Insulin Resistance and Type 2 Diabetes: Effects of Lifestyle," *Obesity Reviews* 10, no. 2 (March 2009): 178–93, https://doi.org/10.1111/j.1467-789X.2008.00544.x.

54. Yki-Järvinen, "Nutritional Modulation of Non-alcoholic Fatty Liver Disease," 9127–38.

55. Grundy et al., "Diagnosis and Management of the Metabolic Syndrome," 2735–52.

56. Peramaiyan Rajendran et al., "The Vascular Endothelium and Human Diseases," *International Journal of Biological Sciences* 9, no. 10 (November 9, 2013): 1057–69, https://doi.org/10.7150/ijbs.7502.

57. R. Jay Widmer and Amir Lerman, "Endothelial Dysfunction and Cardiovascular Disease," *Global Cardiology Science & Practice* 2014, no. 43 (October 16, 2014): 291–308, https://doi.org/10.5339/gcsp.2014.43.

58. Michel Félétou, "Multiple Functions of the Endothelial Cells," in *The Endothelium: Part 1: Multiple Functions of the Endothelial Cells—Focus on Endothelium-Derived Vasoactive Mediators* (San Rafael, CA: Morgan & Claypool Life Sciences, 2011).

59. Widmer and Lerman, "Endothelial Dysfunction and Cardiovascular Disease," 291–308; and Sven Möbius-Winkler et al., "How to Improve Endothelial Repair Mechanisms: The Lifestyle Approach," *Expert Review of Cardiovascular Therapy* 8, no. 4 (April 2010): 573–80, https://doi.org/10.1586/erc.10.7.

60. David Abraham and Oliver Distler, "How Does Endothelial Cell Injury Start? The Role of Endothelin in Systemic Sclerosis," *Arthritis Research & Therapy* 9, Suppl suppl. 2, no. Suppl 2 (2007): S2–S2, https://doi.org/10.1186/ar2186.

61. Andrew Rosenbaum et al., "Outcomes Related to Antiplatelet or Anticoagulation Use in Patients Undergoing Carotid Endarterectomy," *Annals of Vascular Surgery* 25, no. 1 (January 2011): 25–31, https://doi.org/10.1016/j.avsg.2010.06.007.

62. M. L. Flaherty et al., "The Increasing Incidence of Anticoagulant-Associated Intracerebral Hemorrhage," *Neurology* 68, no. 2 (January 9, 2007): 116, https://doi.org/10.1212/01.wnl.0000250340.05202.8b.

63. Zahra Rezaieyazdi et al., "Reduced Bone Density in Patients on Long-Term Warfarin," *International Journal of Rheumatic Diseases* 12, no. 2 (July 2009): 130–35, https://doi.org/10.1111/j.1756-185X.2009.01395.x.

64. G. P. Lambert et al., "Effect of Aspirin Dose on Gastrointestinal Permeability," *International Journal of Sports Medicine* 33, no. 6 (May 29, 2012): 421–25, https://doi.org/10.1055/s-0032-1301892.

65. Kuanrong Li et al., "Associations of Dietary Calcium Intake and Calcium Supplementation with Myocardial Infarction and Stroke Risk and Overall Cardiovascular Mortality in the Heidelberg Cohort of the European Prospective Investigation into Cancer and Nutrition study (EPIC-Heidelberg)," *BMJ* 98, no. 12 (2012): 920–25, https://doi.org/10.1136/heartjnl-2011-300806.

66. Mark J. Bolland et al., "Calcium and Vitamin D Supplements and Health Outcomes: A Reanalysis of the Women's Health Initiative (WHI) Limited-Access Data Set," *The American Journal of Clinical Nutrition* 94, no. 4 (October 2011): 1144–49, https://doi.org/10.3945/ajcn.111.015032; and Mark J. Bolland et al., "Effect of Calcium Supplements on Risk of Myocardial Infarction and Cardiovascular Events: Meta-Analysis," *BMJ* 341, no. 7767 (2010): c3691, https://doi.org/10.1136/bmj.c3691.

67. Jeri W. Nieves, "Osteoporosis: The Role of Micronutrients," *The American Journal of Clinical Nutrition* 81, no. 5 (May 1, 2005): 1232S–1239S, https://doi.org/10.1093/ajcn/81.5.1232.

68. Lin Ling, Shaohua Gu, and Yan Cheng, "Resveratrol Activates Endogenous Cardiac Stem Cells and Improves Myocardial Regeneration following Acute Myocardial Infarction," *Molecular Medicine Reports* 15, no. 3 (March 2017): 1188–94, https://doi.org/10.3892/mmr.2017.6143.

69. Partha Mukhopadhyay et al., "Restoration of Altered MicroRNA Expression in the Ischemic Heart with Resveratrol," *PLoS ONE* 5, no. 12 (2010): e15705, https://doi.org/10.1371/journal.pone.0015705.

70. Denise Wilson, "Arsenic Content in American Wine," *Journal of Environmental Health* 78, no. 3 (October 2015): 16–22.

71. Declan P. Naughton and Andrea Petróczi, "Heavy Metal Ions in Wines: Meta-Analysis of Target Hazard Quotients Reveal Health Risks," *Chemistry Central Journal* 2 (October 30, 2008): 22, https://doi.org/10.1186/1752-153X-2-22; and "23 Abstracts with Myocardial Regeneration Research," GreenMedInfo.com, accessed June 14, 2018, http://www.greenmedinfo.com/keyword/myocardial-regeneration.

72. G. Siegel et al., "Pleiotropic Effects of Garlic" [in German], *Wiener Medizinische Wochenschrift* 149, no. 8–10 (1999): 217–24, https://www.ncbi.nlm.nih.gov/pubmed/10483684.

73. Matthew J. Budoff et al., "Inhibiting Progression of Coronary Calcification Using Aged Garlic Extract in Patients Receiving Statin Therapy: A Preliminary Study," *Preventive Medicine* 39, no. 5 (November 2004): 985–91, https://doi.org/10.1016/j.ypmed.2004.04.012.

74. "157 Abstracts with Chocolate Research," GreenMedInfo.com, accessed October 15, 2019, http://www.greenmedinfo.com/substance/chocolate.

75. Peter Whoriskey and Rachel Siegel, "Cocoa's Child Laborers," *The Washington Post*, June 5, 2019, https://www.washingtonpost.com/graphics/2019/business/hershey-nestle-mars-chocolate-child-labor-west-africa/.

76. "Supplemental Labeling: Roundup—Herbicide by Monsanto," EPA reg. no. 524–445, Environmental Protection Agency, https://www3.epa.gov/pesticides/chem_search/ppls/000524-00445-19920713.pdf, accessed July 27, 2018, PDF.

77. Michael Aviram et al., "Pomegranate Juice Consumption for 3 Years by Patients with Carotid Artery Stenosis Reduces Common Carotid Intima-Media Thickness, Blood Pressure and LDL Oxidation," *Clinical Nutrition* 23, no. 3 (June 2004): 423–33, https://doi.org/10.1016/j.clnu.2003.10.002.

78. "327 Abstracts with Pomegranate Research," GreenMedInfo.com, accessed October 15, 2019, https://www.greenmedinfo.com/substance/pomegranate.

79. Brynmor C. Breese et al., "Beetroot Juice Supplementation Speeds O_2 Uptake Kinetics and Improves Exercise Tolerance during Severe-Intensity Exercise Initiated from an Elevated Metabolic Rate," *American Journal of Physiology—Regulatory, Integrative and Comparative Physiology* 305, no. 12 (December 2013): R1441–50, https://doi.org/10.1152/ajpregu.00295.2013; and Stephen J. Bailey, et al., "Dietary Nitrate Supplementation Reduces the O2 Cost of Low-Intensity Exercise and Enhances Tolerance to High-Intensity Exercise in Humans," *Journal of Applied Physiology* 107, no. 4 (October 2009): 1144–55, https://doi.org/10.1152/japplphysiol.00722.2009.

80. F. S. Fluer et al., "Influence of Various Pectins on Production of Staphylococcal Enterotoxins Types A and B" [in Russian], *Zhurnal Mikrobiologii, Epidemiologii, i Immunobiologii* no. 6 (November–December 2007): 11–6, https://www.ncbi.nlm.nih.gov/pubmed/18277535.

81. M. Agarwal et al., "Hepatoprotective Activity of *Beta vulgaris* against CCl_4-Induced Hepatic Injury in Rats," *Fitoterapia* 77, no. 2 (February 2006): 91–93, https://doi.org/10.1016/j.fitote.2005.11.004.

82. Hanna Szaefer et al., "Evaluation of the Effect of Beetroot Juice on DMBA-induced Damage in Liver and Mammary Gland of Female Sprague–Dawley Rats," *Phytotherapy Research* 28, no. 1 (January 2014): 55–61, https://doi.org/10.1002/ptr.4951; and Marie-Christine R. Shakib, Shreef G. N. Gabrial, and Gamal N. Gabrial, "Beetroot-Carrot Juice Intake Either Alone or in Combination with Antileukemic Drug 'Chlorambucil' as a Potential Treatment for Chronic Lymphocytic Leukemia," *Open Access Macedonian Journal of Medical Sciences* 3, no. 2 (June 15, 2015): 331–36, https://doi.org/10.3889/oamjms.2015.056.

83. Andrew J. Webb et al., "Acute Blood Pressure Lowering, Vasoprotective, and Antiplatelet Properties of Dietary Nitrate via Bioconversion to Nitrite," *Hypertension* 51, no. 3 (March 2008): 784–90, https://doi.org/10.1161/HYPERTENSIONAHA.107.103523.

84. Jonathan M. Oliver et al., "Novel Form of Curcumin Improves Endothelial Function in Young, Healthy Individuals: A Double-Blind Placebo Controlled Study," *Journal of Nutrition and Metabolism* 2016 (2016): 1089653, https://doi.org/10.1155/2016/1089653.

85. Nobuhiko Akazawa et al., "Curcumin Ingestion and Exercise Training Improve Vascular Endothelial Function in Postmenopausal Women," *Nutrition Research* 32, no. 10 (October 2012): 795–99, https://doi.org/10.1016/j.nutres.2012.09.002.

86. Amy C. Ellis, Tanja Dudenbostel, and Kristi Crowe-White, "Watermelon Juice: A Novel Functional Food to Increase Circulating Lycopene in Older Adult Women," *Plant Foods for Human Nutrition* 74, no. 2 (June 2019): 200–3, https://doi.org/10.1007/s11130-019-00719-9.

87. Arturo Figueroa et al., "Influence of L-Citrulline and Watermelon Supplementation on Vascular Function and Exercise Performance," *Current Opinion in Clinical Nutrition and Metabolic Care* 20, no. 1 (January 2017): 92–98, https://doi.org/10.1097/MCO.0000000000000340.

88. Arturo Figueroa et al., "Watermelon Extract Supplementation Reduces Ankle Blood Pressure and Carotid Augmentation Index in Obese Adults with Prehypertension or Hypertension," *American Journal of Hypertension* 25, no. 6 (June 2012): 640–43, https://doi.org/10.1038/ajh.2012.20.

89. N. M. Massa et al., "Supplementation with Watermelon Extract Reduces Total Cholesterol and LDL Cholesterol in Adults with Dyslipidemia under the Influence of the MTHFR C677T Polymorphism," *Journal of the American College of Nutrition* 35, no. 6 (August 2016): 514–20, https://doi.org/10.1080/07315724.2015.1065522.

90. Guoyao Wu et al., "Dietary Supplementation with Watermelon Pomace Juice Enhances Arginine Availability and Ameliorates the Metabolic Syndrome in Zucker Diabetic Fatty Rats," *The Journal of Nutrition* 137, no. 12 (December 2007): 2680–85, https://doi.org/10.1093/jn/137.12.2680.

91. Mee Young Hong et al., "Watermelon Consumption Improves Inflammation and Antioxidant Capacity in Rats Fed an Atherogenic Diet," *Nutrition Research* 35, no. 3 (March 2015): 251–58, https://doi.org/10.1016/j.nutres.2014.12.005.

92. A. Figueroa et al., "Effects of Watermelon Supplementation on Arterial Stiffness and Wave Reflection Amplitude in Postmenopausal Women," *Menopause* 20, no. 5 (May 2013): 573–77, https://doi.org/10.1097/GME.0b013e3182733794.

93. Michel de Lorgeril et al., "Recent Findings on the Health Effects of Omega-3 Fatty Acids and Statins, and Their Interactions: Do Statins Inhibit Omega-3?," *BMC Medicine* 11 (January 4, 2013): 5, https://doi.org/10.1186/1741-7015-11-5.

94. Zhaoping Li et al., "Hass Avocado Modulates Postprandial Vascular Reactivity and Postprandial Inflammatory Responses to a Hamburger Meal in Healthy Volunteers," *Food & Function* 4, no. 3 (2013): 384–91, https://doi.org/10.1039/C2FO30226H.

95. "The Science of HeartMath," HeartMath, accessed October 15, 2019, https://www.heartmath.com/science/.

CHAPTER 7

1. "Overweight & Obesity Statistics," National Institutes of Health—National Institute of Diabetes and Digestive and Kidney Diseases, August 2017, https://www.niddk.nih.gov/health-information/health-statistics/overweight-obesity.

2. Lena M. Thorn et al., "Metabolic Syndrome in Type 1 Diabetes: Association with Diabetic Nephropathy and Glycemic Control (the FinnDiane Study)," *Diabetes Care* 28, no. 8 (August 2005): 2019–24, https://doi.org/10.2337/diacare.28.8.2019.

3. Enrique Z. Fisman et al., "Oral Antidiabetic Therapy in Patients with Heart Disease." *Herz* 29, no. 3 (May 1, 2004): 290–98. https://doi.org/10.1007/s00059-004-2476-5.

4. J. M. Gamble et al., "Insulin Use and Increased Risk of Mortality in Type 2 Diabetes: A Cohort Study." *Diabetes, Obesity and Metabolism* 12, no. 1 (January 1, 2010): 47–53. https://doi.org/10.1111/j.1463-1326.2009.01125.x.

5. E. Fisman et al., "Oral Antidiabetic Therapy in Patients with Heart Disease. A Cardiologic Standpoint," *Herz* 29, no. 3 (May 2004): 290–98, https://doi.org/10.1007/s00059-004-2476-5.

6. Adam G. Tabák et al., "Prediabetes: A High-Risk State for Diabetes Development," *The Lancet* 379, no. 9833 (June 16, 2012): 2279–90, https://doi.org/10.1016/S0140-6736(12)60283-9.

7. C. Morgan et al., "Association between First-Line Monotherapy with Sulphonylurea versus Metformin and Risk of All-Cause Mortality and Cardiovascular Events: A Retrospective, Observational Study," *Diabetes, Obesity and Metabolism* 16, no. 10 (October 2014): 957–62, https://doi.org/10.1111/dom.12302.

8. "29 Abstracts with Beta Cell Regeneration Research," GreenMedInfo.com, accessed October 15, 2019, https://www.greenmedinfo.com/keyword/beta-cell-regeneration.

9. C. Elke Wiseman et al., "Amylopectin Starch Induces Nonreversible Insulin Resistance in Rats," *The Journal of Nutrition* 126, no. 2 (February 1996): 410–15, https://doi.org/10.1093/jn/126.2.410.

10. "Glycemic Index for 60+ Foods," Harvard Health Publishing, February 2015, https://www.health.harvard.edu/diseases-and-conditions/glycemic-index-and-glycemic-load-for-100-foods.

11. Robert H. Lustig et al., "Fructose: Metabolic, Hedonic, and Societal Parallels with Ethanol," *Journal of the Academy of Nutrition and Dietetics* 110, no. 9 (September 2010): 1307–21, https://doi.org/10.1016/j.jada.2010.06.008.

12. David A. Brase et al., "Antagonism of the Morphine-Induced Locomotor Activation of Mice by Fructose: Comparison with Other Opiates and Sugars, and Sugar Effects on Brain Morphine," *Life Sciences* 49, no. 10 (1991): 727–34, https://doi.org/10.1016/0024-3205(91)90105-K; and Fred Lux, David A. Brase, and William L. Dewey, "Antagonism of Antinociception in

Mice by Glucose and Fructose: Comparison of Subcutaneous and Intrathecal Morphine," *European Journal of Pharmacology* 146, no. 2–3 (February 9, 1988: 337–40, https://doi.org/10.1016/0014-2999(88)90312-3.

13. Fred Lux, David A. Brase, and William L. Dewey, "Antagonism of Antinociception in Mice by Glucose and Fructose: Comparison of Subcutaneous and Intrathecal Morphine," *European Journal of Pharmacology* 146, 2–3 (February 1988): 337–40, https://doi.org/10.1016/0014-2999(88)90312-3.

14. Sade Spencer, Michael Scofield, and Peter W. Kalivas, "The Good and Bad News about Glutamate in Drug Addiction," *Journal of Psychopharmacology* 30, no. 11 (November 2016): 1095–98, https://doi.org/10.1177/0269881116655248.

15. Ka He et al., "Consumption of Monosodium Glutamate in Relation to Incidence of Overweight in Chinese Adults: China Health and Nutrition Survey (CHNS)," The American Journal of Clinical Nutrition 93, no. 6 (June 2011): 1328–36, https://doi.org/10.3945/ajcn.110.008870.

16. "66 Abstracts with Monosodium Glutamate (MSG) Research," GreenMedInfo.com, accessed October 15, 2019, http://www.greenmedinfo.com/toxic-ingredient/monosodium-glutamate-msg.

17. De-Kun Li et al., "Urine Bisphenol-A Level in Relation to Obesity and Overweight in School-Age Children," *PLOS ONE* 8, no. 6 (June 12, 2013): e65399, https://doi.org/10.1371/journal.pone.0065399; and "Focused Research Topics Bisphenols & Obesity," GreenMedInfo.com, accessed October 15, 2019, https://www.greenmedinfo.com/greenmed/topic/96253/focus/5066/page.

18. Somlak Chuengsamarn et al., "Curcumin Extract for Prevention of Type 2 Diabetes," *Diabetes Care* 35, no. 11 (November 2012): 2121–27, https://doi.org/10.2337/dc12-0116.

19. Hassan Mozaffari-Khosravi et al., "The Effect of Ginger Powder Supplementation on Insulin Resistance and Glycemic Indices in Patients with Type 2 Diabetes: A Randomized, Double-Blind, Placebo-Controlled Trial," *Complementary Therapies in Medicine* 22, no. 1 (February 2014): 9–16, https://doi.org/10.1016/j.ctim.2013.12.017.

20. Tahereh Arablou et al., "The Effect of Ginger Consumption on Glycemic Status, Lipid Profile and Some Inflammatory Markers in Patients with Type 2 Diabetes Mellitus," *International Journal of Food Sciences and Nutrition* 65, no. 4 (June 2014): 515–20, https://doi.org/10.3109/09637486.2014.880671.

21. Paul A. Davis and Wallace Yokoyama, "Cinnamon Intake Lowers Fasting Blood Glucose: Meta-Analysis," *Journal of Medicinal Food* 14, no. 9 (April 11, 2011): 884–89, https://doi.org/10.1089/jmf.2010.0180.

22. Joanna Hlebowicz et al., "Effect of Cinnamon on Postprandial Blood Glucose, Gastric Emptying, and Satiety in Healthy Subjects," *The American Journal of Clinical Nutrition* 85, no. 6 (June 2007): 1552–56, https://doi.org/10.1093/ajcn/85.6.1552.

23. Martin de Bock et al., "Olive (*Olea europaea* L.) Leaf Polyphenols Improve Insulin Sensitivity in Middle-Aged Overweight Men: A Randomized, Placebo-Controlled, Crossover Trial," *PLOS ONE* 8, no. 3 (2013): e57622, https://doi.org/10.1371/journal.pone.0057622.

24. Riitta Törrönen et al., "Berries Reduce Postprandial Insulin Responses to Wheat and Rye Breads in Healthy Women," *The Journal of Nutrition* 143, no. 4 (January 30, 2013): 430–36, https://doi.org/10.3945/jn.112.169771.

25. Abdullah Bamosa et al., "Effect of Nigella sativa Seeds on the Glycemic Control of Patients with Type 2 Diabetes Mellitus," *Indian Journal of Physiology and Pharmacology* 54 (October 2010): 344–54; and Reza Daryabeygi-Khotbehsara et al., "*Nigella sativa* Improves Glucose Homeostasis and Serum Lipids in Type 2 Diabetes: A Systematic Review and Meta-Analysis," *Complementary Therapies in Medicine* 35 (December 2017): 6–13, https://doi.org/10.1016/j.ctim.2017.08.016.

26. Azabji-Kenfack Marcel et al., "The Effect of *Spirulina platensis* versus Soybean on Insulin Resistance in HIV-Infected Patients: A Randomized Pilot Study," *Nutrients* 3, no. 7 (July 2011): 712–24, https://doi.org/10.3390/nu3070712.

27. Hui Dong et al., "Berberine in the Treatment of Type 2 Diabetes Mellitus: A Systemic Review and Meta-Analysis," *Evidence-Based Complementary and Alternative Medicine* 2012 (October 15, 2012): 591654, https://doi.org/10.1155/2012/591654.

28. Gijs den Besten et al., "The Role of Short-Chain Fatty Acids in the Interplay between Diet, Gut Microbiota, and Host Energy Metabolism," *Journal of Lipid Research* 54, no. 9 (September 2013): 2325–40, https://doi.org/10.1194/jlr.R036012.

29. Jolene Zheng et al., "Resistant Starch, Fermented Resistant Starch, and Short-Chain Fatty Acids Reduce Intestinal Fat Deposition in *Caenorhabditis elegans*," *Journal of Agricultural and Food Chemistry* 58, no. 8 (April 28, 2010): 4744–48, https://doi.org/10.1021/jf904583b.

30. Martin P. Wegman et al., "Practicality of Intermittent Fasting in Humans and Its Effect on Oxidative Stress and Genes Related to Aging and Metabolism," *Rejuvenation Research* 18, no. 2 (April 1, 2015): 162–72, https://doi.org/10.1089/rej.2014.1624.

31. Eun Ju Kim et al., "UV Modulation of Subcutaneous Fat Metabolism," *Journal of Investigative Dermatology* 131, no. 8 (August 2011): 1720–26, https://doi.org/10.1038/jid.2011.106.

32. Ji A. Seo et al., "Association between Visceral Obesity and Sarcopenia and Vitamin D Deficiency in Older Koreans: The Ansan Geriatric Study," *Journal of the American Geriatrics Society* 60, no. 4 (April 2012): 700–6, https://doi.org/10.1111/j.1532-5415.2012.03887.x.

33. "Focused Research Topics Vitamin D & Obesity," GreenMedInfo.com, accessed December 4, 2019, https://www.greenmedinfo.health/greenmed/topic/18782/focus/5066/page.

34. Brian A. Irving et al., "Effect of Exercise Training Intensity on Abdominal Visceral Fat and Body Composition," *Medicine and Science in Sports and Exercise* 40, no. 11 (November 2008): 1863–72, https://doi.org/10.1249/MSS.0b013e3181801d40.

CHAPTER 8

1. "The IUCN Red List of Threatened Species," IUCNredlist.org, accessed October 24, 2018, https://www.iucnredlist.org/.

2. Cor Kwant, "Hiroshima: A-Bombed Ginkgo," The Ginkgo Pages, accessed June 19, 2018, https://kwanten.home.xs4all.nl/history.htm#Hiroshima.

3. Sayer Ji, "Gingko Biloba: A 'Living Fossil' with Life-Extending Properties," GreenMedInfo.com, June 10, 2019, http://www.greenmedinfo.com/blog/gingko-biloba-living-fossil-life-extending-properties.

4. William J. Rowe, "Correcting Magnesium Deficiencies May Prolong Life," *Clinical Interventions in Aging* 2012, no. 7 (February 16, 2012): 51–54, https://doi.org/10.2147/CIA.S28768.

5. David W. Killilea and Jeanette A. M. Maier, "A Connection between Magnesium Deficiency and Aging: New Insights from Cellular Studies," *Magnesium Research* 21, no. 2 (June 2008): 77–82.

6. Damiano Piovesan et al., "The Human 'Magnesome': Detecting Magnesium Binding Sites on Human Proteins," *BMC Bioinformatics* 13, Suppl. 14 (2012): S10, https://doi.org/10.1186/1471-2105-13-S14-S10.

7. S. B. Sartori et al., "Magnesium Deficiency Induces Anxiety and HPA Axis Dysregulation: Modulation by Therapeutic Drug Treatment," *Neuropharmacology* 62, no. 1 (January 2012): 304–12, https://doi.org/10.1016/j.neuropharm.2011.07.027.

8. Neil Bernard Boyle, Clare Lawton, and Louise Dye, "The Effects of Magnesium Supplementation on Subjective Anxiety and Stress— A Systematic Review," *Nutrients* 9, no. 5 (May 2017): 429, https://doi.org/10.3390/nu9050429.

9. K. Held et al., "Oral Mg2+ Supplementation Reverses Age-Related Neuroendocrine and Sleep EEG Changes in Humans," *Pharmacopsychiatry* 35, no. 4 (2002): 135–143, https://doi.org/10.1055/s-2002-33195.

10. Harvard Health Publishing, "Magnesium Content in Milligrams (mg) of Certain Foods," Harvard Women's Health Watch, accessed December 12, 2019, https://www.health.harvard.edu/healthy-eating/magnesium-content-in-milligrams-mg-of-certain-foods.

11. "266 Abstracts with Yoga ResearchYoga," GreenMedinfoGreenMedInfo. com, accessed October 15, 2019, http://www.greenmedinfo.com/therapeutic-action/yoga.

12. Nitya Shree and Ramesh R. Bhonde, "Can Yoga Therapy Stimulate Stem Cell Trafficking from Bone Marrow?," *Journal of Ayurveda and Integrative Medicine* 7, no. 3 (2016): 181–84, https://doi.org/10.1016/j.jaim.2016.07.003.

13. "266 Abstracts with Yoga Research," GreenMedInfo.com."Yoga," GreenMedinfo, http://www.greenmedinfo.com/therapeutic-action/yoga.

14. J.-C. Baumeister, G. Papa, and F. Foroni, "Deeper Than Skin Deep—the Effect of Botulinum Toxin-A on Emotion Processing," *Toxicon* 118 (August 2016): 86–90, https://doi.org/10.1016/j.toxicon.2016.04.044.

15. Chisato Nagata et al., "Association of Dietary Fat, Vegetables and Antioxidant Micronutrients with Skin Ageing in Japanese Women," *British Journal of Nutrition* 103, no. 10 (May 28, 2010): 1493–98, https://doi.org/10.1017/S0007114509993461.

16. Soyun Cho et al., "Dietary Aloe Vera Supplementation Improves Facial Wrinkles and Elasticity and It Increases the Type I Procollagen Gene Expression in Human Skin In Vivo," *Annals of Dermatology* 21, no. 1 (February 2009): 6–11, https://doi.org/10.5021/ad.2009.21.1.6.

17. Soyun Cho et al., "Red Ginseng Root Extract Mixed with Torilus Fructus and Corni Fructus Improves Facial Wrinkles and Increases Type I Procollagen Synthesis in Human Skin: A Randomized, Double-Blind, Placebo-Controlled Study," *Journal of Medicinal Food* 12, no. 6 (December 2009): 1252–59, https://doi.org/10.1089/jmf.2008.1390.

18. Nagata et al., "Skin Ageing in Japanese Women," 1493–98.

19. Els J. M. Van Damme et al., "Potato Lectin: An Updated Model of a Unique Chimeric Plant Protein," *The Plant Journal* 37, no. 1 (January 2004): 34–45, https://doi.org/10.1046/j.1365-313X.2003.01929.x.

20. Willy J. Peumans, Pierre Rougé, and Els J. M. Van Damme, "The Tomato Lectin Consists of Two Homologous Chitin-Binding Modules Separated by an Extensin-Like Linker," *Biochemical Journal* 376, pt. 3 (December 15, 2003): 717–24, https://doi.org/10.1042/BJ20031069.

21. Michael L. Mishkind et al., "Localization of Wheat Germ Agglutinin-Like Lectins in Various Species of the Gramineae," *Science* 220, no. 4603 (June 17, 1983): 1290–92, https://doi.org/10.1126/science.220.4603.1290.

22. David L. J. Freed, "Do Dietary Lectins Cause Disease? The Evidence is Suggestive—and Raises Interesting Possibilities for Treatment," *BMJ* 318, no. 7190 (April 17, 1999): 1023–24, https://doi.org/10.1136/bmj.318.7190.1023.

23. Akram Kooshki et al., "Effect of Topical Application of Nigella sativa Oil and Oral Acetaminophen on Pain in Elderly with Knee Osteoarthritis: A Crossover Clinical Trial," *Electronic Physician* 8, no. 11 (November 25, 2016): 3193–97, https://doi.org/10.19082/3193.

24. Koran 7:71:592.

25. "8 Abstracts with Hormone Replacement Therapy Research," GreenMedInfo. com, accessed October 15, 2019, https://www.greenmedinfo.com/toxic-ingredient/hormone-replacement-therapy.

26. Gillian Flower et al., "Flax and Breast Cancer: A Systematic Review," *Integrative Cancer Therapies* 13, no. 3 (September 8, 2013): 181–92, https://doi.org/10.1177/1534735413502076.

27. Sarika S. Shirke, Sanket R. Jadhav, and Aarti G. Jagtap, "Methanolic Extract of *Cuminum cyminum* Inhibits Ovariectomy-Induced Bone Loss in Rats," *Experimental Biology and Medicine* 233, no. 11 (November 1, 2008): 1403–10, https://doi.org/10.3181/0803-RM-93.

28. Jian Su et al., "Effect of *Curcuma comosa* and Estradiol on the Spatial Memory and Hippocampal Estrogen Receptor in the Post-Training Ovariectomized Rats," *Journal of Natural Medicines* 65, no. 1 (January 2011): 57–62, https://doi.org/10.1007/s11418-010-0457-y.

29. "484 Abstracts with Soy Research," GreenMedInfo.com, accessed July 22, 2018, http://www.greenmedinfo.com/substance/soy.

30. Arlene Weintraub, "FDA to Testosterone Makers: Stop Wooing Average Guys," *Forbes*, March 4, 2015, https://www.forbes.com/sites/arleneweintraub/2015/03/04/fda-to-testosterone-makers-stop-wooing-average-aging-guys/#319a723d1ac5.

31. "359 Abstracts with Endothelial Dysfunction Researc," GreenMedInfo.com, accessed October 15, 2019, http://www.greenmedinfo.com/disease/endothelial-dysfunction.

32. Louise H. Naylor et al., "Exercise Training Improves Vascular Function in Adolescents with Type 2 Diabetes," *Physiological Reports* 4, no. 4 (February 2016): e12713, https://doi.org/10.14814/phy2.12713.

33. Johanna L. Hannan et al., "Beneficial Impact of Exercise and Obesity Interventions on Erectile Function and Its Risk Factors," *The Journal of Sexual Medicine* 6 (March 2009): 254–61, https://doi.org/10.1111/j.1743-6109.2008.01143.x.

34. D. Neves et al., "Does Regular Consumption of Green Tea Influence Expression of Vascular Endothelial Growth Factor and Its Receptor in Aged Rat Erectile Tissue? Possible Implications for Vasculogenic Erectile Dysfunction Progression," *Age (Dordr)* 30, no. 4 (December 2008): 217–28, https://doi.org/10.1007/s11357-008-9051-6.

35. Patricia F. Hadaway et al., "The Effect of Housing and Gender on Preference for Morphine-sucrose Solutions in Rats," *Psychopharmacology* 66, 1 (1979): 87–91, https://doi.org/10.1007/bf00431995.

36. "Video Testimonials: Share Your Story," Kelly Brogan MD, accessed October 15, 2019, https://kellybroganmd.com/video-testimonials/; and Kelly Brogan et al., "Healing of Graves' Disease Thorough Lifestyle Changes: A Case Report," *Advances in Mind-Body Medicine* 33, no. 2 (Spring 2019): 4–11, https://www.ncbi.nlm.nih.gov/pubmed/31476135.

PART THREE

PHASE THREE

1. Joerg Hucklenbroich et al., "Aromatic-Turmerone Induces Neural Stem Cell Proliferation In Vitro and In Vivo," *Stem Cell Research & Therapy* 5, no. 4 (September 26, 2014): 100, https://doi.org/10.1186/scrt500.

2. Nikola Getoff et al., "Photo-Induced Regeneration of Hormones by Electron Transfer Processes: Potential Biological and Medical Consequences," *Radiation Physics and Chemistry* 80, no. 8 (August 2011): 890–94, https://doi.org/10.1016/j.radphyschem.2011.04.001.

3. Zhenxian Han et al., "Effects of Sulforaphane on Neural Stem Cell Proliferation and Differentiation," *Genesis* 55, no. 3 (March 2017): e23022, https://doi.org/10.1002/dvg.23022.

PHASE FOUR

1. Joseph Campbell with Bill Moyers, *The Power of Myth* (New York: Anchor Books, 1991), 4–5.

2. Chia-Wei Cheng et al., "Prolonged Fasting Reduces IGF-1/PKA to Promote Hematopoietic-Stem-Cell-Based Regeneration and Reverse Immunosuppression," *Cell Stem Cell* 14, no. 6 (June 5, 2014): 810–23, https://doi.org/10.1016/j.stem.2014.04.014.

3. Chanchal Deep Kaur and Swarnlata Saraf, "*In Vitro* Sun Protection Factor Determination of Herbal Oils Used in Cosmetics," *Pharmacognosy Research* 2, no. 1 (January–February 2010): 22–25, https://doi.org/10.4103/0974-8490.60586.

4. Yangxin Li et al., "Exosomes Mediate the Beneficial Effects of Exercise," in *Advances in Experimental Medicine and Biology*, vol. 1000, *Exercise for Cardiovascular Disease Prevention and Treatment*, ed. Junjie Xiao (n.p.: Springer, 2017): 333–53, https://doi.org/10.1007/978-981-10-4304-8_18.

5. Masahiko Ayaki et al., "Protective Effect of Blue-Light Shield Eyewear for Adults against Light Pollution from Self-Luminous Devices Used at Night," *Chronobiology International* 33, no. 1 (2016): 1–6, https://doi.org/10.3109/074 20528.2015.1119158.

6. Candace Pert, *Molecules of Emotion* (New York: Scribner, 1999).

7. Eckhart Tolle, The Power of Now (Novato: New World Library, 2004), 221.

8. Alexander G. Panossian, "Adaptogens: Tonic Herbs for Fatigue and Stress," *Alternative and Complementary Therapies* 9, no. 6 (July 5, 2004): 327–31, https://doi.org/10.1089/107628003322658610.

9. Shinichiro Haze, Keiko Sakai, and Yoko Gozu, "Effects of Fragrance Inhalation on Sympathetic Activity in Normal Adults," *The Japanese Journal of Pharmacology* 90, no. 3 (2002): 247–53, https://doi.org/10.1254/jjp.90.247.

10. J. Lehrner et al., "Ambient Odors of Orange and Lavender Reduce Anxiety and Improve Mood in a Dental Office," *Physiology & Behavior* 86, no. 1–2 (September 2005): 92–95, https://doi.org/10.1016/j.physbeh.2005.06.031.

11. Jin Hee Hwang, "The Effects of the Inhalation Method Using Essential Oils on Blood Pressure and Stress Responses of Clients with Essential Hypertension," *Journal of Korean Academy of Nursing* 36, no. 7 (December 2006): 1123–34.

12. Tiago Costa Goes et al., "Effect of Lemongrass Aroma on Experimental Anxiety in Humans," *The Journal of Alternative and Complementary Medicine* 21, no. 12 (September 14, 2015): 766–73, https://doi.org/10.1089/acm.2015.0099.

13. Jocelyn N García-Sesnich et al., "Longitudinal and Immediate Effect of Kundalini Yoga on Salivary Levels of Cortisol and Activity of Alpha-Amylase and Its Effect on Perceived Stress," *International Journal of Yoga* 10, no. 2 (2017): 73–80, https://doi.org/10.4103/ijoy.IJOY_45_16.

14. Britta K Hölzel et al., "Mindfulness Practice Leads to Increases in Regional Brain Gray Matter Density," *Psychiatry Research* 191, no. 1 (January 30, 2011): 36–43, https://doi.org/10.1016/j.pscychresns.2010.08.006.

15. Yi-Yuan Tang, Britta K. Hölzel, and Michael I. Posner, "The Neuroscience of Mindfulness Meditation," *Nature Reviews Neuroscience* 16 (March 18, 2015): 213, https://doi.org/10.1038/nrn3916.

16. Tang, Hölzel, and Posner, "Neuroscience of Mindfulness Meditation," 213.

ACKNOWLEDGMENTS

This book is dedicated to my beloved wife and partner, Kelly Brogan. Without you, and our love, this book would not have been written.

I also want to acknowledge the special role of Heather Jackson, my literary agent and midwife. Your graciousness, patience, and powerful advocacy on my behalf were essential ingredients in bringing this creation into being.

I am deeply grateful for my mother, Dorothy Ji; my sister, Mia Ji; and my father, Sungchul Ji, all three of whom helped deliver me into adulthood in one piece and inspired in me a love of literature and art, which ultimately lead me to become a philosopher. A special thanks to Mia who helped me edit the book in its early stages and supported me with her nieces.

I would like to acknowledge Lisa Ji, the mother of my two beautiful daughters, Sienna and Bella, for her support in this process and for sharing in the powerful commitment to raise these amazing and magical beings of light.

A special acknowledgment goes to Ali Le Vere, who greatly contributed to the writing of this book, and whose brilliance in the biomedical realms goes virtually unparalleled in my experience. I also want to acknowledge my pinch-hitting developmental editor, Julia Serebrinsky, whose patience and powerful support helped to polish the manuscript into something I am proud of.

I want to share my deep love and appreciation for Kate Colter, without whom my many responsibilities to GreenMedInfo would have fallen to the wayside while engaged in the two-year-long book-writing process. You've been a dear friend, godmother to my children, and an exemplary professional who has functioned to about as close as an angel as I think I've experienced in human form thus far.

There are, as is always the case, too many people to name if I were to exhaustively account for those who have inspired me and indirectly helped me to bring this book into existence. But I'm going to list a few:

Joe Wallen, my mentor and supporter early on in my journey into the natural health advocacy realm.

Eli Buren, my mentor who has helped me cultivate awareness, patience, and depth in my day-to-day practice of simply being human.

Bruce and Donna Wilshire, my mentors at Rutgers, who opened me to a world of ideas and ignited my passion to embrace the lifelong commitment to self- and other-exploration that is philosophy.

To my dear friend and former creative partner, Jon Hebel, whose parting from my life helped me to open and heal my heart and understand that death too can be a beautiful gift.

ABOUT
THE AUTHOR

S ayer Ji is founder of GreenMedInfo, the world's largest open-access natural health database. He is also a reviewer at the *International Journal of Human Nutrition and Functional Medicine*, the co-founder and CEO of Systome Biomed, a board member of the National Health Federation, and a steering committee member of the Global Non-GMO Foundation. You can visit him online at www.greenmedinfo.com.

To further explore the practical application of the information within Regenerate, visit the online course: **http://www.regeneratemasterclass.com.**

INDEX

E

zero-point energy and, 88–90

Molecular Medicine Reports, 193–194

Molecules of Emotion (Pert), 140–141

monosodium glutamate (MSG), 160,
211–212

Monsanto, 27

mood disorders
Sickness Syndrome, 239–240
sugar and, 210

Moore, Gertrude, 67

Moselhy, Jim, 128

"mother" and "daughter" cells, 125–
129. *see also* stem cells

Motrin (ibuprofen), 155–156

mushrooms
chaga mushroom, 267
lion's mane mushroom, 169
as radioprotective food, 79–80

music, 175–176

myelin, 152, 159

N

National Cancer Act (1971), 101

National Cancer Institute, 107–108,
120

National Institute of Mental Health
and Neurosciences (India), 166

National Lung Screening Trial (NLST),
117

Nature, 54, 55

nature, connecting with, 282

Neurology, 174

New Biology, 3–39. *see also* Regenerate
Rx
on aging, 225
birth of, 4–11
body's potential and, 3–5
on brain regeneration, 148–151 (*see
also* brain)
epigenetics and, 11–22 (*see also*
epigenetics)

food and, 24–39

foundation principles of, 10–11

on metabolic syndrome, 207

quantum energy field and, 43–44

regenerative capacity and, 22–24

New England Journal of Medicine, 7–8,
32, 109–110, 117

Nixon, Richard, 101

noninvasive follicular thyroid neoplasm with papillary-like nuclear
features (NIFTP), 120

nonsteroidal anti-inflammatory drugs
(NSAIDS), 155–156, 234

nori, 55

*Nuclear Transmutation of Stable and
Radioactive Isotopes in Biological
Systems* (Vysotskii), 93

nutrigenomics, 14

O

"Old Cancer Paradigm" (burn, cut, poison), 124

olive leaf, 216, 269

omega-3 fatty acids, 199

oncogerminative hypothesis, 132

Oncology Reports, 122–123

Oncotarget, 126

Origin of Inorganic Substances (von
Herzeele), 91

origin of life, water cavitation and, 97

Oronsky, Bryan, 102

osteoarthritis, 234–235

Own Your Self (Brogan), 284

P

paleo-deficit disorder
defined, 81–82
evolutionary mismatch and, 19–20
sunlight, grounding, and, 81–85
sunlight, hairlessness, and, 77–78

HAY HOUSE TITLES OF RELATED INTEREST

YOU CAN HEAL YOUR LIFE, the movie,
starring Louise Hay & Friends
(available as an online streaming video)
www.hayhouse.com/louise-movie

THE SHIFT, the movie,
starring Dr. Wayne W. Dyer
(available as an online streaming video)
www.hayhouse.com/the-shift-movie

———

CHRIS BEAT CANCER:
A Comprehensive Plan for Healing Naturally,
by Chris Wark

KETOFAST:
Rejuvenate Your Health with a Step-by-Step Guide
to Timing Your Ketogenic Meals,
by Dr. Joseph Mercola

OWN YOUR SELF:
The Surprising Path beyond Depression, Anxiety, and Fatigue
to Reclaiming Your Authenticity, Vitality, and Freedom,
by Kelly Brogan, M.D.

RADICAL HOPE:
10 Key Healing Factors from Exceptional Survivors
of Cancer & Other Diseases,
by Kelly A. Turner, Ph.D., and Tracy White

———

All of the above are available at your local bookstore,
or may be ordered by contacting Hay House (see next page).

We hope you enjoyed this Hay House book. If you'd like to receive our online catalog featuring additional information on Hay House books and products, or if you'd like to find out more about the Hay Foundation, please contact:

Hay House, Inc., P.O. Box 5100, Carlsbad, CA 92018-5100
(760) 431-7695 or (800) 654-5126
(760) 431-6948 (fax) or (800) 650-5115 (fax)
www.hayhouse.com® • www.hayfoundation.org

———

Published in Australia by: Hay House Australia Pty. Ltd.,
18/36 Ralph St., Alexandria NSW 2015
Phone: 612-9669-4299 • *Fax:* 612-9669-4144
www.hayhouse.com.au

Published in the United Kingdom by: Hay House UK, Ltd.,
The Sixth Floor, Watson House, 54 Baker Street, London W1U 7BU
Phone: +44 (0)20 3927 7290 • *Fax:* +44 (0)20 3927 7291
www.hayhouse.co.uk

Published in India by: Hay House Publishers India,
Muskaan Complex, Plot No. 3, B-2, Vasant Kunj, New Delhi 110 070
Phone: 91-11-4176-1620 • *Fax:* 91-11-4176-1630
www.hayhouse.co.in

———

**Access New Knowledge.
Anytime. Anywhere.**

Learn and evolve at your own pace
with the world's leading experts.

www.hayhouseU.com

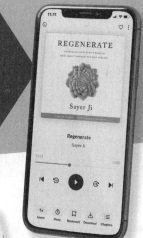
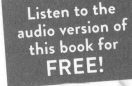